ADVANCES IN RESPIRATORY THERAPY RESEARCH

PUBLIC HEALTH IN THE 21ST CENTURY

Additional books in this series can be found on Nova's website
under the Series tab.

Additional e-books in this series can be found on Nova's website
under the e-book tab.

PUBLIC HEALTH IN THE 21ST CENTURY

ADVANCES IN RESPIRATORY THERAPY RESEARCH

MILOŠ JESEŇÁK, M.D., PH.D.
EDITOR

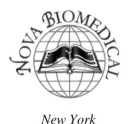

New York

NOTICE TO THE READER

The Publisher has taken reasonable care in the preparation of this book, but makes no expressed or implied warranty of any kind and assumes no responsibility for any errors or omissions. No liability is assumed for incidental or consequential damages in connection with or arising out of information contained in this book. The Publisher shall not be liable for any special, consequential, or exemplary damages resulting, in whole or in part, from the readers' use of, or reliance upon, this material. Any parts of this book based on government reports are so indicated and copyright is claimed for those parts to the extent applicable to compilations of such works.

Independent verification should be sought for any data, advice or recommendations contained in this book. In addition, no responsibility is assumed by the publisher for any injury and/or damage to persons or property arising from any methods, products, instructions, ideas or otherwise contained in this publication.

This publication is designed to provide accurate and authoritative information with regard to the subject matter covered herein. It is sold with the clear understanding that the Publisher is not engaged in rendering legal or any other professional services. If legal or any other expert assistance is required, the services of a competent person should be sought. FROM A DECLARATION OF PARTICIPANTS JOINTLY ADOPTED BY A COMMITTEE OF THE AMERICAN BAR ASSOCIATION AND A COMMITTEE OF PUBLISHERS.

Additional color graphics may be available in the e-book version of this book.

Library of Congress Cataloging-in-Publication Data

ISBN: 978-1-63463-004-7

Library of Congress Control Number: 2014950590

Published by Nova Science Publishers, Inc. † New York

Contents

Preface

Respiratory diseases represent and important part of daily practice of nearly all physicians. Their incidence, prevalence and significant impact on the quality of life require a substantial attention. In last few decades, the understanding of the pathogenesis of particular diseases allowed focusing the research in the field of therapy on exact components and characteristics of the diseases and modern effective therapies have been developed. The close relationship between experimental, pre-clinical and clinical research is very characteristic for respiratory medicine. The prevalence of certain respiratory diseases is increasing very dramatically and their impact on different aspects of healthcare is evident (morbidity, mortality, economic aspects, quality of life, patients' prognosis, associated complications and comorbidities). Unfortunately, precise and effective tools of disease prevention are not widely available. Therefore, the intensive research in the field of therapy and development of new therapeutic strategies and tools are urgently needed.

This new book summarize the most actual and exciting achievements and successes in the respirology (dominantly pediatric pulmonology) and is focused on the current research in the therapy of bronchial asthma, other respiratory diseases with bronchoobstruction, primary ciliary dyskinesia, sleep apnea syndrome and physiotherapy.

Chapter 1 – During the last few years, only a few new medicaments and compounds have been introduced for the treatment of bronchial asthma. However, the research in this area is dramatic and many potential molecules and compounds are currently under experimental, pre-clinical or even clinical investigations. Better understanding or asthma pathogenesis, associated inflammation and chronic remodeling airway changes in the context of genetic background and environmental impacts are opening new perspectives for the development of novel effective therapies. The chapter summarizes the most actual movements in the area of bronchial asthma therapy with the overview of those compounds, which are currently in clinical investigation and thus will probably enlarge current treatment options, especially for the patients with severe persistent and hard-to-treat form of disease.

Chapter 2 – Nitric oxide (NO) is one of the mostly studied signaling molecules in modern medicine. Under physiological conditions, basal production of NO is responsible for neurotransmission, vasodilatation, bronchodilation and bronchoprotection and acts in various immune processes. In pathological circumstances associated with inflammation of various origin, the production of NO is significantly increased and leads to the over-production of mucus, extravasation of plasma with airway edema, acceleration of inflammatory infiltrates (predominantly T_H2-driven) and through increased formation of reactive nitrogen species causes the oxidative damage to DNA and proteins.. Thus, NO plays an important role in many physiological processes, but increased production is typical for certain diseases, e.g. bronchial asthma. Therefore, enzymes associated with the metabolism of NO (inducible NO-synthase, arginase) seem to be an interesting target for anti-asthmatic therapy. In this chapter the authors summarize current knowledge and direction in therapeutic modulation of NO formation and through own original results from animal experiments support the possible application of NO-synthase inhibitors for the treatment of respiratory diseases associated with bronchial hyperreactivity and obstruction.

Chapter 3 – Never-ending story of pediatric gastroenterology and pulmonology is represented by the dilemma about the possible association of bronchial asthma and gastroesophageal reflux (GER). Authors in this chapter provide a critical review of current knowledge based on the recent data from the studies. They analyze, whether there could be any association (and if yes, how it is expressed and how far is it clinically relevant) or if these two entities only coexist with each other. It should be admitted, that causal relationship between GER and asthma has not been clearly explained and still remains unclear, whether the reflux causes asthma, asthma (and certain anti-asthmatic medications) triggers reflux, or both coexists simultaneously in one patients. The chapter provides rationale view on the current diagnostic approach and therapeutic strategy in those asthmatics, in which GER could participate on the respiratory symptoms and disease worsening. The crucial remains the presence of clinical symptoms of GER. Recent double-blinded studies showed that the treatment of asymptomatic GER did not improve asthma control in children. Moreover, long-term use of proton pump inhibitors could have side effects. Therefore, the association of GER and asthma as well therapeutic strategy should be evaluated very carefully in each particular patient.

Chapter 4 – Cough is the most common chronic respiratory symptom across all the age categories and could be associated with a broad spectrum of respiratory and extra-respiratory diseases and conditions. The understanding of different modes of cough induction and the identification of various cough receptors is crucial for developing of effective anti-cough therapies. Moreover, the empirical use of many, especial over-the-counter preparations should have the scientific basis and the understanding of mode of action of each compound is important not only for efficacy confirmation but also for the selection of suitable patient for such therapy. The chapter supplies up-to-date description of different cough receptors and their localization and analyzes the possibilities of the pharmacological modulation of cough reflex through different over-the-counter medications.

Chapter 5 – Syndromes of primary ciliary dyskinesia (PCD) represent an emerging and enlarging area of pulmonology with explosion of knowledge, especially regarding the genetic background of particular form of PCD. In last few years, several PCD causal genes were detected and the morphological and/or functional clinical correlates were described. The chapter provides an interesting view on the clinical picture, genetic reasons and diagnostic approach to the patients with suspected ciliary dyskinesia. The closing part of the chapter analyses current and future possibilities of the therapy of these severe diseases with substantial impact on quality of life and patients' prognosis.

Chapter 6 – Sleep medicine studies the pathological situations emerging during various phases of sleep. Polysomnography has developed into the validated and relevant diagnostic tool for sleep disorders. The chapter analyses the topic of obstructive sleep apnea syndrome in children and showed current diagnostic strategy. Authors present their own experiences with obstructive sleep apnea syndrome and its screening among children. The last part clearly describes current and perspective therapeutic possibilities for affected children.

Chapter 7 – Animal models of respiratory diseases and pathological statuses provide an important mode of research in respirology, regarding etiology, pathophysiology, diagnostic and therapeutic modalities of particular diseases. Chest physiotherapy is an important part of complex respiratory therapy of different acute and chronic diseases. The chapter analyses experimental studies assessing the efficacy and safety of chest physiotherapy techniques and characterizes the challenges in the assessment of mucus clearance *in vivo*. Authors present also their original results and experiences.

The book brings current view on the characteristics, diagnosis and therapy of the most important entities of pediatric respiratory medicine. The chapters provide a concise view on the current movement in the area of novel therapies. In each chapter, the authors present critical review of the literature data in the context of their own experiences and original results.

Assoc. prof. Miloš Jeseňák, M.D., Ph.D. et Ph.D., MBA.
Editor
Department of Paediatrics
University Hospital in Martin
Kollarova 2, 036 59 Martin
Slovak Republic
Email: jesenak@gmail.com

Acknowledgment

This work was supported by project "Virtual and Simulation Tuition as a New Form of Education at JFM CU in Martin", ITMS: 26110230071, co-funded from EU sources and European Social Fund.

In: Advances in Respiratory Therapy Research
Editor: Miloš Jeseňák

ISBN: 978-1-63463-004-7
© 2015 Nova Science Publishers, Inc.

Chapter 1

Current Challenges and Perspectives in Bronchial Asthma Therapy

Miloš Jeseňák*

Department of Pediatrics,
Centre of Experimental and Clinical Respirology,
Comenius University, Jessenius Faculty of Medicine, Martin, Slovakia

Abstract

Bronchial asthma is the most common chronic respiratory disease in children and adults. It is characterized by chronic ongoing inflammation with significant changes to the structure and function of the airways. As a result of its symptoms and severity, it can significantly affect the quality of life of the affected patients with the determination of their prognosis. The step-based approach of the therapeutic algorithm for bronchial asthma in children and adults has recently been elaborated and introduced into daily practice. However, despite this significant progress and improvements, there are still patients with insufficient control over the disease and with significant deterioration of their daily and nocturnal life activities. Admittedly, only a few new drugs and medicaments have appeared for use in asthma therapy over the last few years. One of the most evident successes, anti-IgE monoclonal antibody (omalizumab), was added as the 5th or 6th step of asthma therapy. However, there is an urgent need for new medicaments, with potential and strong efficacy and an excellent safety profile, especially in children. The development of new drugs and therapeutic options is strongly dependent on the understanding of the bronchial asthma pathogenesis and persistence of the chronic inflammation. Another important issue is the therapeutic modulation of the chronic progression of the diseases with preventive effects for the future. Recently, many new inventions have been made in the field of the pathogenesis of bronchial asthma. The

* Corresponding Author address: Assoc. Prof. Milos Jesenak, M.D., Ph.D., Ph.D., MBA, Department of Pediatris, Centre of Experimental and Clinical Respirology, Jessenius Faculty of Medicine in Martin, Comenius University in Bratislava, University Hospital, Kollarova 2, 036 59, Martin, Slovak Republic, e-mail: jesenak@gmail.com

understanding of so-called neurogenic inflammation, involvement of the oxidative damage of the macromolecules, a description and characterization of many new signaling molecules in the airways and immune system, and the understanding of the genetic background of the different aspects and characteristics of bronchial asthma create the best proposals and grounds for the new therapies in asthmatic patients.

Keywords: Bronchial Asthma, Pharmacotherapy, Personalized Medicine, Targeted Therapy

1. Introduction

Bronchial asthma (BA) is the most common chronic airway disease in childhood and its prevalence has substantially increased worldwide, particularly in pre-school children. It is associated with significant morbidity and economic aspects. The disease is characterized by *chronic airway inflammation*, which is responsible for *bronchial hyperresponsiveness* leading to the classic clinical symptoms of asthma (cough, wheezing, dyspnea, chest tightness) [222]. Bronchial hyperresponsiveness is both specific (to certain allergen or specific triggers) and non-specific (changes of air temperature, bronchoconstrictive agents, exercise) stimuli. Chronic airway inflammation has many characteristics and discriminates between the different asthmatic phenotypes (atopic vs. non-atopic, eosinophilic vs. neutrophilic) of asthma [24, 227, 333, 369, 370]. A substantial contribution to the chronic changes in the airways and lungs is presented by *oxidative stress,* which leads to the damage of biomolecules. Whether oxidative stress is the consequence of, or the reason for, chronic changes in asthmatic airways is still being discussed [16, 17].

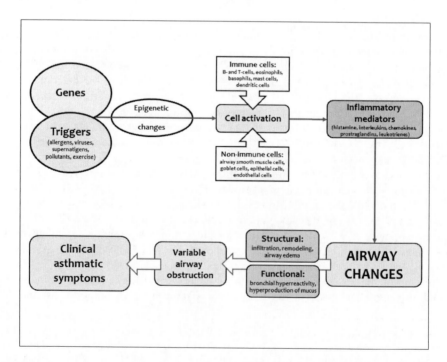

Figure 1. Different aspects and stages of bronchial asthma development (Modified and enlarged according to Harmanci et al., 2007).

Recently, *neurogenic inflammation* in bronchial asthma has been described as playing an important role in the hyperreactivity of airway nerves and smooth muscles. Inflammation, neurogenic changes and oxidative stress are responsible for the development of chronic structural changes in the airways – *remodeling*, which is also presented in the very early stages of asthma (Figure 1) [26, 92]. To date, no convincing therapeutic strategy has been developed that could significantly reverse the already initiated remodeling; however, early controlled anti-inflammatory therapy could significantly contribute to the stabilization of inflammatory changes in the airways with substantial achievement of clinical control over the asthmatic symptoms [27]. The prevalence of asthma is increasing worldwide, and untreated or mistreated disease has a severe impact on the quality of life of affected individuals. Moreover, the impact of the economics of asthma aspects on the whole population level cannot be ignored. Therefore, an effective, safe and widely available therapy is crucial in the management of this most common chronic airway disease.

2. Anti-Asthmatic Therapy

Current anti-asthmatic therapy is based on the step-up/down approach in respect of achieved control over the disease and frequency and degree of persistent clinical symptoms. Several factors and methods allow for the evaluation of each asthma stage in patients with a modification of therapy (Table 1).

Table 1. Available methods for asthma monitoring in clinical practice

Monitoring Tools for Bronchial Asthma		
Clinical Aspects	**Functional Examination**	**Inflammometry**
Daily and nocturnal symptoms frequency	Spirometry	Fractional exhaled nitric oxide (FENO)
Exacerbations rate	Bronchoobstruction reversibility (bronchodilator test)	Allergic markers in blood: eosinophils, total IgE, periostin*, eosinophilic cationic protein
Admission to hospital and unplanned visits of physician	Degree of bronchial Hyperreactivity (bronchoconstrictive test)	Exhaled breath condensate analysis*
Impact on the daily activities due to asthma	Peakflowmetry	Other markers in exhaled breath*: carbon monoxide, pH, ethane, 8-isoprostanes, H_2O_2, exhaled air temperature m etc.
Questionnaires: Asthma control test, Tests for Quality of life in asthmatics	Cough receptor sensitivity testing *	Induced sputum analysis
Use of rescue therapy (short-acting β_2-mimetics)		

* Experimental use

The strategy is similar both in adults and in children and differs only in the doses and principles of use of some medicaments. Anti-asthmatics can be divided into relievers (for acute relief of the symptoms) and controllers (allowing long-term control over the asthma due to suppression of the airway inflammation). Today, there are several categories of anti-asthmatic therapies with acceptable safety profiles and good clinical efficacy. The two classes of drugs most commonly used for treating childhood and adult asthma are inhaled corticosteroids (ICS) and β_2-agonist bronchodilators (SABA – short-acting β_2-agonist and LABA – long-acting β_2-agonist). However, only a few new drugs have been introduced into clinical practice in the last few decades. One of the most important newly introduced groups of anti-asthmatics is represented by leukotriene-receptor antagonists (antileukotrienes). Based on a better understanding of the pathophysiological processes within asthmatic inflammation in the airways, new targets of potential anti-asthmatic therapy have been identified.

3. Call for Novel Anti-Asthmatic Therapies

Despite existing effective medicaments for asthma, new therapies are still needed. A combination of inhaled corticosteroids (ICS) together with long-acting β_2-agonists allows good therapeutic response and achievement of disease control in most (approximately 90%) but not all asthmatics.

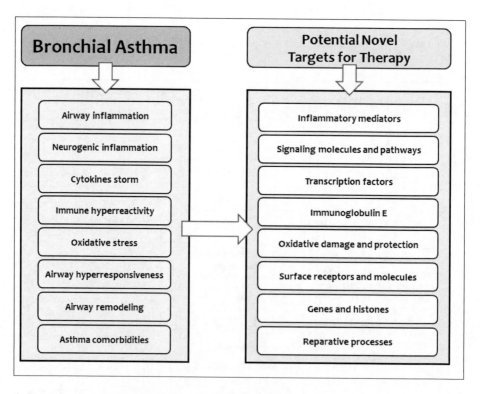

Figure 2. Detecting the novel targets for anti-asthmatic therapy.

In addition, patients with good clinical control and response to the currently available therapies could *benefit from newer and more effective compounds*. Another important factor that supports the development of new therapies is to gain a better understanding of different *asthmatic phenotypes and endotypes* that significantly determine the therapeutic response. Detection of *various associated co-morbidities* (e.g. allergic rhinitis, nasal polyposis, drug allergy, obesity) also requires the adaptation of applied strategy [266].

Furthermore, different subtypes of *asthma occur in children and in adults*, resulting in distinctive patterns of treatment sensitivity. The future direction of asthma therapy is based on understanding each patient's genome, proteome and kinome, which could lead to a *personalized approach* for each individual regarding the choice of a particular compound with the possible estimation of therapeutic response and possible adverse events [6]. Therefore, novel therapies are especially important in the management of severe poorly controlled asthma. The detection of novel targets of anti-asthmatic therapies is based on the increasing knowledge of the asthma pathogenesis and a better understanding of the different aspects of asthma development (Figure 2).

4. New Bronchodilators

Bronchodilators represent one of the most important groups of medicaments used for the relief of acute asthmatic symptoms (rescue therapy) as well as long-term therapy for maintenance of disease control (controllers). They are important for preventing and relieving bronchoconstriction. The major advance has been the introduction of the long-acting β_2-agonists (LABA) *salmeterol* and *formoterol*, the effects of which last for over 12 hours. However, research in the field of bronchodilation agents is still ongoing. There is a new group of long-acting β_2-agonists with a rapid onset of clinical action and long-lasting effects for more than 24 hours. Several of these ultra-long-acting β_2-agonists are in clinical testing, e.g. *indacaterol, carmoterol, vilanterol, olodanterol* and *GSK159797*. They are effective for more than 24 hours, are fast acting and are useful for once-daily dosing (Figure 3) [299]. These agents are also very suitable to be used in fixed combination with long-lasting corticosteroids (e.g. mometasone furoate) with improved compliance. Combined formulations of LABA and ICS in one inhaler have been found to confer synergistic effects in terms of controlling airway inflammation and improving lung function [88]. Recently, a new combined formulation was developed that allows once-daily dosing, combining the corticosteroid fluticasone furoate with the long-lasting β_2-agonists vilanterol. Studies showed that this combination was well tolerated, significantly improving lung function, when compared to treatment with the single drugs alone [73, 335]. Moreover, this combination effectively inhibited both early and late asthmatic responses to an allergen challenge [339].

The bronchodilation effectiveness of β_2-agonists is influenced by the functional antagonism of bronchoconstricting agents, e.g. muscarinic receptor agonists or histamine. This reduced β_2-adrenergic responsiveness may be due to cross talk between C_q-coupled muscarinic M_3 or histamine H_1 receptors and G_s-coupled β_2-adrenoreceptors [21]. This provides a strong rationale for combination treatment with β_2-agonists and muscarinic receptor antagonists, as muscarinic receptor antagonists both attenuate bronchoconstriction and potentiate β_2-agonist-induced bronchodilation by relieving the cholinergic restraint on β_2-

adrenoreceptor function. Therefore, several *combinations of long-lasting β₂-agonists (LABA) and long-lasting muscarinic antagonists (LAMA)* are under development. There were also some attempts to develop a triple inhaler containing LABA + LAMA + ICS [36].

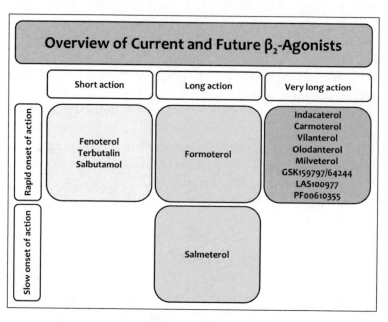

Figure 3. Overview of currently available and future β₂-agonistis regarding the onset and duration of action (Adapted from Sedlak & Koblizek, 2010).

Another interesting concept is presented by *bi-directional dual-acting molecules that link a muscarinic receptor antagonist and β₂-adrenoreceptor agonist* (MABA) [21, 40, 124]. A once-daily muscarinic antagonist, *tiotropium bromide*, is less effective as a bronchodilator in asthma patients than β₂-agonists and is used predominantly in chronic obstructive pulmonary disease (COPD), but appears to be a useful add-on therapy in some patients with severe asthma [341, 346]. There are also some other potential bronchodilator agents, such as vasoactive intestinal peptide analogues, neuropeptide analogues or potassium-(K^+)-channel openers, which were also studied as potential anti-asthmatic drugs. However, they also have potent vasodilator effects causing unwanted side effects that complicate their clinical applicability [33, 300]. Recently, agonists of bitter taste receptors (TAS2R), e.g. quinine, chloroquine and saccharine, have been identified as a novel class of bronchodilators [125] (Figure 4).

Bronchodilators are important for preventing and relieving bronchoconstriction in asthmatic patients. The current trend is the use of ultra-long-acting β₂-agonists with a rapid onset of clinical action and a long-lasting effect of more than 24 hours, which are now also available in fixed combinations with inhaled corticosteroids allowing once-daily dosing. There is also increasing evidence for the usefulness of combinations of long-lasting β₂-agonists and long-lasting muscarinic antagonists in severely asthmatic patients. Another interesting concept is represented by bi-directional molecules that link a muscarinic receptor antagonist and a β₂-adrenoreceptor agonist (MABA).

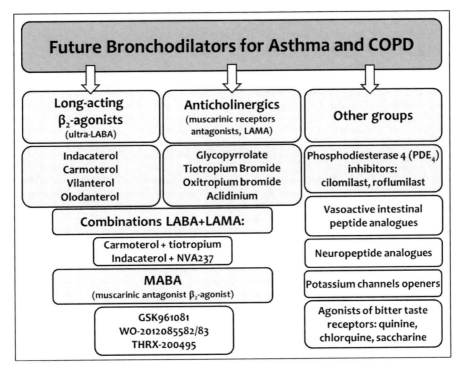

Figure 4. Future trends in development of bronchodilators for asthma and chronic obstructive pulmonary disease.

5. Novel Glucocorticosteroids

Current therapeutic strategies for bronchial asthma with the use of modern anti-asthmatic drugs allow the effective management of the majority of asthmatic patients. However, in certain patients, control of the disease cannot be achieved despite the optimal strategy. The reasons can lie in the specific phenotype of the asthma, a genetically determined response to a particular anti-asthmatic drug, or in associated co-morbidities. Glucocorticosteroids are one of the most important drugs in clinical use and they are mainly used to suppress disease-related inflammation. The invention of inhalant corticosteroids should be considered a crucial milestone in the treatment of bronchial asthma in children and in adults.

Glucocorticosteroids (GC) are steroidal hormones synthesized from cholesterol and they enable the organism to respond adequately to physical and emotional stress. The name glucocorticosteroid (glucose + cortex + steroid) is derived from their role in the regulation of glucose metabolism, their synthesis in the adrenal cortex and their steroidal structure [122]. Besides their pluripotent physiological and pathological effects and roles in organisms in different circumstances and conditions, their immunomodulatory and anti-inflammatory actions are the most important biological effects applicable for the therapeutic use of glucocorticosteroids [238]. In recent years, the mechanisms of the action of GC were clarified and several important inventions have been made.

The mechanisms of GC action can be divided into genomic and nongenomic [95, 121, 180, 279]. Genomic mechanisms of GC action include their direct or indirect influence on gene transcription and translation. Genomic effects do not appear until after twenty to thirty minutes, but the time to reach maximal effectiveness can be as much as two weeks. The cytoplasmatic GC receptor (GCR) is present in non-active form in complex with chaperones. After the activation of GCR by CS, the dissociation of the chaperone-GCR complex and GCR together with GCs can translocate to the nucleus, where it dimerizes. A homodimer can subsequently bind to the DNA regulatory sequences, which are called GC response elements (GRE) and are found in the promoter regions of glucocorticoid-regulated genes. If this binding leads to gene activation, the GRE sequence is termed as positive GRE and this action is called trans-activation. By *trans-activation*, GCs are able to induce the expression of pro-inflammatory, anti-inflammatory and regulatory factors and mediators (nuclear action of GC). This genomic action is responsible for the unwanted side effects of GC. Negative GRE leads to gene suppression (*direct repression*); however, the presence of negative GRE in the promoter region was proven only for a few genes. Many genes may be influenced by GCs without direct interaction with DNA. This effect is mediated through the binding of factors important for inflammatory process development (usually co-activators or co-receptors of other genes' transcription). The complex GC-GCR interacts with many proteins, such as signaling pathways kinases, transcription factors (e.g. activator protein 1, nuclear factor kappa B), and co-activator proteins, preventing their interactions within the nucleus area and DNA. This process of gene transcription inhibition without direct DNA binding is called *indirect trans-repression* and is responsible for the most important anti-inflammatory properties of GCs (cytoplasmatic action of GC) (Figure 5).

Trans-repression of the nuclear factor κB is believed to be a major mechanism by which GCs reduce inflammatory gene transcription. However, recent data indicates that this effect is not the primary mechanism of GC-mediated repression of inflammatory gene transcription in pulmonary epithelial cells and airway smooth muscles, post-translational or translational mechanisms of inflammatory genes regulation play a role in the mediation of GC anti-inflammatory effects as well [87, 121].

Nongenomic mechanisms of GC action are mediated through a GC receptor placed in the cell membrane, and more rarely in cytoplasm. This action has very rapid onset and cannot be inhibited by GCR antagonists. In this mechanism, GCs activate secondary messengers (calcium ions, inositol triphosphate, diacylglycerol, cyclic nucleotides such as cAMP, cGMP) followed by the activation of different protein kinases with influence on the cellular processes and signaling pathways (Figure 5).

Inhaled corticosteroids (ICS) are considered the most important drug category used in bronchial asthma management and treatment. Different molecules differ in anti-inflammatory potential, incidences of unwanted side effects, systemic availability and other pharmacological properties. During regular evaluation of the bronchial asthma status, the dose of ICS is usually increased gradually with the aim of reaching full clinical control over the disease. An important issue associated with increasing the ICS dose is the increasing frequency of side effects in patients with high doses of corticosteroids (inhalant or systemic). However, at a certain point the increasing dose of ICS reaches the maximal anti-inflammatory action (plateau) with a subsequent gradual increase of the side effects, which are usually the result of systemic availability (Table 2).

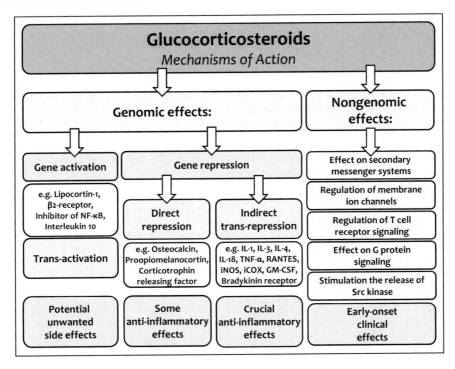

Figure 5. Schematic principles of glucocorticorticosteroid mechanisms of action and their clinical meaning (Modified from Grzanka et al., 2011). *Legend*: GM-CSF – granulocytes macrophages colony stimulating factor, iCOX – inducible cyclooxygenase, IL – interleukin, iNOS – inducible nitric oxide synthase, NF-κB – nuclear factor kappa B, TNF-α – tumor necrosis factor alpha.

Table 2. Systemic availability of different inhalant corticosteroids (Adapted from Kalish et al., 2009)

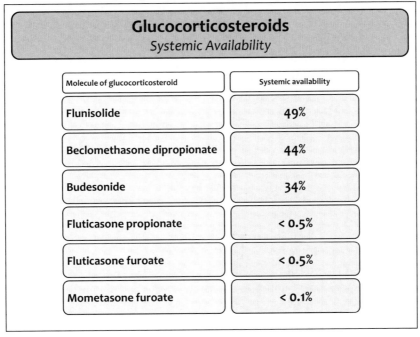

Molecule of glucocorticosteroid	Systemic availability
Flunisolide	49%
Beclomethasone dipropionate	44%
Budesonide	34%
Fluticasone propionate	< 0.5%
Fluticasone furoate	< 0.5%
Mometasone furoate	< 0.1%

Therefore, the development of novel anti-inflammatory drugs is of maximal interest. The research is strongly dependent upon the understanding of asthma pathophysiology and its complications and consequences [132]. Unfortunately, most of the "steroid-sparing" medications were either poorly effective in the studies and/or have intolerable side effects. Another aspect is the price and availability of the drugs. Many of these agents showed some positive effects in only a small number of studies, and well-designed randomized trials are usually lacking [375]. Therefore, development of new corticosteroid molecules is of increasing interest.

Development in the field of inhaled corticosteroids is still ongoing. The first research stream is the modification of old molecules or the development of completely new molecules. The new modern ICS molecules are represented by *mometasone furoate* and *ciclesonide* and they demonstrated excellent efficacy in both children and adults [365]. The once-daily application significantly improves compliance and adherence to the therapy [159]. Ciclesonide presents a new concept in inhaled therapy and belongs to the so-called "soft steroids". These drugs are either inactive pro-drugs that are enzymatically activated at their site of action, or active drugs that exert their desired effect at a specific site of action and are then broken down by esterification or other enzymatic action to produce an inactive metabolite [44]. Ciclesonide is applied in the form of a pro-drug that is activated by esterases within the lungs to form the active compound – des-ciclesonide. Both molecules have very low systemic availability, which is reflected by an excellent safety profile. Several pediatric studies have demonstrated that mometasone applied once daily yielded minimal long-term velocity effect [398]. Today, fixed combinations of ciclesonide/mometasone with formoterol or even once-daily ultra-LABA (e.g. indacaterol, vilanterol) are also tested in clinical trials with the potential for a once-daily fixed combined therapy [89].

Recently, non-glucocorticoid steroids were developed as novel anti-asthmatic drugs. EPI-12323 (Naturasone) is an inhaled small non-glucocorticoid steroid molecule that showed positive pre-clinical data and has entered Phase I of clinical trials. It possesses long-term anti-inflammatory activity (inhibits T_H2 inflammatory response, reduces adenosine hypersecretion in asthmatic lungs, suppresses neutrophils) with an excellent safety profile (no bone demineralization) [354]. Another concept is represented by the use of self-assembling nanoparticles that target the drug to sites of interest and protect them from degradation and inactivation. They have the capacity to improve drug efficacy and decrease undesirable systemic side effects. Dexamethasone in nanoparticles yielded a better effect on bronchial hyperresponsiveness and lung functions in animal models than dexamethasone alone with a better safety profile [245]. The final effect of the glucocorticoid molecule could be modified by adding an NO-donating group (to prednisolone – *NCX1015* or to budesonide – *NCX1020*). This modification of classic molecules showed improved corticosteroid efficacy against lipopolysaccharide-induced inflammatory responses and prevented lipopolysaccharide-induced airway hyper-responsiveness, eosinophilia, and neutrophilia in animal models. Classic molecules had only a small effect on eosinophilia [323, 342]. NO groups were also added to β_2-agonists [270] (Table 3).

Another possible direction in the field of inhaled corticosteroids is the development of new molecules with potentiated anti-inflammatory effects and diminished side effects. The development of these new "dissociated" molecules is based on the recent findings describing a different mode of action of corticosteroids in the organisms [35, 38].

Table 3. Current directions in inhaled corticosteroids and glucocorticoid receptor modulators

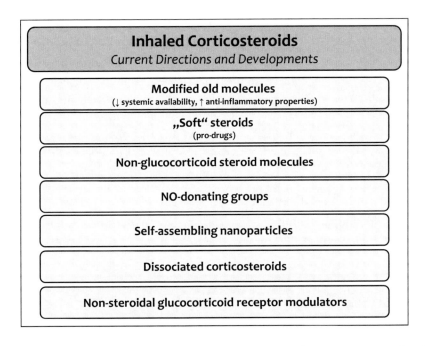

Insight into how trans-activation mechanistically differs from trans-repression is crucial for the development of dissociated ligands for GC receptors (SEGRA, Selective glucocorticosteroid receptor agonists) – so-called dissociated corticosteroids. Novel ligands were developed aiming to separate or dissociate trans-activation from trans-repression, which leads to the improved therapeutic index. If this concept is proven by clinical studies, it will also allow the use of high doses of ICS (or possibly even oral forms) in severe asthmatics with a good safety profile. There is a growing number of such improved GCR ligands, currently still undergoing pre-clinical testing. Three *steroid molecules with dissociated characteristics* were being tested (*RU24782, RU24858, RU40066*). Some trans-activation activity was retained (between 9% and 35% of that of dexamethasone) in combination with a trans-repressive activity on activator protein-1, but with similar activity to prednisolone (*RU24858* was two times more active in the skin inflammation model than prednisolone) [441]. Despite the initial optimism, these three molecules were not proven as effective in other studies and they yielded some side effects typical of classic GC [43]. Another possibility is represented by *non-steroidal dissociated GCR modulators*, e.g. *AL-438, ZK216348, ZK245186, LGD5552* or *maprocorat*, which showed a better clinical and safety profile than steroidal GCR agonists [87, 354]. Particular dissociated steroid molecules differ in certain structural characteristics (e.g. by having C21-thiomethyl and C21-cyanide moieties), which significantly determine the degree of dissociated function and therapeutic index [126]. A recent study demonstrated, in animal models, which C21-mercapto derivatives of hydrocortisone act as a dissociated steroid with an improved safety profile based on the optimal lung deposition, efficacy against pulmonary inflammation, improvement of lung function tests and dissociated side effects (thymolysis) (Table 4) [49]. *In vitro* assays using these compounds appear to show good dissociation. However, *in vivo*, the dissociation appears to be at least partially lost and these molecules still produce many of the side effects associated with conventional GCs [87]. The solution lies in a better understanding of the molecular mechanisms behind GS-induced effects. It would allow the design of better novel selective GCR modulators with an improved therapeutic index, also confirmed in vivo and in clinical trials [87]. It was also suggested that, for full trans-repression effect on inflammatory gene expression, some degree of trans-activation (e.g. trans-activation of anti-inflammatory protein such as DUSP1 or annexin-1 – lipocortin 1) is also required and necessary [1, 87].

Further investigation in this field is required with the aim of an improved therapeutic index of GCR ligands. There are several possibilities: compounds with increased interaction with repressive co-factors, targeted the affinity of GC to particular promoters based on the type of GRE, cell or tissue-specific GCR ligands or selective activators of the nuclear enzyme histone deacetylase-2 (HDAC-2), which inhibits already activated inflammatory genes [32, 34, 87].

Table 4. Potential clinical benefits of dissociated glucocorticosteroids and non-steroidal glucocorticoid receptor modulators (Adapted from De Bosscher et al., 2010)

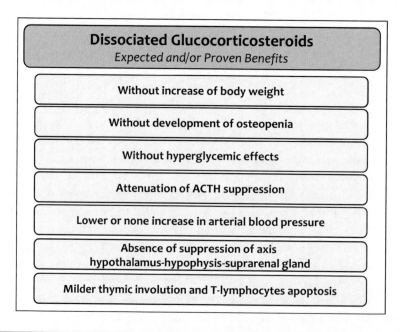

Dissociated Glucocorticosteroids
Expected and/or Proven Benefits

- Without increase of body weight
- Without development of osteopenia
- Without hyperglycemic effects
- Attenuation of ACTH suppression
- Lower or none increase in arterial blood pressure
- Absence of suppression of axis hypothalamus-hypophysis-suprarenal gland
- Milder thymic involution and T-lymphocytes apoptosis

Glucocorticoids represent the most important therapeutic modality for bronchial asthma. The invention of inhaled corticoids is considered to be the most important and crucial milestone in asthma therapy. However, side effects can also be observed, especially in high-dose therapy or in oral corticotherapy in severe asthmatic patients. Over the past decade, remarkable progress in understanding the mechanisms of corticosteroids action was made, which allowed the development of modern molecules. Current directions in this field are: the development of novel molecules with low or zero systemic availability, softer steroids, non-glucocorticoid steroids and an emerging class of corticosteroids – dissociated corticoid receptor ligands. However, it seems that the simple dissociation of trans-repression from trans-activation seems to be insufficient to develop the glucocorticoid receptor agonist of the new generation with an excellent therapeutic index and safety profile.

6. Targeting Lipid Mediators

Lipid mediators play an important role in the pathogenesis of bronchial asthma, and therefore it is rational to use drugs that influence lipid mediators' production or action in asthma treatment. To date, more than 100 mediators were identified as being involved in the complex inflammatory processes in asthma. Whether the blockage of the synthesis or a receptor for a single mediator could be therapeutically effective, should be discussed. The only mediator receptor antagonists currently used in asthma treatment are the cysteinyl-leukotriene receptor antagonists – $CysLT_1R$ (LTRA, leukotriene modifiers, antileukotrienes), which play an important role especially in preschool asthmatic children with virus-induced bronchospasms and in patients with exercise-induced asthma [37, 38]. Most of the knowledge about the pathophysiological role of leukotrienes in asthma is currently limited to $CysLT_1R$ receptor-mediated effects, whereas the role of the $CysLT_2R$ and other emerging receptors (e.g. $CysLT_3R$ – GP17) are largely unknown [314]. $CysLT_2R$ showed some similarities regarding its distribution in tissues and cells with $CysLT_1R$, but the expression in the heart, brain and adrenals appears to be peculiar to $CysLT_2R$ [374]. Leukotriene modifiers are in general less effective than ICS; however, they are also able to influence the pathways that are not fully inhibited by corticosteroids. Cysteinyl leukotrienes (cLTs) significantly contribute to the pathogenesis of asthma and other allergic diseases and participate in the development of airway inflammation [278, 334] (Table 5).

Table 5. Biologic effects of leukotrienes in bronchial asthma pathogenesis (Adapted from Peters-Golden and Henderson, 2007)

Leukotrienes in Bronchial Asthma
Biological Effects and Mechanisms

Type of Cell	Biological Effects
Leucocytes	↑ recruitment of T lymphocytes, eosinophils and mast cells
Dendritic cells	↑ recruitment and activation
Epithelial cells	↑ mucus secretion and ↑ proliferation of goblet cells
Fibroblasts and myofibroblasts	↑ collagen release and fibrotization → airway re-modelling
Smooth muscle cells	↑ contractility and proliferation, muscles hypertrophy
Endothelial cells	↑ vascular permeability and oedema formation

Cysteinyl leukotrienes are derived from membrane phospholipids after the liberation of arachidonic acid by phospholipase A_2. Arachidonic acid is converted by 5'-lipoxygenase to leukotriene A_4, which is metabolized into LTC_4, LTD_4 and LTE_4 (they were formerly known as slow reacting substances of anaphylaxis). These three compounds interact with cysteinyl-leukotriene receptor 1 ($CysLT_1$) (Figure 7).

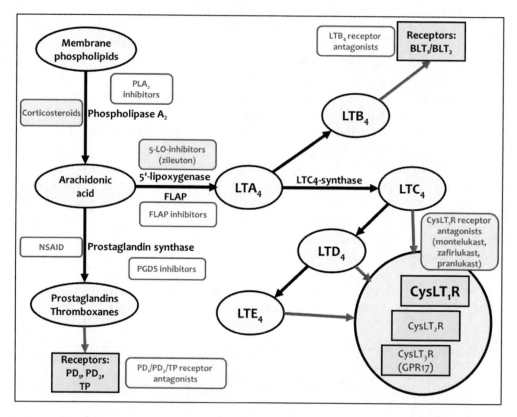

Figure 7. Schematic metabolism of lipid mediators and potential therapeutic targets in bronchial asthma.

The clinical response to the LTRA is significantly modified by specific genetic factors. It was shown that allelic variation in the promoter region of 5'-lipoxygenase gene resulted in decreased expression of this enzyme and reduced the response to LTRA [129]. The selected single nucleotide polymorphisms in the promoter region of LTC4-synthase gene also modify the clinical response to zafirlukast [377]. It is clear that polymorphisms of the leukotriene synthetic pathway underlie at least some of the heterogeneity of the response to LTRA [78, 117, 421]. Leukotriene receptor antagonists yielded *pluripotent anti-inflammatory properties* in many clinical trials with asthma and some other allergic diseases (allergic rhinitis, urticarial, atopic dermatitis). Moreover, since the production of leukotrienes is not significantly affected by inhaled, oral or intravenous corticosteroids, LTRA enlarge the spectrum of anti-inflammatory anti-asthmatic drugs [207]. Leukotriene receptor antagonists effectively inhibit bronchoconstriction in patients with asthma undergoing an allergen, exercise, cold air, or aspirin challenge. Clinical trials showed that LTRA are able to reduce exacerbation rate, improve lung functions, decrease the nighttime and daytime symptom score, improve asthma control and suppress allergic inflammation (decrease of eosinophils in sputum and peripheral blood, sputum eosinophilic cationic protein, fractional exhaled nitric oxide) [6, 296]. The most widely used is *montelukast*, but some other molecules are also in use (*zafirlukast, pranlukast*). According to recent studies, montelukast has been reported to possess secondary anti-inflammatory properties unrelated to conventional antagonism of cysteinyl leukotriene receptors (e.g. through the inhibition of transcription factor NF-κB). These activities enable montelukast to target eosinophils, monocytes, and in particular, the corticoid-insensitive activities than originally thought. According to the studies, montelukast is able to inhibit 5'-lipoxygenase, phosphodiesterase, inhibit eosinophils' adhesion to the endothelium and suppress the activity of several signaling receptors (e.g. P2Y receptor) [427]. With the rising number of diseases with leukotrienes involvement in their pathogenesis, the development of new antileukotrienes and 5'-lipoxygenase inhibitors becomes more and more important [407].

Given the efficacy of LTRA, their anti-inflammatory activity, oral administration once daily and safety, this group has become an important tool in the treatment of children with asthma. The current evidence indicates that the first-line monotherapy with antileukotrienes is not generally recommended in asthmatics, with the exception of those who have aspirin-induced asthma and exercise-induced asthma and children with virus-induced wheezing. Its efficacy and cost-effectiveness in comparison with ICS for the management of mild persistent asthma is inferior, but there are studies supporting the addition of LTRA in patients whose symptoms remain uncontrolled by ICS. Antileukotrienes may also be suitable for those asthmatics who find it difficult to use inhaled medications. The effect of LTRA is complementary to current corticosteroid treatment [193]. Moreover, montelukast seems to be beneficial in asthmatics who smoke [272]. Recently, intravenous application of montelukast was studied in acute asthmatics. It had an additive benefit in terms of early improvement in lung function as an adjunct to the standard therapy for acute asthma, especially in those with less severe exacerbations. Some data suggest that certain patients may also benefit from the repressive effect of intravenous montelukast on the progression of an asthma exacerbation [80, 187].

There are some naturally occurring endogenous antileukotrienes in the organisms, e.g. lipoxin A_4. Its levels are significantly reduced in severe bronchial asthma. It would also be possible to use lipoxin A_4 as therapy for severe asthmatics [283].

Several other drugs that inhibit receptors or the synthesis of various lipid mediators are currently in development (Table 6). Phospholipase A2 (PLA_2) is important in the regulation of lipid mediator generation. There is uncertainty as to whether to block the secretory or cytosolic isoforms of PLA_2 and, to date, no safe or highly selective PLA_2 inhibitor has been developed [291].

5-lipoxygenase (5'-LO) is an important enzyme involved in the production of leukotrienes and works through the 5'-LO-activating protein (FLAP). Several inhibitors of 5'-LO (*zileuton* – Zyflo[TM]) and FLAP (*MK-886, BAY x1005*) are in clinical development as potential medicaments for asthma treatment. Due to the blockage of leukotriene B_4 (LTB_4) synthesis, they seem to be more effective, especially among patients with neutrophilic asthma. 5'-LO inhibitors are able to inhibit neutrophilic chemotaxis and activation. Zileuton, the first and only approved 5'-LO inhibitor, blocks the synthesis of cysteinyl leukotrienes and leukotriene B_4. It is used mainly in the U.S.A. However, it has several drawbacks: it exhibits liver toxicity and has an unfavorable pharmacokinetic profile with a short half-life [59]. Thus, it requires liver-function tests and several daily doses. There is an extended-release version with zileuton (Ziflo CR) available, which is applied twice daily instead of four times. A recent study with *zileuton extended-release tablets* showed that zileuton was more effective for the treatment of mild to moderate chronic persistent asthma compared to montelukast based on the greater improvement of asthma symptoms and lung function tests in the zileuton arm [268]. There are several possible alternatives to zileuton for asthma therapy under clinical development (e.g. *setileuton* – Phase II completed, *PF-4191834* – Phase II completed) [407]. Another interesting possibility brings the inhibition of leukotriene A_4 hydrolase, which is now undergoing clinical trials.

The FLAP inhibitors (e.g. *DG031* – *veliflapon* – Phase III suspended participant recruitment, *AM103* – Phase I completed, *GSK-2190915/AM803* – Phase II completed) could be useful in patients with distinct genetic and phenotypic backgrounds, especially as a steroid add-on therapy in the treatment of asthma exacerbations [347]. Leukotriene B_4 is a chemoattractant for neutrophils, eosinophils, monocytes and macrophages. The number of cells expressing its receptor (BLT_1) is increased in asthma [306]. However, LTB_4 receptor antagonist (BLT_1) was not effective in a small group of asthmatic patients with mild asthma, although this has not been tested in patients with neutrophilic asthma [139].

Table 6. Current anti-asthmatic therapies targeting lipid mediators

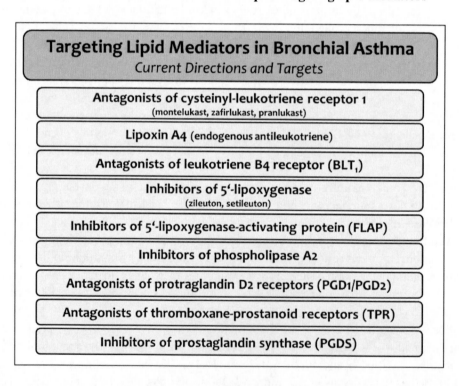

Other target molecules among lipid mediators are prostaglandins and their receptors. Prostaglandin D_2 is released from mast cells and activates its receptor (DP_2, CRT_H2), which is important in chemotaxis of T_H2 lymphocytes and eosinophils. There are several DP_2 receptor antagonists in clinical development for asthma (e.g. *AMG-853*, *OC000459*, *MK-2746*). They showed early clinical efficacy as oral therapy for asthma and rhinitis [28, 38]. Compound

TM30089 was effective in the animal model of asthma and a once daily oral molecule, *ODC9101*, is now in Phase IIa of clinical trials for asthma [350]. It would also be possible to develop dual inhibitors of both DP_1/DP_2 receptors for prostaglandin D_2, since the activation of DP_1 leads to vasodilatation and enhanced T_H2 polarization of dendritic cells. The inhibitors of prostaglandin synthase (PGDS) could also prevent the bronchoconstriction mediated via thromboxane-prostanoid receptors [38].

To date, only cysteinyl leukotriene receptor antagonists (antileukotrienes) are approved for asthma treatment. According to the current guidelines, antileukotrienes are recommended in the long-term treatment of asthma. They reduce the clinical symptoms (including cough), improve lung function, reduce airway inflammation and decrease the frequency of asthma exacerbations. They may allow the dose of steroids to be reduced. Zileuton (inhibitor of 5'-lipoxygenase) is another approved compound from the therapy targeting lipid mediators. Since the role of different lipid mediators is increasing not only in asthma but also in other distinct diseases, the development of novel drugs targeting lipid mediators is of increasing interest. Certain compounds currently under clinical investigation could potentially expand the possibilities of anti-asthmatic therapy, especially in certain asthmatic phenotypes (e.g. neutrophilic asthma).

7. Histamine Receptors and Antihistamines

Histamine is one of the most important mediators of allergic reactions and its inhibition has been used for several decades to prevent, treat and attenuate allergic symptoms. To date, four histamine receptors have been discriminated (H_1R, H_2R, H_3R, H_4R). Histamine receptor 1 (H_1R) was discovered in 1937 and is the major histamine receptor in allergies. Histamine receptor 4 is implicated in the induction of pruritus and its inhibitors are currently in clinical trials aimed at the treatment of pruritic diseases (urticaria, eczema).

H1-antihistamines are considered the inverse agonist of H_1R, because they are able to shift the homeostasis between active and inactive isoforms of H_1R towards the inactive one. H1-antihistamines are the major anti-allergic drugs and they are in the three most common prescribed drug groups all over the world. In high doses, antihistamines are able to reduce mast cell functions, acting as mast cell stabilizers [264, 282].

The modern generation of antihistamines with immunomodulatory and anti-inflammatory effects also possesses, besides classic H_1R antagonism, several other important effects that increase their clinical efficacy and spectrum of actions (Table 7).

Histamine also plays an important role in allergic asthma (Table 8). Histamine produces bronchoconstriction by direct muscle stimulation as well as indirect stimulation of airway parasympathetic afferent nerves. It increases vascular permeability with mucosal edema and promotion of cellular allergic infiltration.

By direct stimulation of H_1R on sensory nerves, histamine provokes coughing, and via H_2R on mucosal glands it increases mucus production. Histamine has significant immune and pro-inflammatory properties mediated through various cells such as macrophages, T lymphocytes, epithelial and endothelial cells. It induces the expression of E-selectin, intracellular adhesion molecule 1 (ICAM-1), lymphocyte function antigen-1 (LFA-1), various lipid mediators (prostacyclin, platelet activating factor and leukotrienes) and the production of different interleukins (IL-1, 6, 8, 10, 18) [54, 170].

Table 7. Immunomodulatory effects of modern generation of antihistamines

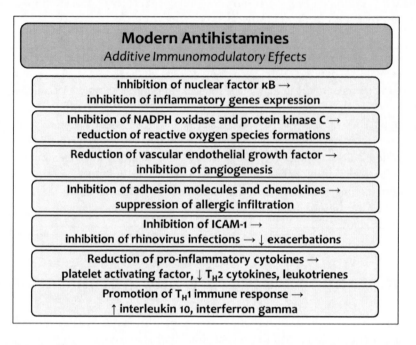

Table 8. Histamine role in asthma (Adapted from Borade et al., 2006)

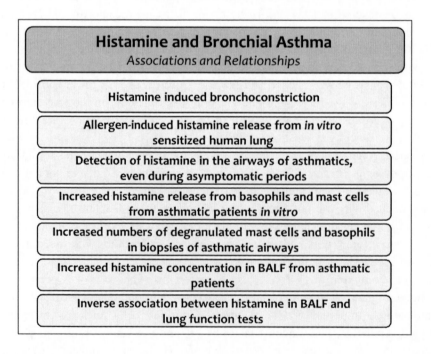

Although antihistamines are not involved in current therapeutic algorithms for bronchial asthma, their use in allergic asthma and asthma with other allergic comorbidities is rational and can support the efficacy of other anti-asthmatic therapies. Allergic rhinitis (AR) is commonly associated with asthma and is one of the multiple risk factors identified for asthma development. Therefore, patients with persistent AR should be evaluated for asthma and, vice versa, patients with asthma should be properly evaluated for rhinitis. The combined strategy of treating both upper and lower airways could significantly improve the clinical control of respiratory allergic symptoms [115].

Many studies investigated the effect of rhinitis treatment on the course of bronchial asthma. Both nasal corticosteroids and antihistamines might reduce the asthma exacerbation rate, improve respiratory symptoms and spirometry, and reduce bronchodilators [18, 100]. Desloratadine and montelukast were equally effective in reducing asthma symptoms and bronchodilator use in patients with seasonal AR and concomitant asthma [19].

Antihistamines possess many important characteristics with a potential effect on asthma treatment. Most antihistamines produce *acute bronchodilation*, especially second-generation molecules. They are also able to *reduce early and late bronchoconstrictor response* in an allergen challenge, but some differences between different molecules have been described. Some protective effects were also observed in *exercise-induced bronchoconstriction*, especially in increased conventional dosing. Cetirizine, desloratadine, terfenadine and some other compounds are able to *improve asthma symptoms and lung functions* when given to mild-to-moderate asthmatics. Modern molecules are capable of *attenuating bronchial hyperresponsiveness* and *reducing the use of rescue bronchodilator therapy* [54]. Antihistamines protect lower airways from the bronchoconstrictive effects of allergic reactions [456]. Clinical efficacy is increased in combination with leukotriene receptor antagonists (montelukast) [39].

Several studies were aimed at the possible *preventive effect of antihistamines in reversing the atopic march*. Preventive administration of *ketotifen* in children with a positive atopic family history had a significant protective effect on the asthma development compared to a placebo [76]. Another important preventive study (ETAC – Early Treatment of the Atopic Child) evaluated the effect of cetirizine in children with atopic eczema and a positive family history for atopy. Although there was no protective effect of cetirizine in the entire population, cetirizine showed significant protective effects against asthma in children with high IgE to grass pollen and house dust mites. These effects were maintained after therapy discontinuation [9].

Current evidence of potent anti-inflammatory and immunomodulatory effects of modern antihistamines make them an attractive proposition in the treatment of asthma. They can be recommended for treatment of seasonal or mild-to-moderate asthma with concomitant allergic rhinitis or urticaria. Their action supports the effects of other anti-asthmatic drugs, especially antileukotrienes and corticosteroids. The therapeutic potential of these agents in asthma without coexistent allergic rhinitis and severe persistent or perennial asthma needs further evaluation.

8. Mast Cell Stabilizers and Cromones

Activation and degranulation of mast cells and eosinophils is a fundamental process in the pathophysiology of allergic diseases. Cromones (*sodium nedocromil, disodium cromoglycate*) possess different anti-inflammatory properties and are used in an inhaled form for the treatment of bronchial asthma as a controller therapy. They act as *mast cell stabilizers* but also have an effect on other inflammatory cells participating in allergic inflammation [293]. They suppress inflammatory cell activation and decrease the production of various cytokines and mediators, e.g. (leukotrienes, prostaglandins, thromboxanes, platelet-activating factor) [466]. In the studies, cromones decreased airway hyperresponsiveness in allergen and exercise challenges [349, 406, 472]. Cromones also showed efficacy in children with non-atopic asthma [148]. However, studies clearly showed that inhaled corticosteroids are superior to cromones in controlling bronchial asthma, exacerbation prevention and lung function improvement. The anti-inflammatory potential of cromones is weaker compared to corticosteroids, and to achieve its full spectrum, several doses per day are necessary [259]. They were useful only in mild-to-moderate asthmatics, but their role decreased significantly after the introduction of inhaled corticosteroids into asthma management. The use of ICS was shown to be more cost effective compared to sodium cromoglycate [11]. Cromones can only be used in mild forms of asthma and in those with side systemic effects to inhaled corticosteroids, especially in children or young patients [237, 240].

Since stabilization of the mast cells seems to be a suitable therapeutic approach, there are several new targets for such therapeutic strategies. Currently, there are several new compounds in pre-clinical development e.g. agonist of inhibitory surface receptors (CD300a, IgG receptors – FcγRI/II/III, Siglec-8), antagonists of thymic stromal lymphopoietin receptor (TSLPR), modulators of endocannabinoid receptors (CD1/2) and neutralizing specific antibodies against CD48. These strategies have been studied in animal models and *in vitro* studies; however, more research is needed to assess their effects and potential efficacy in different human diseases mediated by mast cells or basophils [196].

> Although cromones have been used for many years in childhood asthma treatment, most evidence suggests that they now play only a small role. Cromones could serve only in mild and intermittent asthmatics, especially in children and young patients.

9. Cytokine Targeted Therapy

Cytokines are critical players in different processes in chronic inflammation and airway remodeling in bronchial asthma. Increasing knowledge about their functions, regulations and common relationships allows the development of specific targeting strategies aimed more specifically at the blockage of particular cytokines.

To date, more than 50 cytokines have been implicated in bronchial asthma and specific inhibitors of certain cytokines have been tested in pre-clinical and clinical studies (Figure 8). However, the novel drugs that are designed to manipulate the immune system and its functions in asthma need to prove their safety against acute and long-term side effects. There is a real risk of potentially serious hazards of pharmacological modulation of immune system functions in humans. New targeted therapies are closely linked to the appropriate selection of a specific asthmatic phenotype and the possible side effects should be outweighed by the therapeutic benefits [104, 385]. There are several possibilities for blocking the cytokines' action (Figure 9).

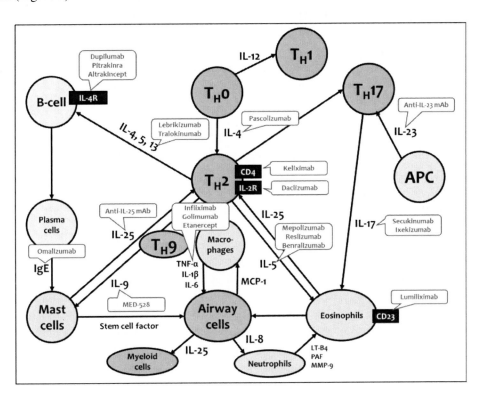

Figure 8. Schematic pathogenesis of bronchial asthma, the relationships between involved participating molecules and possible therapeutic targets (Modified according to Trevor & Deshane, 2014 and Pelaia et al., 2012).

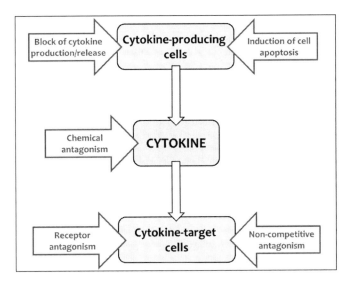

Figure 9. Current available strategies for blocking cytokine actions (Adapted from Simon, 2006).

9.1. Cytokine Blockade

The most commonly studied cytokines for possible therapeutic blockade are T_H2 cytokines, which play a critical role in promotion of eosinophilic allergic inflammation in the airways (Table 9). These cytokines could be targeted by specific monoclonal antibodies or fusion receptor proteins. Their inhibition could have an interesting therapeutic effect on corticosteroid-resistant pathways. The potential side effects of this therapy are anaphylactic reactions and immune dysregulation that may increase risk of sepsis or even cancer. Due to the cytokine storm in asthma, in certain patients targeting only one cytokine may be ineffective as previous redundant cytokine pathways can continue to promote the inflammation [48].

There are only a few peroral inhibitors of cytokine synthesis under clinical investigation. *Suplast tosilate* is a selective inhibitor of IL-4 and IL-5 production from Z cells. It attenuated allergen-induced goblet cells' metaplasia and reduced blood and serum eosinophilia with decrease of airway hyperresponsiveness in mild-to-moderate asthmatics [81]. In a small placebo-controlled trial, suplast was as effective as beclomethasone in improving lung function and was corticoid sparing in patients with moderate asthma [81]. *AVP-13358* is a peroral inhibitor of IgE, CD23 and T_H2 cytokine responses *ex vivo* and *in vitro* in mouse models and human cell assays [364]. Early safety data from clinical trials are favorable.

Interleukin 4 (IL-4) is typical of T_H2 cytokines. Its inhibition by different approaches (monoclonal antibodies against IL-4, inhaled soluble receptor for IL-4) yielded unfortunately disappointing results in the clinical trials. A humanized monoclonal antibody against IL-4 – *pascolizumab* (*SB240683*) showed beneficial effects in preclinical studies on T_H2 inflammation suppression, but clinical studies were unsuccessful [194]. A single dose of nebulized IL-4R therapy demonstrated its safety [56]. A 12-week multiple-dose, placebo-controlled study in corticosteroid-dependent asthmatics showed some effects on lung function and symptom score; however, due to the corticosteroid withdrawal prior to randomization, a high rate of withdrawal from the trial was observed [55]. *Altrakincept* (*Nuvance*) is a recombinant soluble IL-4 receptor antagonist that inactivates IL-4 and decreases IL-13 production with activated T_H2 cells. Although the early clinical findings were very promising (improvement of lung function, improved symptom score), a Phase III trial did not confirm these positive results [7]. *Dupilumab*, an IL-4Rα monoclonal antibody, in clinical trials, was able to reduce asthma exacerbations in subjects on high-dose ICS/LABA and with sputum eosinophilia [453]. Therefore, it seems that *dupilumab* could be a crucial treatment for difficult-to-treat asthma, but further studies are needed [449].

Despite disappointing results with the inhibition of IL-4, the blockade of related cytokine regulating IgE formation – interleukin 13 – is of increasing interest. Interleukin 4 and 13 share the same receptor and both are involved in driving T_H2 inflammation. A recombinant IL-4 variant – *pitrakinra* (Aerovant) – which targets the IL-4R-α component, has been designed as a competitive antagonist of both IL-4 and IL-13 action. Two Phase II studies showed some positive therapeutic effect of pitrakinra: inhibition of late allergic reaction, some effects on lung function and decrease of exhaled nitric oxide [454]. Several IL-13 and IL-4Rα blocking antibodies are now in clinical development, but so far, clinical studies with severe asthma have been disappointing. The right responder phenotypes are probably crucial for the clinical responsiveness, e.g. patients with very high IL-13 concentration in the sputum. In a recent study with mild atopic asthmatics, IL-13 blockade (*IMA-638, IMA-026*) attenuated respiratory late phase allergic response, but did not influence the airway hyperresponsiveness or sputum eosinophils [167].

Table 9. Cytokine targeted therapy and bronchial asthma – short overview of the most important compounds

Cytokine Blocking Therapy		
Molecule	Mode of Action	Clinical Efficacy
Interleukin 4		
mAb against IL-4	Pascolizumab	Uncertain clinical efficacy
Inhaled rs-IL-R4 antagonist	Altrakincept	Uncertain clinical efficacy
mAb against IL-R4α	Dupilumab	Clinical trials
Recombinant IL-4 variant	Pitrakinra	Clinical trials
Interleukin 13		
mAb against IL-13	Lebrikizumab	Clinical trials
mAb against IL-13	Tralokinumab	Clinical trials
mAb against IL-13	Antrukinzumab	Clinical trials
IL-13Rα2 fusion protein	Pitrakinra	Preclinical development
Interleukin 5		
mAb against IL-5	Mepolizumab	Clinical trials
mAb against IL-5	Reslizumab	Clinical trials
mAb against IL-5	Benralizumab	Clinical trials
mAb against IL-5Rα	MEDI-563	Clinical trials
Interleukin 9		
mAb against IL-9	MED-528	Uncertain clinical efficacy
Interleukin 17		
mAb against IL-17	Secukinumab	Clinical trials
mAb against IL-17	Ixekizumab	Clinical trials
mAb against IL-17RA	Brodalumab	Clinical trials
Tumor necrosis factor alpha		
Fusion receptor protein TNF-α	Etanercept	Clinical trials
mAb against TNF-α	Infliximab	Clinical trials
mAb against TNF-α	Golimumab	Serious side effects
Other target molecules:		
mAb against TSLP	AMG157	Preclinical development
mAb against OX40L		Clinical trials
mAb against CD4	Keliximab	Clinical trials
mAb against IL-2Rα	Daclizumab	Serious side effects
mAb against GM-CSF	MT-203	Clinical trials
mAb against IL-25		Preclinical development
mAb against IL-33		Preclinical development

Lebrikizumab is a humanized anti-IL-13 monoclonal antibody that was successful in Phase II clinical trials. It blocks the pro-inflammatory effects of IL-13, reduces bronchial hyperactivity and prevents airway remodeling. The laboratory markers indicating a good response to lebrikizumab could be periostin, which is a marker of T_H2 inflammation [425] but also of higher levels of fractional exhaled nitric oxide (FENO) [105]. Periostin is a newly recognized T_H2 inflammation marker and is probably a key molecule linking airway remodeling and T_H2/eosinophilic inflammation [301]. *Lebrikizumab* in a clinical trial with adult asthmatics reduced serum T_H2 cytokines and total IgE, decreased FENO and improved lung function [105]. Another human monoclonal antibody against IL-13 is *CART-354*, which prevents the expression of the FcεRII receptor, IL-13-proliferation of mast cells and release of histamine. In Phase I trials, this compound prevented the development of airway hyperresponsiveness by suppression of eosinophil recruitment and reduction of serum IgE [395]. There are also other anti-IL-23 blocking monoclonal antibodies in the clinical investigation for bronchial asthma (*tralokinumab, antrukinzumab*) [345].

Another possibility is the inhibition of STAT6 (signal transducer and activation of transcription), which is a common transcription factor for both IL-4 and IL-13. Its inhibitor (*AS1517499*) showed some positive results in a murine model of asthma [93].

Interleukin 5 (IL-5) is closely associated with eosinophilic inflammation. IL-5 promotes eosinophil differentiation and activation, as well as trafficking into the lungs and airways. Several monoclonal antibodies have been developed to target eosinophilic inflammation (anti-IL-4 monoclonal antibodies, anti-IL4R antagonists, inhibitors of IL-13, inhibition of IL-5). There are several monoclonal antibodies against IL-5, working on two principles: *mepolizumab* blocks binding of human IL-5 to the α-chain of the IL-5 receptor (IL-5R) expressed on the surface of eosinophils, whereas *SCH55700* binds IL-5 and thereby blocks its ability to interact with IL-5R [134, 194]. In the clinical trial, *Mepolizumab* reduced eosinophils in peripheral blood and induced sputum, so the drug is actively able to suppress eosinophilic lung inflammation [195, 273]. However, studies on mild asthmatics, who are probably not the target population for *mepolizumab*, did not show any changes of bronchial hyperresponsiveness after anti-IL-5 treatment [150]. Another study with symptomatic patients showed, despite ICS therapy, some effects of *mepolizumab* on lung function and non-significant reduction of exacerbation rate compared to the placebo [151]. The application of *mepolizumab* was well tolerated in all the studies. There is a theoretical increased risk for parasitic infections with anti-eosinophil therapies, but to date, there have been no reports of this phenomenon. Further studies and clinical trials are now ongoing to assess the target asthmatic population for *mepolizumab* and to evaluate its role, as an adjunct therapy to the ICS, in uncontrolled patients with eosinophilic asthma. Target patients would be those with persistent eosinophilic inflammation despite corticosteroids [74]. *Reslizumab* is another monoclonal antibody against interleukin 5. It was studied in patients with poorly controlled eosinophilic asthma. Patients receiving reslizumab showed greater reduction in sputum eosinophils accompanied by improvement of lung function and a trend towards better asthma control compared to the placebo. The therapy was in general well-tolerated [84]. Another anti-IL-5 humanized monoclonal antibody – *benralizumab* – was also tested in the treatment of persistent asthma with frequent exacerbations. *Benralizumab* inhibits the binding of IL-5 to IL-5Rα. The clinical effect was achieved only in subjects with significant pathophysiological contribution of eosinophils (assessed by elevated fractional exhaled nitric oxide or peripheral blood eosinophils). Benralizumab led to a decreased exacerbation rate and improved lung function (FEV$_1$). The clinical effect was more evident among subjects with higher eosinophils counts. Lower doses of the drug did not cause any significant clinical effect [252].

Interleukin 9 (IL-9) has pleiotropic effects on inflammatory cells and airway structural cells and thereby is involved in the complex pathogenesis of bronchial asthma. In animal models, blockade of IL-9 resulted in inhibition of pulmonary infiltration of inflammatory cells and cytokine production, especially IL-17. Therefore, blockade of IL-9 is suitable for further research in IL-17-mediated airway diseases [247]. Another IL-9-specific monoclonal antibody (*MEDI-528*) is being studied in Phase II trials. This treatment inhibits airway inflammation and hyperresponsiveness [7]. In a recent large study, the addition of *MEDI-528* to existing controlled medications was not associated with an improved asthma control score, asthma exacerbation rate, FEV$_1$, health-related quality of life, or any major safety concerns [338].

Interleukin 17 (IL-17) is another interesting cytokine involved in allergic inflammation, especially in severe neutrophilic asthma [217]. In recent years, T$_H$17 cytokine – IL-17 has received considerable attention due to its key role in different inflammatory and autoimmune diseases. Mast cells are the predominant cell type producing this cytokine. The family of IL-17 cytokines contains six members (IL-17A, B, C, D, IL-17E = IL25 and IL-17F). IL-17F was shown to play a crucial pro-inflammatory role in asthma (Figure 10) [244]. Monoclonal antibodies against IL-17 (*secukinumab, ixekizumab*) or IL-17 receptor (*brodalumab*) are currently being investigated in patients with psoriasis, psoriatic arthritis, uveitis and rheumatoid arthritis [196].

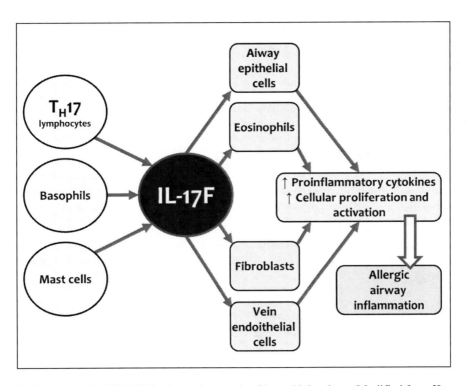

Figure 10. Complex role of IL-17F in the pathogenesis of bronchial asthma (Modified from Kawaguchi et al., 2009).

A recent double-blind study of a large population of asthmatic patients did not confirm any significant therapeutic effects of *brodalumab*. Some clinical effects were seen only in high-reversibility (post-bronchodilator FEV_1 improvement $\geq 20\%$) subgroups in asthma symptoms score and control [71]. Upstream blocking of IL-17 production by T_H17 cells using an anti-IL-23 antibody was also effective in reducing recruitment of neutrophils, eosinophils and lymphocytes into the airways [340]. Use of both anti-IL-17 and anti-IL-23 antibodies in humans is currently being investigated in clinical trials for other immune-mediated diseases such as Crohn's disease and rheumatoid arthritis. Based on the results from clinical trials with asthma, this therapeutic approach is likely to represent a future target in the treatment of this disease. Interleukin 25 is a member of IL-17 family. Animal models of asthma yielded the attenuation of airway hyperresponsiveness, goblet cell hyperplasia and decreased inflammatory cytokines [23]. Anti-IL-25 monoclonal antibody suppressed T_H2-dependent allergic airway inflammation in mice [420]. In humans, it has been shown that eosinophils and basophils represent the primary source of IL-25 [448]. Therapeutic blockade of IL-25 may inhibit acute exacerbations of asthma [348].

Tumor necrosis factor alpha (TNF-α) is another pro-inflammatory cytokine with pluripotent activities participating in the asthma pathogenesis (Figure 11). Previously, the blockade of TNF-α was studied in chronic inflammatory autoimmune diseases, such as rheumatoid arthritis, where it was incorporated into the therapeutics guidelines. The discovery of increased TNF-α expression in BALF and bronchial and lung biopsies in severe asthmatics pointed the attention to its modulation in the treatment of bronchial asthma.

Etanercept (soluble fusion protein of TNF-α receptor and Fc component of human IgG_1) acts as a competitive inhibitor for TNF-α-binding to cell surface receptors. It possesses an affinity to TNF-α of 50-1000-times higher than naturally occurring monomeric forms of soluble TNF-α receptor [318]. Its immunogenicity is very low. Uncontrolled and placebo-controlled studies showed the significant effect of etanercept on improvement of lung function, symptoms score, quality of life and bronchial hyperreactivity in severe refractory asthmatics [46, 63].

The effect is probably mediated through the inhibitory action of etanercept on mast cells. *Infliximab* (a monoclonal chimeric antibody against TNF-α) binds directly soluble and membrane-bound TNF-α in plasma and tissues. In a placebo-controlled clinical study, the application of infliximab did not result in improvement of lung function, although a decreased exacerbation rate was observed [138]. Long-term application of TNF-α-blocking agents could cause reactivation of chronic infections (e.g. latent tuberculosis) and there are some concerns about the increased risk of malignancy. A recent large multicenter study with human monoclonal antibody against TNF-α – *golimumab* – showed no beneficial effect on lung function, symptom score or exacerbation rate, but there were increased reports of cancer and pneumonia [452].

Therefore, this approach will probably be reserved only for patients with severe refractory asthma. In the literature, a case report of the induction of bronchial asthma as a side effect of anti-TNF-α-targeted therapy (*etanercept*) in psoriatic patients was also reported. Although this side effect is rare, it should be considered especially in patients with positive family history of asthma and atopy. *Ustekinumab* may be considered a first line treatment in the patients with psoriasis instead of TNF-α-blocking agents [431].

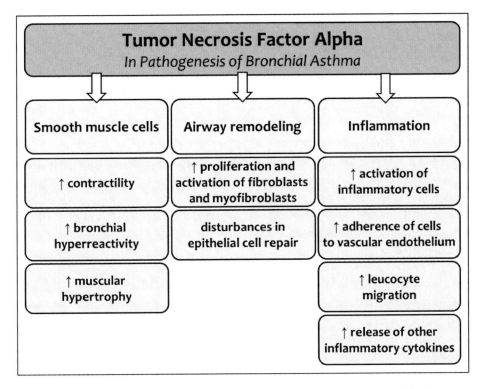

Figure 11. Involvement of tumor necrosis factor alpha in different aspects of bronchial asthma pathogenesis (Modified from Bhowmick & Singh, 2008).

9.2. Other Cytokines and Signaling Molecules Blockade

Currently, several other cytokine and signaling molecule blockers are being tested in different stages of clinical trials with bronchial asthma, including IL-9, IL-17, IL-27, IL-33, GM-CSF or TSLP.

Thymic stromal lymphopoietin (TSLP) is a cytokine derived from epithelial cells and is important in the initiation of allergic inflammation. It is crucial in allergen-induced airway responses and persistent airway inflammation in allergic asthma. In a recent study, human monoclonal antibody against TSLP (*AMG157*) was studied in a group of asthmatic patients. Treatment resulted in attenuated late allergic response measured by FEV_1 decline and reduced blood and sputum eosinophils. Inhibition of TSLP looks to be very promising for asthma treatment in the future [169]. TSLP influences the expression of co-stimulatory molecules on dendritic cells, particularly the OX40 ligand (OX40L). The OX40/OX40L interaction contributes to an optimal T cell response following allergen stimuli and plays an important role in the maintenance and reactivation of memory T effector cells. Pharmacological blockade with monoclonal antibody against OX40L in a small group of asthmatics reduced airway sputum eosinophils and decreased total IgE in serum, but there was no effect on allergen-induced airway responses. However, treatment duration was short (four doses over three months) [168].

Transforming growth factor beta (TGF-β) is a multifunctional cytokine that participates in initiation and resolution of inflammatory responses and contributes to the pathophysiology of asthma. It has important roles in inflammation regulation, cell growth and differentiation and wound and tissue healing. The TGF-β gene is over-expressed in asthmatic airways and lung tissue and probably participates in the processes of remodeling. TGF-β is able to enhance the production of the extracellular matrix and airway smooth muscle cells are the target cells for this cytokine [362]. Evidence from animal models suggests that airway remodeling may be reversed or even prevented by agents targeting TGF-β [208]. Human studies are missing.

Keliximab is a primatized anti-CD4 monoclonal antibody that has been studied in patients with steroid dependent asthma, as a single infusion with a four-week follow up. The dose-dependent decrease of CD4 counts in peripheral blood and decline in mitogen-induced T-cell proliferation was observed during the application of keliximab. The highest dose resulted in an increase of morning and evening peak expiratory flow rates, however, the asthma symptom score was not influenced [255, 256].

Daclizumab is a humanized monoclonal antibody against high-affinity soluble IL-2 receptor and is used in transplantology for protection against graft rejection. It acts through the inhibition of pro-inflammatory cytokine production from activated T lymphocytes. In a group of moderate partially controlled asthmatics, daclizumab improved lung function and decreased symptom score and rescue medication use. However, some serious adverse events were described (anaphylactic shock, varicella meningitis, breast cancer), which limits the use of this compound in the treatment of asthma [70]. Another anti-IL-2Rα (CD25) inhibitor of potential interest is *basiliximab*.

Interleukin 27 (IL-27) is secreted from monocytes and macrophages and is probably involved in the pathogenesis of severe, corticosteroid-resistant asthma. In severe neutrophilic asthma, IL-27 levels are increased in the airways [285]. IL-27 may represent a potential target for new therapeutic strategies aimed at providing a better control of severe, steroid-refractory asthma [164].

Blocking of IL-33 is another novel therapeutic approach to treating allergic airway inflammation. In murine models, this therapy significantly reduced the marker of eosinophilic inflammation (lung eosinophils, total serum IgE, IL-4, IL-5 and IL-13 concentrations in BALF) [287].

Interleukin 1 (IL-1) is a well-known pro-inflammatory cytokine participating in inflammatory processes of different origins (allergic, non-allergic, infectious etc.). Antagonist of IL-1R is an endogenous counter-regulator of IL-1 and limits allergic inflammation. It is able to reduce inflammatory responses caused by genetically determined high levels of IL-1 [388]. Recombinant IL-1 receptor antagonist reduced airway hyperresponsiveness in experimental models [371].

Granulocyte macrophage colony stimulating factor (GM-CSF) is an important factor over-expressed in asthmatic airways, where it plays a key role in eosinophil differentiation and survival [344]. In a murine model, intranasal administration of anti-GM-CSF exerted a significant inhibitory effect on airway inflammation, mucus production and bronchial hyperresponsiveness [465]. A human anti-GM-CSF monoclonal IgG$_1$ antibody – *MT203* – was shown to reduce survival and activation of peripheral human eosinophils significantly [265].

Vascular endothelial growth factor A (VEGF) is thought to be involved in tissue remodeling associated with chronic inflammation, e.g. asthma. It is released by many cells, especially mast cells and basophils. However, studies with its blockade in humans have not been done and this theory of targeting of VEGF in asthma management should be confirmed through studies [196].

Vascular cell adhesion molecule-1 (VCAM-1) is another important receptor implicated in the recruitment of eosinophils and lymphocytes to the sites of pathological inflammation. In animal models, human anti-VCAM-1 monoclonal antibody decreased the production of inflammatory cytokines, goblet cell hyperplasia and peribronchial fibrosis. Targeting VCAM-1 could represent a potential anti-asthma treatment option [274].

9.3. Cytokines as Therapy

Certain cytokines (especially T_H1 cytokines) also possess immunoregulating and anti-inflammatory properties and therefore they have been studied as a possible anti-asthmatic therapy.

Interleukin 10 (IL-10) displays a broad spectrum of anti-inflammatory effects and is defective in bronchial asthma, especially in more severe forms [103]. The therapeutic application of IL-10 was effective in animal models, but its efficacy has not yet been demonstrated through clinical trials.

Interferon gamma (IFN-γ) is a typical T_H1 cytokine with pluripotent anti-inflammatory and antiviral activities. Moreover, IFN-γ is able to suppress T_H2 response [162]. Subcutaneous application of IFN-γ had no clinical benefit for asthmatics [53]. Inhaled IFN-β or IFN-γ may be useful in treating or preventing viral exacerbations of asthma. IFN-α therapy increased T_H1 cells, decreased asthma symptoms and reduced the need for glucocorticosteroids in severely asthmatic patients, perhaps due to increased corticosteroid sensitivity [178]. It seems that IFN-α could be effective in corticosteroid-resistant asthma, but its use should be restricted to this patient group only and monitored by an experienced clinical immunologist [393].

Another possibility is the induction of endogenous production of IFN-γ by exogenous IL-12, which is crucial in determining the T_H1/T_H2 homeostasis through the production of IFN-γ [198]. Repeated injections of IL-12 in asthmatics decreased circulating eosinophils, but did not reduce airway hyperresponsiveness or allergen-specific hyperreactivity compared to IL-5 inhibitors. On the other hand, the application of exogenous IL-12 was associated with a high rate of side effects, especially flu-like symptoms and abnormal liver function tests [190].

Glycosaminoglycan heparin is co-released from mast cells together with histamine and is able to prevent exercise-induced bronchoconstriction [281]. A Phase II trial of IVX0142, a novel heparin-derived oligosaccharide, in the treatment of mild asthma, has just been completed [6].

9.4. Chemokine Blockade

Chemokines are involved in the recruitment of different cells into an area of inflammation. This influx could be suppressed by the antagonists of G-protein-coupled chemokine proteins. These small molecule cytokines attract inflammatory cells (e.g. mast cells, eosinophils, T_H2 cells). The most relevant chemokine receptor involved in asthma is CCR3, because it is able to control eosinophil recruitment by eotaxin and is expressed on many immune cells. CCR3 is expressed on eosinophils and mediates chemotactic response to CXCL11 (eotaxin). An inhaled mixture of two antisense oligonucleotides (*TPI AMS-8*) is targeted against CCR3 and common β-chain of receptors of the pro-inflammatory cytokines (IL-3, 5, GM-CSF) that are participating in T_H2 inflammation [166]. These antisense nucleotides bind to complementary mRNA with subsequent suppression of gene expression. This mixture was able to suppress T_H2 inflammation. In a small placebo crossover study, TPI ASM-8 inhibited early allergic response, whereas the suppression of late response was not significantly decreased. The compound also suppresses post-challenge eosinophilia and mRNA levels of target molecules [166]. Other chemokine receptors involved in asthma development are CCR2 (on monocytes, T-cells), CXCR2 (on neutrophils, monocytes), CCR4, CCR8 and CXCR4 (on T_H2 cells). In animal models, blockade of CCR4 resulted in depletion of T_H2 cells and reduced lung inflammation. In patients with neutrophilic asthma, an increased concentration of CXCL8 (Interleukin 8), which acts through a CXCR2 receptor, was described. Small molecule antagonists of CXCR2 (e.g. *SCH527123*) were studied for COPD, but may also be effective in neutrophilic asthma. Oral *SCH527123* administration is effectively able to prevent the increases in sputum neutrophils induced by ozone [205]. Further studies are needed.

Cytokines are key players in the initiation, development and persistence of bronchial asthma. Increasing knowledge about the function of particular cytokines and their common relationships and regulations allow identification of new therapeutic targets, which could be blocked in various ways (predominantly via monoclonal antibodies). Due to their anti-inflammatory potential, some cytokines could also be used as potential therapies in asthma treatment. New targeted therapies are closely linked to the appropriate selection of specific asthmatic phenotypes, and the possible side effects should be outweighed by the therapeutic benefits.

---

10. Immunoglobulin E Modulators

Immunoglobulin E (IgE) is a crucial player in the 1st type of allergic reactions and it acts through its high-affinity and low-affinity receptors. Targeting IgE production and function is an optimal strategy for IgE-mediated diseases, e.g. atopic (allergic) bronchial asthma.

CD23 is a low-affinity IgE receptor, which is important in the regulation of IgE production. It is expressed in many inflammatory cells (e.g. eosinophils, T and B cells, neutrophils), is significantly over-expressed in allergic disease [455] and correlates with disease severity and control [25]. Monoclonal antibody against CD23 (*IDEC-152, lumiliximab*) in intravenous application was studied in the treatment of IgE-mediated bronchial asthma [371]. A single dose-escalating placebo-controlled *study* in asthmatics showed that *lumiliximab* caused a dose-dependent reduction in serum IgE. Further studies aimed at its clinical efficacy should be performed [372].

Humanized monoclonal antibody against IgE – *omalizumab* (OMA) – is actually a unique monoclonal antibody that has been integrated into the official guidelines for treatment of asthma in adults and in children over six years of age (in some countries over 12 years of age). There are several recognized mechanisms of OMA action (Figure 12). Besides binding of circulating and bound IgE molecules, omalizumab also targets the high-affinity IgE receptors (FcεRI) and stabilizes the mast cells and other inflammatory cells against degranulation. The binding of OMA to IgE forms immune complexes that are subsequently cleared by the reticuloendothelial system and are not able to activate the complement system. Because OMA binds to the same site that IgE molecules use to attach to FcεRI, it cannot cross-link cell surface-expressed IgE. OMA does not bind to receptor-bound IgE. During OMA treatment, due to increased clearance of free IgE and suppressed IgE production, the amount of cell-bound IgE also decreases [58]. During the application of OMA, the rapid and substantial decline of serum-free IgE can be noted. A 99% reduction of serum-free IgE has been noted within two hours of OMA administration [284]. Due to decreased expression of FcεRI, OMA might have a significant effect on the sensitization phase of the allergic response. OMA also reduces blood and sputum eosinophils. During the treatment, a decrease of tissue eosinophils and cells expressing FcεRI receptor (CD3$^+$, CD4$^+$, CD8$^+$, CD19$^+$) is observed. During the therapy with OMA, a significant reduction of blood basophil populations was also observed [202]. During the treatment with OMA, decreased production of cytokines involved in T_H2 polarization (thymic stromal lymphopoetin, thymus and activation-regulated chemokine, OX40 ligand) was noted. In children with severe atopic dermatitis, increased IL-10 was observed during OMA therapy [218] (Table 10). However, the effect of OMA on airway hyperresponsiveness is unclear based on the clinical studies [144, 329, 353]. The dosing of the drug is dependent on body weight and the pre-application level of total serum IgE. To date, the exact duration of the OMA application is not known, but with the high exacerbation rate and control worsening after withdrawal or a decreased dose of OMA, it is intended to be a life-long treatment until updated data becomes available from the studies and clinical observations. Reducing OMA doses below those in the dosing table cannot be recommended, because the resulting increase in free IgE would cause deterioration in asthma control [399].

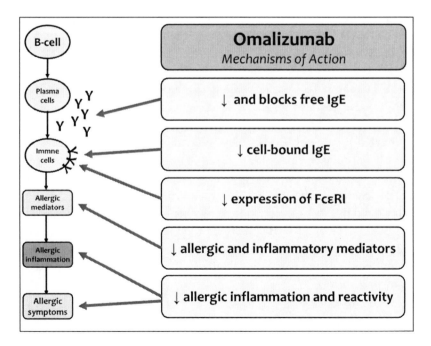

Figure 12. Mechanism of omalizumab action (Modified from Incorvaia et al., 2014).

Table 10. Effects of omalizumab on immune system in the context of its clinical actions

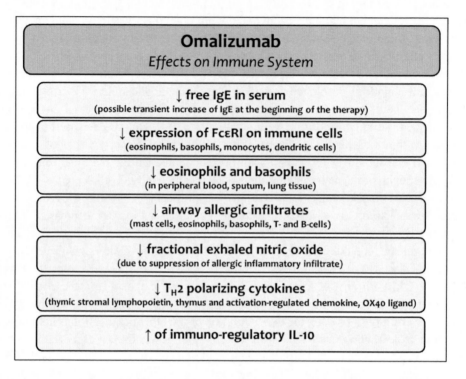

Some authors also showed data with a persisting clinical effect, post dose reduction, based on serum IgE level monitoring after the decline of IgE to a normal range [408].

Omalizumab in adults: A number of well-designed studies in both adults and children demonstrated the efficacy of OMA in the treatment of moderate-to-severe persistent IgE-mediated asthma. OMA reduced the asthma exacerbation rate, emergency department visits and hospital admissions, and the use of rescue medication; it improved clinical symptom scores and asthma control, and in a substantial proportion of patients, it allowed withdrawal of peroral corticotherapy [83]. In several studies, the decline of other applied therapy (e.g. inhaled corticosteroids) was also noted. In adolescents and adults, OMA caused a small but significant improvement of FEV_1 and peak expiratory flow rates [401]. Patients with features suggestive of greater disease severity appeared to obtain the most benefits from the addition of OMA to their therapeutic regimens [83] (Table 11).

Omalizumab in children: Data for children of preschool age are not available; however, several studies of school age children have been published. The most consistent finding from the available childhood study is a reduction in asthma exacerbation frequency [352, 366]. In their ICATA study, Busse et al. (2011) demonstrated the benefits in total asthma symptoms days, and an apparent loss of seasonal effects on symptom days, exacerbation frequency and ICS dose administered (Table 12) [72]. Omalizumab also yielded a corticosteroid-sparing effect in pediatric trials [64].

The preventive effect of OMA was also maintained during the autumn and winter, when the exacerbation rate in children due to viral infectious is higher when compared to other periods of the year.

Table 11. Omalizumab in adults – summary and meta-analysis of the clinical studies (according to Norman et al., 2013 and Normansell et al., 2014)

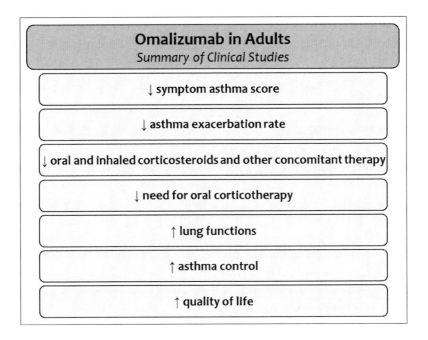

Table 12. Omalizumab in children – summary and meta-analysis of the clinical studies (according to Norman et al., 2013 and Normansell et al., 2014)

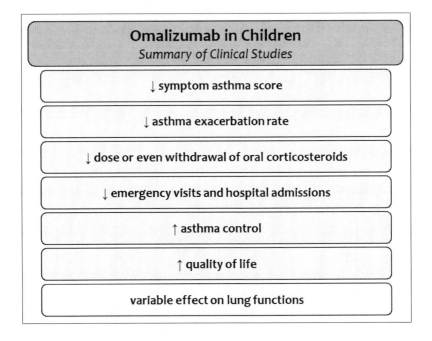

In pediatric studies, in contrast to adult studies, no clear effect of OMA treatment on lung function was detected. However, many child asthmatics do not experience serious and irreversible structural changes to the airways with the deterioration of lung function. A significant portion of children and adolescents particularly suited for omalizumab because of asthma severity may be ineligible due to IgE > 1300 IU/mL [402]. The role of OMA in children who fulfill the criteria but who have total IgE levels above 1300 IU/mL remains unclear at present. On the other hand, the effectiveness of OMA in patients with very low total IgE was also questioned, but some data showing the potential role of OMA in such patients with negative specific IgE (which may be induced by long-term corticosteroid administration) already exist [302].

Some other humanized monoclonal antibodies against IgE were studied. *TNX-901* was evaluated in patients with a peanut allergy and a significant improvement of the threshold dose was noted in a proportion of the patients (25% of the patients had no improvement) [280]. Recently, a novel high affinity monoclonal antibody against IgE (*MEDI4212*) was developed to allow anti-IgE treatment for patients with very high IgE levels, who are currently contraindicated for the use of omalizumab. *MEDI4212* potently inhibited responses through FcεRI and also prevented the binding of IgE to CD23. When used *ex vivo* in identical concentrations, *MEDI4212* depleted free-IgE from human sera to levels ≈1 log lower than omalizumab. The results from the recent study documented that *MEDI4212* binds specifically to IgE and prevents IgE from binding to its high- and low-affinity receptors. This compound effectively depleted free-IgE from human sera *ex vivo* to a level (1 IU/mL) anticipated to provide optimal IgE suppression in severe asthmatic patients. Further clinical studies are needed [102].

To date, no single clinical or laboratory marker has been determined for the evaluation and prediction of therapeutic response to omalizumab. The current therapy effectiveness is provided through *global evaluation of treatment efficacy* (GETE), which involves laboratory, clinical and spirometric parameters. According to the ICATA study, response to OMA was strongest in those sensitized to cockroach antigens, with increased serum eosinophils (> 2%) or increased FENO (> 20 ppb) [72]. Early changes in IgE may be used as a predictor of future responders to OMA in terms of exacerbation rate (elevation of total serum IgE after three months was significantly associated with the exacerbation rate over the 1-year survey) [118]. Other authors suggested the use of basophil CD203c levels [171] or peripheral blood eosinophils [75] as a predictive tool for the effectiveness of OMA therapy.

Omalizumab in other allergic and non-allergic diseases: Currently, OMA is shown to be effective in the treatment of chronic idiopathic urticaria. OMA is more likely to be of therapeutic benefit in patients with chronic urticaria, with autoantibodies to IgE or FcεRI [83]. From off-label indications, OMA was studied and proven to be effective in selected patients with anaphylactic reactions to foods and drugs, allergic persistent rhinitis, nasal polyposis, allergic bronchopulmonary aspergilosis, atopic eczema, bullous pemphigoid, Churg-Strauss syndrome, latex allergy, Hyper-IgE syndrome, cystic fibrosis, hypereosinophilic syndromes and anaphylaxis [20, 82, 288, 441]. The combination of OMA and specific allergen immunotherapy might be an effective strategy to permit more rapid and higher doses of allergen immunotherapy to be given more safely and with greater efficacy to patients with allergic diseases [82].

Omalizumab and side effects: OMA is well tolerated and the most common adverse events are local reactions at the injection sites. Anaphylaxis was reported in clinical trials at a frequency of 0.1%, and therefore OMA should be applied in healthcare settings, where anaphylaxis can be managed [72]. Previous concerns about the risk of malignancy during anti-IgE treatment were not confirmed [69].

> Omalizumab is indicated for the treatment of severe persistent IgE-mediated bronchial asthma where symptoms are not well controlled by a medium-to-high dose of inhaled corticosteroids and long-acting β_2-agonists. Despite current cost-effectiveness concerns, a trial for at least six months' duration of omalizumab in atopic asthmatics fulfilling the respective national criteria should be recommended.

11. Immunosuppressants

Immunosuppressants were studied particularly in the treatment of severe and steroid-resistant asthma; however, the studies brought conflicting and inconsistent results. The main problem was the high rate of different side effects that in some patients led to a withdrawal from the treatment. Some options could be presented by the modified analogues of the old molecules. A typical example is *cyclosporin A*, which is used especially in transplantology, and which can be used for several conditions involving inflammation (such as arthritis). It is clearly efficacious in the inhibition of T-cell proliferation with the subsequent decline of inflammatory processes and responses. Since bronchial asthma is associated with chronic unregulated inflammation with an important contribution of T-cells, it was suggested that cyclosporin A, could help in the treatment of the most severe cases. Its potential beneficial effects are outweighed by its toxicity (especially nephrotoxicity) [31].

Several studies showed that the use of cyclosporin could reduce the need for systemic corticosteroids; however, side effects were weighed against these possible benefits for asthma [320]. It was shown that the inhalation of small doses of cyclosporin strongly inhibited the influx of inflammatory cells into the airways during acute allergic reactions, even though associated bronchospasm and airway hyperreactivity were undiminished [317]. According to the meta-analysis, there was a small but significant treatment effect of cyclosporin in terms of steroid dose reduction and a small but significant improvement of lung function testing [140]. Cyclosporin seems to be effective in only a proportion of patients with oral corticosteroid-dependent asthma, when it may improve disease severity and/or enable oral steroid dosage reduction [107]. Several studies used *novel cyclosporin analogues* as promising new therapies for asthma, but the results of the studies were inconclusive [133].

Another immunosuppressant, the macrolides *tacrolimus* (FK506) and *sirolimus* (*rapamycin*) have similar effects on asthma treatment as cyclosporin. Some other drugs were also studied (e.g. *methotrexate, hydrochloroquine, dapsone, gold salts*), but the potential therapeutic effects were, in the majority of patients, outweighed by quite frequent side effects [132]. The use of *methotrexate* (MTX) usually showed only marginal steroid reduction [241]. Although some authors observed the possibility of a reduction of peroral corticosteroid therapy with the reduction of corticosteroid-related side effects [128, 400] and the therapy of MTX was well tolerated without any significant side effects [199], the meta-analysis concluded that MTX may have a small steroid-sparing effect in adults with corticodependent-asthma, but overall reduction in daily steroid use is probably not large enough to also reduce the corticosteroid-induced side effects [120].

The main reason for these studies was the search for new steroid-sparing therapeutic strategies, but none of the studied immunosuppressants yielded a sufficient and acceptable benefit/risk ratio [405]. They demonstrated some positive effects in a small number of studies and subjects. Most of them are, however, minimally effective in large series and/or have intolerable side effects in these chronically ill patients [375].

The use of different immunosuppressants in asthma management is limited due to several reasons [107]:

- Not all patients respond, and response cannot be predicted a priori
- The high incidence of unwanted side effects makes it difficult to assess overall benefit/risk ratios
- There are many absolute and relative contraindications to therapy
- There is a lack of knowledge about the long-term effects, beneficial or otherwise, of therapy

Based on the available trials, the therapeutic effect of cyclosporin in severe bronchial asthma is small and of questionable clinical significance. Regarding the side effects of cyclosporin, the available evidence does not recommend routine use of this drug in the treatment of bronchial asthma, even in its corticoid dependent forms.

12. Methylxanthines

Methylxanthines are commonly used in the treatment of bronchial asthma and chronic obstructive pulmonary disease (COPD) in adults; however, their usefulness in children was not proven. Meta-analysis of 34 pediatric randomized controlled trials showed that theophylline at standard dosing is less effective compared to inhaled corticosteroids [387]. Other important issues were its narrow therapeutic index requiring serum level monitoring, along with its negative effect on children's behavior and concentration. Today, theophylline is again at the center of interest, but *in low dosage* (serum levels 5 – 10 mol/L vs. conventional 10-20 mol/L) [366]. It was shown that *in vitro*, low-dose theophylline has several beneficial complementary effects with potential application in asthma treatment, e.g. *down-regulation of inflammatory gene expressions, activation of neutrophil apoptosis* and *prevention of down-regulation of β-receptors induced by β$_2$-agonists* [366]. In patients with COPD, the use of theophylline is associated with *decreased corticosteroid resistance* [109]. However, studies confirming the beneficial effect of low-dose theophylline in pediatric asthma are still lacking. In two small trials with mild-to-moderate asthma, adding theophylline did not result in any clinical benefits and was inferior to add-on therapy with montelukast [257, 413]. A recent study of children with mild persistent asthma showed that application of low-dose theophylline in the form of sustained-release dry syrup formulation improved the daytime and nighttime asthma symptoms score accompanied by decreased inflammatory markers (e.g. eosinophilic cationic protein) [276]. Data in more severe asthmatics are missing. There are also some new methylxanthines, such as doxofylline, with a better side effects profile compared to theophylline, but pediatric data are missing [378]. The potential target subgroup of asthmatic children suitable for low-dose theophylline seems to be children with inadequately controlled asthma on maximal or near-maximal therapy [366].

> Methylxanthines are commonly used in adult asthmatics; their usefulness in children is still being discussed, especially regarding their safety profile. Theophylline in a low-dose manner could potentially be used in those child asthmatics with maximal or near-maximal therapy and poor control over the diseases. More pediatric studies are needed. Another option presents newer methylxanthines, e.g. doxofylline.

13. Intravenous Immunoglobulins

Intravenous immunoglobulin (IVIG) represents an important therapeutic tool in modern immunology. Despite many studies, the exact mode of its action has not yet been clarified [261]. Intravenous immunoglobulin is a polyspecific, polyvalent immunoglobulin preparation purified from plasma pools of several thousand healthy donors. It contains predominantly human IgG molecules (with the proportional contribution of four subclasses similar to the plasmatic profile) with a small amount of IgA and IgM [424].

IVIG has become an accepted mode of therapy in immune mediated diseases with the potential to act as an immune enhancer, immunomodulator or even immunosuppressant in a dose-dependent manner. Several studies were aimed at the establishment of potential anti-allergic mechanisms of IVIG action. It was demonstrated that IVIG *inhibits IgE production in human B-lymphocytes*, which can be one of the causal mechanisms of action in allergic diseases [391]. Besides this effect, the application of IVIG in sensitized individuals is able to *decrease immune cell proliferation, to decline T$_H$2 response* and to *induce T regulatory cell differentiation and proliferation* [184, 243, 290]. A reduction in skin prick reactivity after IVIG infusion was also observed [220], although it was not accompanied by RAST inhibition *in vitro* [304]. Some effects of IVIG could probably be attributed also to an interaction with cytochrome p450 and NO-synthase systems in the liver [261]. The suppressive effect on inflammation of various origins is mediated by the interference with different receptors on the surfaces of the immune cells [290, 424] (Figure 13).

Bronchial asthma is accompanied by chronic inflammation in the airways with the dysregulation of the cytokine network and with the accumulation of different inflammatory cells. Therefore, IVIG would be expected to act as a potential anti-inflammatory therapeutic strategy in asthmatics. Intravenous immunoglobulin was considered especially for the treatment *of severe bronchial asthma* requiring the use of systemic (oral) corticosteroids. Unfortunately, most reports are anecdotal and there are few placebo-controlled studies available.

The efficacy of IVIG was proven in *specific subgroups of asthmatic patients*, e.g. with associated IgG subclass deficiency [383]. The substitution of IVIG in a group of severe asthmatic patients with associated mild or severe antibody deficiency led to remarkable clinical benefits: reduction of morbidity, number of hospitalizations, steroid therapy and number of respiratory infections. IVIG application in this specific subgroup of asthmatics probably allows the achievement of asthma prevention rather than an amelioration of inflammation [384]. The efficacy of IVIG on the improvement of clinical symptoms and reduction of the required steroid dose was also observed. The IVIG replacement therapy may thus help to control asthma symptoms in patients with simultaneous antibody deficiency [446].

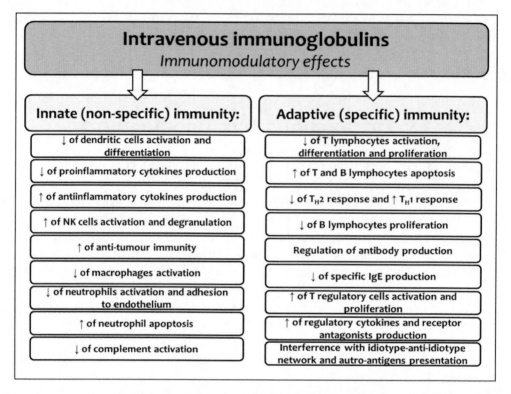

Figure 13. Different immunomodulatory effects of intravenous immunoglobulins in the immune system (adapted from Tha-In et al., 2008 and Wahn et al., 2008).

Studies with non-immunodeficient asthmatics also showed some effect of IVIG administration on the clinical symptoms and control over the disease [149, 444]. In a murine model of bronchial asthma, IVIG markedly attenuated perivascular and peribronchial pulmonary inflammation, followed by a decrease of bronchial hyperresponsiveness [243]. The IVIG application allowed oral prednisone dose reduction with a decreased number of hospital admissions. A decreased symptom score and clinical stabilization of the diseases were also noted (Table 13) [254]. However, the effect of IVIG on lung function was inconsistent [192, 254]. Different IVIG doses were used. Several authors applied a high-dose regimen (2 g/kg of body weight/month) with potential persistence of therapeutic effect after completion of this therapy [254]. Unfortunately, some authors and well-designed placebo-controlled studies concluded that the use of high-dose IVIG is associated with significant incidence of serious adverse events, and the therapeutic advantages over the placebo were not confirmed in steroid-dependent asthmatics [250, 326]. It should be assumed that the number of subjects in the existing clinical trials with IVIG and asthma is usually very low, and therefore it is very difficult to establish any valid conclusions regarding the usefulness of IVIG in asthma management. Moreover, the economic aspect of such therapeutic intervention should also be taken into account [106]. The role of IVIG is also diminished by the increasing number of different biologicals and anti-cytokine therapy. However, it is possible that some specific subgroups of asthmatic patients would profit from IVIG application (Table 14).

Table 13. Observed effects of intravenous immunoglobulins in the studies with asthmatic patients

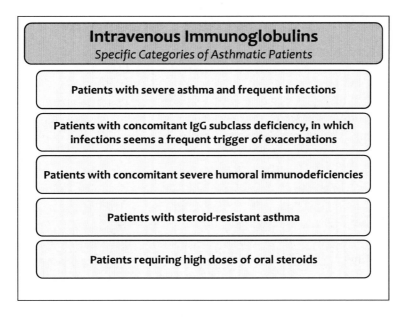

**Table 14. Specific categories of asthmatic patients with considerable indication for intravenous immunoglobulins
(Adapted from Rabinovitch et al., 1999 and Salmun et al., 1999)**

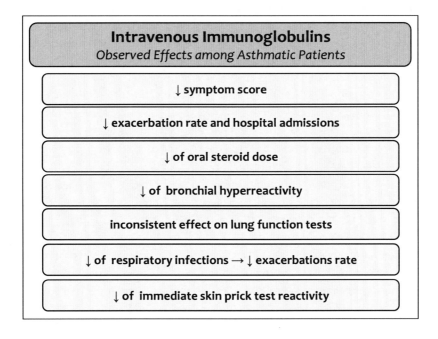

Based on the current studies, use of IVIG could at best be suggested for some specific subgroups of asthmatic patients. However, more studies are needed. Available data are insufficient to conclude that IVIG could be generally recommended for severely asthmatic patients.

14. Specific Allergen Immunotherapy

Current strategies in allergology are aimed at the prevention of allergic diseases, including the prevention of allergic hyperreactivity and development of allergic diseases, as well as the prevention of the worsening of allergic symptoms and new sensitizations. However, to date only a *few preventive strategies* have been successful and research in this area is still ongoing. The universal preventive strategy is the *exclusion of passive smoking* in both the prenatal and postnatal periods. Besides this approach, *specific allergen immunotherapy* (SAIT) is another effective option for preventing the development of bronchial asthma in patients with already established allergic rhinitis and for minimizing the risk of new sensitization development. The effectiveness of SAIT in the treatment of allergic rhinitis was proven by many well-designed studies. However, its utility in the treatment of bronchial asthma with or without concomitant allergic rhinitis is still being discussed. Specific allergen immunotherapy is considered a disease-modifying therapy that is effective in the treatment of allergic rhinitis, rhinoconjunctivitis, allergic asthma and insect venom hypersensitivity [2, 77, 373].

The mechanisms of the clinical effects of SAIT are complex and involve changes in specific immunity, but they are not yet completely understood. The most evident and confirmed mechanism is the *shift from T helper cell type-2 (T_H2) immune responses*, which are associated with the development of IgE sensitization (so-called atopy) and allergic symptoms, to T_H1 immune with subsequent *suppression of specific IgE production*. It was shown that the increase of T_H1 response secondary to SAIT might be associated with *increased resistance to apoptotic signals* [98]. Another important mechanism is the *induction of T regulatory cells* ($CD4^+CD25^+$) that produce anti-inflammatory and immunoregulatory cytokines, e.g. interleukin 10 (IL-10) or transforming growth factor β (TGF-β). These cytokines are able to *suppress the production of allergen-specific IgE* (specific IgE levels initially increase and then gradually decrease), support the *formation of protective IgG_1, IgG_4 and IgA* (none of these changes in antibody levels have been shown to consistently correlate strongly with clinical improvement), and *reduce the release of pro-inflammatory cytokines* from eosinophils, mast cells, basophils and T-lymphocytes. SAIT is associated with the *suppression of allergic cellular inflammation* in the target organs (eyes, nasal and bronchial mucosa) with a reduced release of allergic mediators from these cells [113, 236].

The crucial factor determining the efficacy of SAIT is the detection of causal allergens, which is applied in increasing doses through various modalities of SAIT (e.g. subcutaneous injections, sublingual drops or tablets). The causal allergen is detected by skin prick tests or serum studies (specific IgE measurement, component resolved diagnosis). The observed positivities should be evaluated in context with the clinical symptoms of particular patients. Skin prick tests are in general considered more sensitive and cost-effective than allergen-specific IgE tests [158]. Patients with allergic respiratory disease are suitable for SAIT in these cases [232]:

- Allergic symptoms are persistent
- Clear causal allergen/allergens were detected
- Allergic symptoms are not well controlled by pharmacotherapy or allergen avoidance measures
- Patient requires high doses of medication or multiple and combined medications to maintain control of his diseases and symptoms
- Presence of adverse effects of medication
- Patient wishes to avoid the long-term use of pharmacotherapy

However, *in polysensitized patients* the SAIT can also be administered after a rational evaluation of the causal contribution of particular allergens. SAIT was proven effective and safe in polysensitized patients as well [99].

The number of clinical studies and medical evidence for the use of SAIT in the treatment of bronchial asthma is increasing. Immunotherapy has been shown to be effective in the treatment of allergic bronchial asthma caused by grasses, ragweed, house dust mites, cats and *Alternaria* [315, 475]. According to the Cochrane meta-analysis of 75 randomized controlled trials, SAIT in the management of bronchial asthma has demonstrated these effects [3, 236] (Figure 14):

- Reduction of symptoms score;
- Reduction of pharmacotherapy (e.g. inhaled corticosteroids);
- Improvement of bronchial hyperresponsiveness;
- Improvement of other concomitant allergic diseases (allergic rhinitis, atopic dermatitis);
- Improvement of quality of life.

The effect of SAIT in asthma management *was proven for both subcutaneous* (SCIT) *and sublingual* (SLIT) *applications.* Due to the very limited evidence from head-to-head comparative studies between SCIT and SLIT and variability of the end-point used in different studies, it is not possible to establish the superiority of either route of immunotherapy administration [236]. There is also increasing evidence that SAIT can even *prevent the onset of asthma both in atopic subjects* [325, 179] and *in subjects with already treated allergic rhinitis* [440]. Immunotherapy can also *modify the progression of already established asthma in children* [231]; however, such results were not confirmed in adults. SAIT can be used prior to application of inhaled corticosteroids (ICS) in patients with very mild allergic asthma and concomitant allergic rhinitis or as add-on therapy in patients using ICS alone [475]. It can also be used in patients with combined anti-asthmatic therapy (ICS with leukotriene receptor antagonists and/or long-acting β_2-agonists) or even in patients treated with omalizumab (monoclonal antibody against IgE), if asthma symptoms are controlled. To reduce the risk of severe adverse events and reactions, asthma symptoms must be controlled and spirometric indices should be stable (forces expiratory volume in 1 second – $FEV_1 \geq 70\%$ predicted) [315].

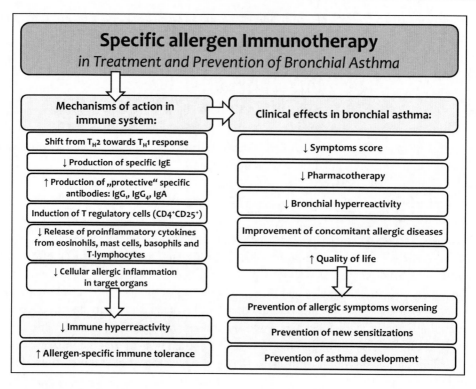

Figure 14. Specific allergen immunotherapy: Mechanisms of action and proven effects in the treatment and prevention of bronchial asthma.

Based on the current knowledge, it can be expected that specific allergen immunotherapy will be used in the management of bronchial asthma more frequently, especially due to its complex immunomodulatory effect and preventive potential in the disease progression. Due to its etiological aimed mode of action and disease-modifying effect based on its immunomodulatory properties, SAIT is considered to be the only real curative modality for the treatment and prevention of bronchial asthma.

15. Therapeutics Targeting Intracellular Signaling and Survival Pathways

15.1. Kinase Inhibitors and Modulators

Kinases represent important intracellular (and partially extracellular) signaling transducers, which are able to activate specific transcription factors with subsequent influence on the expression of different inflammatory cytokines and mediators. Kinases play a critical role in regulating the expression of inflammatory genes in asthma. Between various kinase pathways, intensive cross talk has been described. They have a critical role in the expression and activation of inflammatory mediators in the airways with a subsequent broad mode of action of different aspects of bronchial asthma pathogenesis (inflammation, cellular inflammatory infiltration, epithelium activation, reactive oxygen species production, remodeling) [5, 6, 215]. In asthmatics, changes in kinase activity have been described, especially among severe asthmatics. The changed kinase activity could also be responsible for reduced glucocorticoid responsiveness [4]. Steroid-insensitive asthma is associated with enhanced activation of different kinases, such as c-Jun N-terminal kinase (JNK), p38 mitogen-activated protein kinase (MAPK), Janus kinase/signal transducers and activation of transcription (JAK/STAT) or extracellular signal-related kinase (ERK) (Figure 15) [284, 435]. Patients with severe bronchial asthma usually respond poorly to the anti-inflammatory effect of corticosteroids (few are completely resistant), and therefore there is an urgent need for nonsteroidal anti-inflammatory therapeutic strategies for these patients.

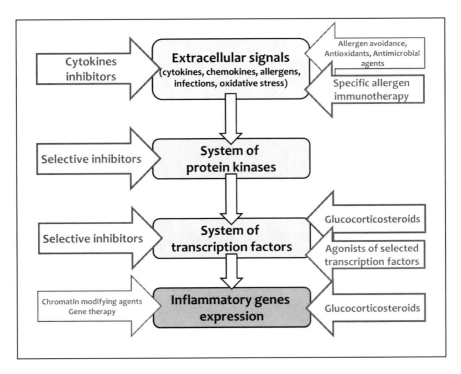

Figure 15. New possible therapeutic targets in intracellular signaling and genes expression.

Inhibitors of p38 MAPK are being studied in association with the reversal of the remodeling changes. Activation of MAPK signaling cascade is associated with differentiation, proliferation, activation, degranulation and migration of various cell types such as immune cells, airway epithelial and smooth muscle cells. In animal models, the use of p38 MAPK inhibitor *SB2439063* reduced the release of inflammatory markers and suppressed allergic inflammation [5]. Another MAPK inhibitor – *SB239063* – induced apoptosis of eosinophils from the BALF of guinea pigs [437]. The combination of dexamethasone with MAPK inhibitor reversed corticoid-insensitivity of peripheral blood cells and bronchoalveolar lavage fluid macrophages [47]. Novel enhydrazione ester CEE-1 also showed potential anti-inflammatory activity. The compound inhibited degranulation and leukotriene C4 release from activated human eosinophils and IgE-dependent degranulation of mast cells from mice. The drug significantly inhibited MAPK. In the mouse asthma model, CEE-1 inhibited bronchial inflammation and eosinophil accumulation in BALF and abolished airway hyperresponsiveness to methacholine [143]. Another possibility is to *inhibit MAPK-associated transcription factor MAPKAP2* (MAPK activated protein kinase 2) [262]. Regarding the potential side effects due to long-term application, an inhalant form of MAPK inhibitor is also being considered. MAPK plays a key role in the activation of GATA3, a transcription factor that regulates T_H2 cell proliferation and cytokine production. Corticosteroids block GATA3 activation and are mimicked by p38 MAPK inhibitors [294].

Nuclear factor kappa B (NF-κB) is one of the most famous and important transcription factors and it is activated by NF-κB kinase (IKK2). Small molecular inhibitors of IKK2/IKKβ block inflammatory response induced by NF-κB and are now in preclinical testing [242].

Extracellular signal-related kinase (ERK) has been found to be elevated in asthmatic mice. Inhibitor of ERK1/2 – *U0126* – inhibited inflammatory cellular infiltrates and decreased the production of various cytokines in the BALF of ovalbumin-challenged mice. This compound also inhibited eosinophils, hyperplasia of goblet cells and reduced expression of vascular cell adhesion molecule 1 (VCAM-1) and attenuated bronchial hyperresponsiveness to methacholine [130].

c-Jun N-terminal kinase (JNK) is another potential target for inhibition in patients with corticoid-insensitivity. In the animal models of bronchial asthma, JNK inhibitor *SP600125* resulted in reduction of eosinophils and lymphocyte accumulation in bronchoalveolar lavage fluid, decreased cytokine production and serum total IgE concentrations and attenuated smooth muscle proliferation [141, 142, 322]. However, this intervention did not attenuate the allergen-induced airway hyperreactivity. Therefore, the utility of JNK inhibitors in the treatment of asthma is limited [141]. *Orazipone* and its derivatives *OR-1958* and *OR-2370* are compounds with a unique mechanism of action. They form reversible conjugates with thiol groups (-SH) of protein and glutathione. *Levosimendan* is a pharmacological agent used in the treatment of heart failure. It acts by sensitizing troponin C to calcium with subsequent improved contraction. *Levosimendan* and *orazipone* have both previously shown anti-inflammatory effects. They enhanced spontaneous eosinophil apoptosis and reversed IL-5-induced eosinophil survival. Their mechanism of action seems to involve JNK and caspases. They also reduced lung eosinophilia in animal models of asthma and are potential novel drug candidates for treating eosinophilic conditions such as asthma [213].

Spleen tyrosine kinase (SAK) is very important in the degranulation of mast cells via high affinity receptors for IgE (FcεRI) and it is also involved in B- and T-lymphocytes antigen receptor signaling and supports eosinophil survival [110]. Animal models showed interesting effects of potent selective and selective SYK inhibitor *BAY-61-3606*. The use of this compound led to the inhibition of lipid mediator release and cytokine synthesis, reduced mast cell degranulation and inhibited human eosinophils, basophils and monocytes [464]. Another SYK inhibitor *R112* rapidly resolved symptoms of allergic rhinitis in topical application, and another compound *R343* is being tested in a clinical trial with bronchial asthma [310]. However, *R112* failed in the Phase II clinical study with allergic rhinitis [297]. Because SYK is widely distributed in immune and neuronal cells, there are concerns about side effects; therefore inhalation administration should be considered [38]. *R343*, an inhaled SYK inhibitor, has been tested in patients with allergic asthma but failed in the clinical Phase II study [185].

Cyclin-dependent kinases (CDK) are key enzymes involved in the cell cycle via phosphorylation of transcription factors and tumor suppressor proteins. Inhibitors of CDK should therefore be able to enhance apoptosis. Archetypal CDK inhibitor (*R-roscovitine*) and selective inhibitor of CDK – *AT7519* are able to enhance spontaneous apoptosis of eosinophils. Both induced a rapid apoptosis compared to that induced by other common factors (e.g. glucocorticoids). CDK inhibitors also increased neutrophil apoptosis. However, *in vivo AT7519* reduced also a number of other infiltrating cells, which may be secondary to reduced eosinophilia. These compounds are potentially useful for eosinophilic conditions such as asthma, but further studies are needed [213].

Another important intracellular kinase involved in the regulation of cell growth and proliferation, cell apoptosis and survival, and which is important in the mediation of cellular response to various cytokines, antigens and co-stimulatory molecules, is phosphoinositide 3-kinase (PI3K) [146]. PI3K is also important in chemotactic responses. It is also involved in the pathogenesis of asthma by affecting smooth muscle proliferation and eosinophil recruitment [146, 215]. However, the need for isoform specificity is still a limiting factor for the use of currently available PI3K inhibitors in asthma [6]. Wortmannin, a PI3K inhibitor, significantly attenuated eosinophil activation and proliferation in animal models of asthma [239]. *LY294002* and *TG-100-115* are other PI3K inhibitors that in animal models, inhibited the inflammatory response, cellular infiltration, expression of various inflammatory mediators (IL-5, IL-13, eotaxin) and suppressed eosinophilia, goblet cell hyperplasia and airway hyperreactivity [131]. *Theophylline* is a selective PI3Kδ inhibitor, and theophylline derivatives that lack PDE inhibition or selective PI3Kδ may therefore be of therapeutic value [38]. Tricyclic antidepressant *nortriptyline* also inhibited PI3Kδ and could reverse corticosteroid resistance [309]. Selective PI3Kδ inhibitors are now in clinical development for asthma. *IC87114* is a highly selective inhibitor of PI3Kδ with potential for the treatment of bronchial asthma [275]. Oral inhibitors of PI3Kδ – *CAL-101* and *CAL-263* - completed Phase I clinical trials for allergic rhinitis [51, 52]. A combined oral inhibitor of PI3Kδ/γ – *IPI-145* - is in Phase II for treatment of allergic asthma [331].

SHIP-1 (Src homology 2 domain-containing inositol 5' phosphatase 1) is a lipid phosphatase that leads to the dephosphorylation of phosphatidylinositol triphosphate (PIP3). The reduction of PIP3 levels leads to inhibition of calcium influx followed by gene transcription and down-regulated cytokine production. Allosteric a small molecular agonist of SHIP-1 – *AQX-1125* – which induces SHIP-1 activity, inhibited activation of mast cells and chemotaxis of leukocytes. Furthermore, it also inhibited lipopolysaccharide-induced pulmonary neutrophilic infiltration and ovalbumin-mediated airway inflammation [411, 412]. This molecule showed good tolerability and anti-inflammatory activity in Phase II clinical trials with mild to moderate bronchial asthma [196].

Rho-associated coiled coil-containing protein kinase (ROCK) is one of the most studied downstream signaling molecules of the monomeric GTP-binding protein Rho (Rhas human ortholog). The major physiological functions of this pathway include the migration, contraction and proliferation of different cells, and ROCK/Rho have been implicated in the pathogenesis of asthma [269]. Blocking of Rho/ROCK inhibits inflammation and airway smooth muscle contraction. *Y-27632*, a ROCK inhibitor, suppressed the release of inflammatory cytokines from T-lymphocytes and attenuated bronchial hyperreactivity [470]. In an *in vivo* model of allergic asthma, the same compound reduced airway eosinophilia and improved airway hyperresponsiveness to allergens or viral challenges [200, 380]. Another ROCK inhibitor, *fasudil (HA-1077)* also inhibited allergen-induced airway inflammation and hyperreactivity in animal models of asthma [419, 459].

Bruton tyrosine kinase (BTK) is an important target downstream of SYK and is significant in antigen-activated mast cells and basophils 196. *Ibrutinib* has been shown to block mast cell degranulation [403] and inhibit IgE-mediated activation of B-cells [289]. However, studies with bronchial asthma are missing and this compound was dominantly successfully studied in the treatment of rheumatoid arthritis and other autoimmune diseases [196]. Tyrosine kinase inhibitor *AB1010* (*mastinib*) is currently being studied in oral form for the treatment of severe persistent corticosteroid-dependent asthma in a Phase II clinical trial. Its efficacy was observed in a murine asthma model – reduced BALF eosinophilia, improved airway inflammation and edema and increased lung function [277].

15.2. Ion Channel Inhibitors

Ion channels are important and essential in many cellular processes and functions and they mediate extracellular and intracellular signaling. Among different ions, calcium ions are important in different allergic reactions and diseases. It was shown that calcium ions are essential in the activation and degranulation processes of mast cells and basophils. The intracellular influx of calcium ions from extracellular space is mediated via calcium-release-activated calcium channels (CRAC), which seem to be an interesting target in the treatment of diseases associated with mast cell or basophil activation and degranulation, e.g. allergic asthma or rhinitis. Several compounds blocking CRAC channels have been developed, e.g. *2-aminophenylborane* or *SFK96365*. These channels can also be blocked by *low concentrations of trivalent cations* Gd^{3+} or by *Synta compound 66*, which do not interfere with potassium channels or ATPase pumps [355]. In animal models, the CRAC antagonist (3-fluoropyridine-4-carboxylic acid, FPCA, Orai 1) significantly reduced asthma allergic inflammation and reduced the cough response and airway resistance [414]. Long-term application of the CRAC antagonist had more strongly expressed effects [415]. To resolve too low specificities of CRAC inhibitors, it has been suggested that CRAC channels could be inhibited by low concentrations of CRAC channel inhibitors and leukotriene receptor antagonists [127]. Animal models showed good inhibitory effects of *BPT2* (*YM-58483*) in allergic asthma [471]. Membrane potential and calcium signaling is, in mast cells, also regulated by the calcium-activated potassium channel KCa3.1. Its blocker (*ICA-17043*) was well tolerated in human subjects; however, the clinical Phase II trial did not confirm any significant therapeutic effect in asthmatic patients [460].

15.3. Inhibitors of Transcription Factors

Different transcription factors are essential parts of different intracellular signaling pathways and they mediate the transduction of information from different kinases to the nuclear DNA. Since different signaling pathways share the same transcription factors, it would be interesting to develop blockers of specific transcription factors with a potential modulatory effect on different signaling pathways involved in allergic responses and inflammation in bronchial asthma.

Nuclear factor kappa B (NF-κB) is induced by many factors involved in asthmatic inflammation, e.g. allergens, cytokines, chemokines, bacterial and viral infections, and it induces the expression of many mediators, signaling molecules, growth factors, receptors or enzymes important in the inflammatory cascade with feed-forward enhancement of inflammation [6]. Over-activation of NF-κB is associated with bronchial asthma [161]. Small molecular inhibitors of NF-κB stimulating kinase (IKK2) completely suppressed inflammatory response in animals and in macrophages from the BALF of asthmatic patients [50, 108]. IKK2 inhibitors also have some beneficial effects on the corticosteroid-insensitive release of CXCL10, which is induced by interferon gamma [436]. Since NF-κB is involved in many physiological processes, potential side effects (e.g. increased susceptibility to infections) are likely [6]. To decrease this risk, delivery by inhalation could be applied. NF-κB is a major target for corticosteroids, and therefore downstream of its co-activators and co-repressors may be potential therapeutic targets as steroid-sparing agents. Recruitment of histone deacetylase 2 (HDAC2) is involved in the glucocorticoid receptor-mediated suppression of NF-κB and its expression and activity are reduced in some corticosteroid-insensitive diseases [216]. *Theophylline* and *curcumin* are able to enhance HDAC2 activity under conditions of oxidative stress, which leads to a restoration of corticosteroid responsiveness [108, 307]. This could be an explanation of the clinical observation that adding a low dose of theophylline is more effective than increasing the dose of ICS in patients with poorly controlled asthma [32].

Transcription factor GATA-3 is increased in T-cells and bronchial biopsies from asthmatic patients [321]. This transcription factor is involved in the regulation of early T-cell development in the thymus, the differentiation of natural killer T-cells and the control of T regulatory cells. It also has a critical role in the differentiation of T_H2 response from naïve CD4 T-cells [6]. *Antisense oligonucleotides* may be an excellent novel anti-asthmatic therapy [111].

Nuclear factor of activated T-cells (NF-AT) is participating with other transcription factors (GATA-3 and AP-1) in the release of cytokines and mediators from T_H2 cells. Immunosuppressant drugs (*cyclosporin A*, *tacrolimus*, *pimecrolimus*) block calcineurin-dependent dephosphorylation of NF-AT, thus preventing its activation. An inhaled derivative of these drugs – MLD987 - should prevent the side effects of calcineurin inhibitors [111]. Inhibitors of NF-AT-calcineurin association (INCA) could be another possibility [111].

Signal transducers and activators of transcription (STAT) are the primary signal-specific mediators of cytokine-regulated gene expression activated by receptor-associated JAKs. Targeting JAK/STAT pathways could be an effective strategy for asthma therapy. STAT1 decoy oligonucleotide *AVT-01* was effective in animal models of asthma [356] and is now being tested in Phase IIa clinical trials. From several STAT proteins, only STAT6 is unique to the asthma-related cytokines IL-4 and IL-13 [81].

Transcription factor Forkhead box 3 (FOXP3) of T regulatory cells is crucial in the activity and functions of these cells. Therefore, respecting their functions and meaning in the complex immune response, T regulatory cells are very attractive candidates for immunotherapy. Over-expression of FOXP3 could be achieved by *retinoic acid*, which can be used for modulation of asthmatic allergic inflammation [91].

15.4. Agonists of Transcription Factors

Peroxisome proliferator-activated receptors (PPARs) are nuclear receptors activated by polyunsaturated fatty acid derivatives, oxidized fatty acids and phospholipids, which typically increase under conditions of acute or chronic inflammation and associated oxidative stress [45]. They belong to the thyroid hormone receptor-like transcription factor class. PPARs after activation by different signals and ligands decrease antigen-induced airway hyperresponsiveness, inflammation, eosinophilic infiltration, cytokine production and expression of certain transcription factors (e.g. GATA-3) [45]. PPARγ agonists can bind to the other transcription factors (NF-κB, STATs, AP-1), preventing their association with DNA sequences. PPARγ agonists have a number of anti-inflammatory effects in addition to the inhibition of GATA-3 levels that could be beneficial for the treatment of allergic diseases [83]. PPARγ agonist – *rosiglitazone* – reduced proliferation of allergen-specific T-cells and induced the production of tolerogenic and anti-inflammatory interleukin 10 [45]. A panel of regulated inflammatory genes by PPARγ agonists differs from those modulated by corticosteroids, and therefore the combination of these drugs may reach greater anti-inflammatory potential than either drug alone [337]. Interestingly, corticosteroids are also able per se to induce PPARγ expression [438]. Diabetic patients with concomitant asthma taking *thiazolidinediones* (*rosiglitazone* - activators of PPARγ) had decreased asthma symptoms and improved lung function [197]. PPARγ agonists - *rosiglitazone* – gave a small improvement in lung function in smoking asthmatics for which ICS were ineffective [404].

15.5. Regulators of Survival/Apoptosis Signals

Dysregulation of cell apoptosis and survival seems to be an important part of allergic processes. Mast cells express proteins of the B-cell lymphoma 2 family (BCL2), which participate in cell apoptosis regulation. The family consists of proteins with pro-apoptotic and anti-apoptotic functions, and the balance between these proteins determinates cellular fate through protein-protein interactions [135]. Members of the BCL2 family share one or more of the four characteristic domains of homology-named BCL2 homology domains (BH). BH3-only proteins (e.g. BIM, PUMA, BAD, NOXA) are capable of inducing apoptosis by binding to and neutralizing the anti-apoptotic proteins (e.g. MCL-1, BFL-1) [461]. Preclinical data suggest that BH3-only mimetic compounds are good candidate drugs for treatment of mast cell-associated diseases, such as mastocytosis, allergy and asthma [196].

15.6. Chromatin Modifying Agents

Chromatin modifying agents may be used in the future as a novel drug category that is based on the control of gene transcription. Chromatin is a protein-DNA complex, and histones are the major protein component. The changes and modification of chromatin are able to influence gene expression and this control of gene transcription is called *epigenetic control*. It is possible that in the future, through the therapeutic modification of chromatin, the expression of genes involved in inflammatory but also tolerogenic processes could be regulated and therapeutically modified. Histone acetylation by histone acetyltransferases is associated with transcription activations, whereas histone deacetylation (via histone deacetylases) is associated with transcription repression. Chromatic modification plays an important role in inflammatory response in asthma pathogenesis. Histone acetylation and pro-inflammatory gene transcription activation could be seen in passive smoking children (e.g. prenatally in smoking pregnant mothers), which explains the increased risk of bronchial hyperreactivity and asthma development in these children. Inhibitors of histone acetylation could potentiate some glucocorticoid receptor actions and support the anti-inflammatory effect of glucocorticosteroids. Modulation of the activity of histone acetyltransferase and histone deacetylases may be important new targets for anti-asthmatic drug development. However, they should be used with caution, because they alter the transcription of many genes and exert pan-cellular effects [354].

15.7. Inhibitors of Adhesion Molecules

Adhesion molecules (e.g. very late antigen-4, VLA-4) are important in the recruitment of inflammatory cells from circulation into the airways. They are involved in leucocyte migration, exocytosis, cytokine production and respiratory burst. Their inhibition could therefore influence the formation of allergen cellular infiltration [306]. Inhibitors of VLA-4 (VLA-4 is involved in the recruitment of eosinophils and T-lymphocytes) were effective in animal models, but unfortunately did not yield similar therapeutic response in asthmatic patients [397]. Inhaled *bimosiamose* (pan-selective selectin inhibitor) showed some inhibitory effects in allergen challenges, but further clinical studies did not repeat these results [41]. Nebulized bimosiamose suppressed sputum neutrophilia, suggesting its possible role in the neutrophilic phenotype of asthma [249].

> Influencing the intracellular signaling pathways seems to be an interesting approach to future anti-asthmatic therapy. The most studied targets are kinases, system of transcription factors, regulators of apoptosis and adhesion molecules. The biggest advances have been made in the field of inhibitors of kinases and transcription factors. However, in many compounds, the initial enthusiasm from animal and *in vitro* studies was not confirmed in clinical trials and human studies. A general concern about novel kinase or transcription factor inhibitors is that they may also have undesired side effects because they target mechanisms that are found in many cell types and essential physiological processes. It may therefore be necessary to develop an inhaled formulation or highly selective kinase or transcription factor inhibitors to decrease the potential unwanted side effects.

16. Modulation of Transient Receptor Potential Channels

Transient receptor potential (TRP) families of ion channels are cation-selective transmembrane proteins. It was shown that TRP prefer calcium (Ca^{2+}) ions. They monitor changes in the cellular microenvironment and respond through the transport of cations followed by changes in membrane potential and intracellular pathways. Their expressions have also been associated with various respiratory diseases [21, 29]. The TRP family consists of 28 members in six families, and e.g. TRPA1, TRPV1, TRPC1 and TRPV4 are expressed in airway smooth muscles, airway macrophages and inflammatory cells (T-lymphocytes, neutrophils) [21]. Targeting these receptors may present an interesting mode of asthma therapy. The most important members of the TRP family with regard to the pathogenesis of asthma are TRPA1 and TRPV1. Activation of these two receptors is associated with asthma-like symptoms and environmental triggers causing asthma-like symptoms to activate the TRPA1 receptor [389]. The TRPA1 receptor is associated with bronchoconstriction in late allergic response and the use of its antagonists in animal models attenuated this reaction. Allergens activate TRPA1 channels in the airways with a subsequent nerve trigger, a neuronal response and bronchoconstriction [359]. The role of the TRPV1 channel in airway hyperresponsiveness is not as clear as in TRPA1. Modulation of this channel resulted in inhibition of inflammation, airway hyperresponsiveness and airway remodeling [316]. Further studies could result in targeting of the function of these channels and the development of novel therapies.

> Transient receptor potential channels are involved in bronchoconstriction and other features of asthma. Modulating their action could lead to the development of novel anti-asthma therapies.

17. Cannabinoid Receptor Agonists

Cannabinoids are a direct class of psychoactive substances with various effects on organisms. Their biological effects are mediated by specific cell surface receptors – cannabinoid receptors, CB_1 and CB_2, in the central nervous system (CB_1) and in peripheral tissues (CB_2) [209]. It was shown that cannabinoids are decreased and dysregulated in neurogenic inflammation in bronchial asthma and stimulation of their receptors is able to inhibit the function of calcium channels. Their role in controlling airway responsiveness seems to be bidirectional and depends on the concomitant stimuli and factors [79]. Therefore, cannabinoid receptor agonists were studied as a potential novel therapy for various inflammatory disorders such as bronchial asthma [469].

In animal studies, several cannabinoid receptor 2 agonists (e.g. *WIN 55212-2, anandamide*) were studied. In general, the agents were able to *block the release of pro-inflammatory mediators* (e.g. substance P), *attenuated neurogenic inflammation, reduced allergen-induced oxidative stress damage, inhibited electrical field stimulation-induced bronchial smooth muscle contractions,* and *prevented capsaicin-induced bronchoconstriction and airway edema* [116, 174, 409, 468, 469]. The preventive effect of anandamide against bronchoconstriction was also demonstrated in the inhaled route of administration [410]. Another cannabinoid receptor 2 agonist (*HU-308*) yielded antioxidant, anti-inflammatory and anti-apoptotic effects in mouse models of ischemia/reperfusion injury [361]. However, studies with humans are lacking.

> Cannabinoid receptor agonists represent an interesting and perspective category of novel anti-asthmatic drugs. However human studies are lacking.

18. Endothelin System Antagonists

Endothelin-1 (ET-1) is an important endogenous factor with regulatory functions in the cardiovascular and respiratory systems. Endothelin-1 is produced by vascular endothelial cells and epithelial cells, T-lymphocytes and phagocytes. In asthmatics, ET-1 is over-expressed in the airway epithelium and supports bronchoconstriction. Moreover, endothelin-1 is important in the development of lung inflammation in asthma [160]. *In vitro*, ET-1 stimulates mucus secretion, activates pro-inflammatory cells (macrophages, mast cells) and serves as a mitogenic stimulus for fibroblasts and smooth muscle cells [258]. Compared to healthy subjects, asthmatic patients have increased levels of ET-1 during an exacerbation and following stabilization. Regarding bronchial asthma, ET-1 antagonist – *sitaxentan* (*thelin*) is undergoing a clinical trial for treatment of acute asthma [145]. In a murine asthma model, the ET-1 antagonist (*BQ123*) up-regulated lymphocytes infiltration and reduced eosinophils, airway hyperreactivity and mucus production [271]. Moreover, *montelukast* is also able to decrease the plasmatic level of endothelin-1, which increases its anti-asthmatic pluripotent mechanisms of action [258]. Another possibility is represented by the antagonist of endothelin-1 receptors, e.g. *bosentan*. *Thyme extract* in animal models inhibited endothelin-induced bronchoconstriction. The interaction/combination with bosentan was additive, but not supra-additive, indicating an interaction with the endothelin system. The authors concluded that thyme extract could be used as a complementary treatment for asthma or COPD due to the effect on endothelin hyper-reagibility typically observed in these diseases [136]. Bosentan in animal models of eosinophilic airway inflammation substantially inhibited the concentrations of TNF-α, IL-4, IL-1β, IFN-γ and ET-1 in BALF [147]. In murine asthma models, another selective ET-1-receptor antagonist, *atrasentan* (*ABT-627*), inhibited the influx of macrophages and eosinophils in allergen-challenged mice [177]. A bifunctional ET1/2-receptor antagonist (*IRL3630A*) was able to inhibit the ET-1 induced changes in respiratory resistance and compliance [292]. Unfortunately, a 4-week clinical trial with *bosentan* in patients with poorly controlled asthma did not improve lung function, use of rescue medication or asthma symptoms [114]. Further, the main side effect of this compound is hepatotoxicity and the potential to induce liver failure [163].

> Endothelin-1 plays an important role in the complex pathogenesis of bronchial asthma. However, despite initial positive results with both endothelin-1 antagonists and endothelin-1-receptor inhibitors in animal asthma models, the use of this compound was not proven to be sufficiently effective in human asthmatic patients. Further research is needed to detect potential candidates for this treatment among asthmatic patients.

19. Dendritic Cell Modulation

Dendritic cells are involved in allergen presentation and in interactions between various immune cells. Dendritic cells play a critical role in the regulation of chronic inflammation in asthma through the release of cytokines and chemokines. Modulation of their function represents a new approach in asthma therapy. Inhibition of already activated dendritic cells by their inhibitor (sphingosine-1-phosphate receptor antagonist – *fingolimod* – *FTY720*) strongly attenuated lung inflammation in mice and prevented migration of dendritic cells to regional lymph nodes [212]. Selective prostaglandin D receptor agonists (e.g. *BW245C*) also suppressed dendritic cell function followed by decreased airway inflammation and hyperresponsiveness through the induction of FOXP3-expressing T regulatory cells [188]. Similar effects also yielded prostacyclin analogue – *iloprost* [189]. To decrease the potential side effects of these compounds, inhalation may be an alternative approach.

Other possibilities for influencing and regulating the function of dendritic cells are agonists of Toll-like receptor 9. Dendritic cells interact with antigens through a number of important mechanisms, including pattern recognition receptors such as Toll-like receptors (TLR). A large number of animal studies have demonstrated that TLR-9 is activated through the CpG rich unmethylated DNA segments commonly found in various bacteria. These stimuli are also known as immunostimulatory DNA sequences (ISS) and can manage to skew the immune response towards T_H1 [288]. Human studies showed that using TLR-9 agonists along with causal allergens in specific allergen immunotherapy could significantly improve the therapeutic response and help in establishing immune tolerance. Currently, clinical trials with the TLR-9 agonist either alone or conjugated to an allergen are planned to investigate the potential role of TLR-9 agonists in asthma treatment [251]. Other TLR agonists are currently being studied as a possibility in the treatment of rhinitis and asthma (TLR-4 agonist – *MPL*, TLR-7 agonist – *AZD8848*, TLR-8 agonist – *VTX-A463*) [13].

Other possibilities for regulation and modulation of dendritic cells functions are represented by blocking of the target molecules – thymic stromal lymphopoetin, OX40 ligand or interleukin 33.

> Dendritic cells play a central role in the regulation and promotion of allergic inflammation in asthma. Therefore, modulating their activity represents a perspective innovative approach in the future treatment of bronchial asthma.

20. Inhibitors of Phosphodiesterase

Phosphodiesterases (PDE) are a superfamily of enzymes regulating various cellular functions and they have been shown to be significantly involved in the pathogenesis of bronchial asthma. Phosphodiesterases regulate airway muscle tone and significantly contribute to the processes of remodeling [67, 429]. Dysregulation of cAMP-PDE pathways was observed in asthmatics and elevated PDE activity could be one of the principal players in the chronic structural changes in the asthmatic airways. A better understanding of PDE isoenzymes and their function and possible roles in bronchial asthma and COPD allowed the development of optimal therapeutic strategies aimed at the inhibition of these enzymes, particularly PDE_4. PDE_4 is dominantly expressed in the airway smooth muscle cells [327]. The gene for PDE_4 is considered one of the asthma susceptibility genes [203]. Therefore, the blockage and modulation of PDE_4 activity seems to be a possible approach in the treatment of bronchial asthma.

PDE_4 inhibitors (e.g. *roflumilast, cilomilast*) are the most advanced nonsteroidal anti-inflammatory agents in the treatment of airway diseases. *Theophylline*, which was used in asthma treatment for many years, is a non-specific PDE inhibitor with bronchodilator, anti-inflammatory and anti-proliferative effects. However, its use has been hampered by its adverse effects. Preclinical laboratory studies showed that the PDE_4 inhibitor *roflumilast* is able to decrease bronchial hyperreactivity in both animal models [66] and human airways [357, 382]. Other described effects of roflumilast are reduction of airway smooth muscle proliferation, reduced inflammatory infiltrate and decreased inflammatory mediators [67, 157, 433]. The anti-inflammatory, immunomodulatory and suppressive activity of PDE_4 inhibitors in asthma involves cytokines, inhibition of generation of oxidants and pro-inflammatory mediators, inhibition of eosinophil migration, attenuation of their degranulation, reduction of smooth muscle proliferation and migration, suppression of pro-inflammatory activity of epithelial cells and attenuation of airway wall edema (Table 15) [6, 96].

Table 15. Pluripotent effects of PDE_4 inhibitors and their results in treatment of bronchial asthma

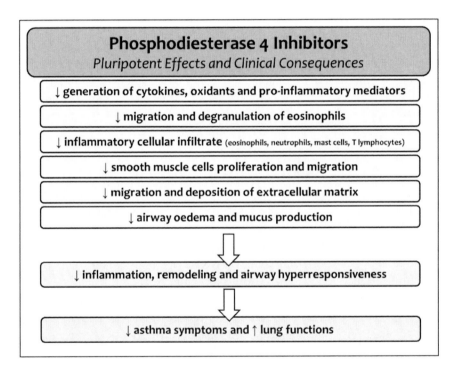

Interesting results arose from a recent study, which observed the decrease of respiratory syncytial virus infection in the airways, a common trigger for asthma exacerbations [298]. Clinical studies also confirmed the potential of PDE_4 inhibitors to be involved in the therapeutic algorithm of asthma. Treatment with PDE_4 inhibitors resulted in improvement of lung function, decreased late phase of allergic response and reduced inflammatory cell numbers (eosinophils, neutrophils) [165]. PDE_4 inhibitors are able to suppress neutrophilic and eosinophilic inflammation and exert distinct anti-inflammatory effects compared to corticosteroids, suggesting that PDE_4 inhibitors could be useful in severe asthma [96]. PDE_4 inhibitors showed comparable effects on lung function and symptom score as low-dose ICS [57]. Both roflumilast and cilomilast show dose-dependent inhibition of early- and late-phase responses to allergens and exercise [96]. Roflumilast yielded a better effect on lung function improvement than cilomilast [57]. There are also some limiting side effects of PDE$_4$ inhibitors such as nausea, vomiting, diarrhea and headache. Therefore, despite their established position in the treatment of chronic obstructive pulmonary diseases, PDE$_4$ inhibitors are currently not approved for bronchial asthma. It seems that selective inhibition of PDE$_4$B might be better tolerated, since nausea and vomiting are mediated via PDE$_4$D. To achieve a broader therapeutic effect, another possibility could be simultaneous combined inhibition of different PDE receptors. In animal models, concomitant use of inhibitors of PDE$_4$ and PDE$_7$ yielded stronger anti-inflammatory effects compared with the effects on smooth muscle and cough [311, 312]. Inhalant administration of PDE$_{3/4}$ inhibitors is being considered, and better bronchodilatation can be achieved through inhibition of PDE$_3$ [33]. In a recent study in healthy volunteers and patients with asthma and COPD, inhaled dual PDE$_{3/4}$ inhibitor was well tolerated and showed very good bronchodilator, bronchoprotective and anti-inflammatory effects [156].

> Phosphodiesterases play an important role in chronic changes in asthmatic airways. PDE$_4$ inhibitors are the most advanced nonsteroidal anti-inflammatory agents and showed many interesting anti-inflammatory and clinical effects in the treatment of asthmatic patients. Because of their side effects, PDE$_4$ inhibitors are currently not approved for bronchial asthma. However, the development of newer forms of PDE$_4$ inhibitors (e.g. selective PDE4B blockers, inhalant PDE$_{3/4}$ inhibitors) could expand current anti-asthmatic therapies.

21. Neurokinin Inhibitors

Bronchial asthma is associated with a specific kind of inflammation called neurogenic inflammation, where a number of neurokinins are involved. Neurogenic inflammation is mediated by a different cellular population, especially released neurokinins such as substance P (SP), neurokinin A (NKA), neurokinin B (NKB) or brain-derived neurotrophic factor (BDNF). These substances activate tachykinin receptors NK1, NK2 and NK3. Neurogenic inflammation is associated with bronchial hyperresponsiveness, mucus production and vasodilatation with airway edema [221, 233, 235]. Several clinical studies were aimed at the efficacy of different neurokinin inhibitors. An antagonist of NK1/NK2 receptor – *FK224* – had no effect on NKA-induced BHR [234]. A selective antagonist of NK2 receptor – *SR48968* (*saredutant*) – yielded some protective effect against NKA-induced BHR [439]. Another dual NK1/NK2 receptor antagonist (*DNK333*) showed only transient bronchoprotective effect in a small cohort of mild-to-moderate asthmatics [235], whereas a triple tachykinin receptor antagonist (*CS-003*) produced a potent and lasting protective effect against NKA-induced bronchoconstriction [381]. In another study, the dual receptor antagonist *AVE5883* paradoxically increased allergen-induced airway responsiveness.

> Neurogenic inflammation seems to be an ideal object for anti-asthmatic therapies. There are many discrepancies between animal and human studies regarding the therapeutic use of neurokinin inhibitors. Current knowledge does not support the use of these drugs in asthma therapy.

22. NO-Synthase and Arginase Inhibitors

Nitric oxide (NO) is an important signaling molecule that plays many important roles in the respiratory, nervous and cardiovascular systems. It is produced by three isoforms of the enzyme NO-synthase (NOS): neuronal (nNOS) and endothelial (eNOS), which are constitutive isoforms continually producing NO for physiological processes, and inducible NOS (iNOS), which is activated and over-expressed in the airway epithelium and cells of inflammatory infiltrate (eosinophils, macrophages, neutrophils) in asthmatic patients [25]. Over-production of NO in pathological circumstances (e.g. bronchial asthma) leads to increased production of mucus, extravasation of plasma with airway edema, promotion of cellular infiltrate (especially T_H2 polarized cytokine production) and increased formation of reactive nitrogen species with oxidative damage of biomolecules (DNA, proteins) (Figure 16).

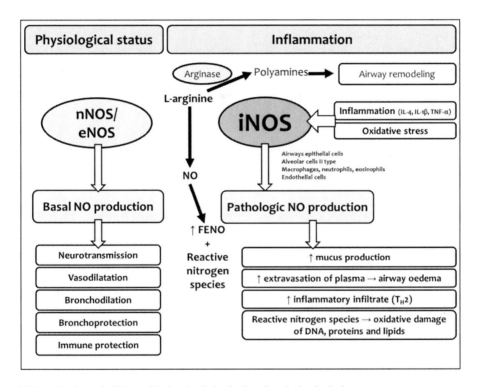

Figure 16. Production of nitric oxide in physiological and pathological circumstances.

Targeting iNOS as the source of NO over-production with its pathological consequences in asthma has been studied as a potential strategy for asthma therapy. Both non-selective iNOS inhibitors (e.g. *L-NAME*) and selective iNOS inhibitors (e.g. *GW274150, BYK402750*) were studied as potential anti-asthmatic drugs [8, 191, 422, 423]. The use of L-NAME did not affect allergen responsiveness, but it did increase AMP and histamine reactivity. These unwanted effects could be attributable to the non-selectivity of L-NAME to iNOS. Inhibition of nNOS/eNOS also reduced physiological basal NO production with reduction of its bronchoprotective effect [422, 423]. Selective iNOS inhibitors decreased inflammation in a cigarette-smoke exposure mouse model [201]. The use of the highly selective iNOS inhibitor

GW274150 resulted in a significant reduction of fractional exhaled nitric oxide in exhaled breath (FENO); however, early and late allergic responses and lung function were not affected [396]. Selective blockage of iNOS decreases NO levels in exhaled air, but is definitely not an effective therapeutic strategy in asthma [173].

Arginase I and II are enzymes that are also involved in the pathogenesis of bronchial asthma and that participate in the metabolism of nitric oxide. They metabolized L-arginine (substrate for NOS for NO production) into polyamines, which participate in the remodeling processes. The blockage of arginase with nor-NOHA attenuated airway hyperreactivity and eosinophilia with the reduction of pro-inflammatory cytokines (IL-4, 5, 13, eotaxin) and goblet cell numbers [418]. The specificity and potency of arginase inhibitors seem to be crucial in the final therapeutic response in asthma and the onset of unwanted side effects (e.g. increased production of nitrogen reactive species) [101].

Current knowledge does not support the use of non-selective or selective inhibitors of inducible NO-synthase in the treatment of bronchial asthma. However, several studies showed some positive results, especially in patients with bronchial hyperreactivity. Nonselective iNOS inhibitors could also exhibit some unwanted side effects due to removal of the bronchoprotective effect of NO produced by neuronal or endothelial NO-synthase. Another possible target is arginase and its inhibition.

---

23. Matrix Metalloproteinase Inhibitors

Matrix metalloproteinases (MMPs) are enzymes involved in the degradation of various components of the extracellular matrix. They are regulated by their inhibitors – tissue inhibitors of MMPs (TIMPs). Dysregulation of the regulation of MMP functions leads to the development of pulmonary diseases. Targeting MMPs and their inhibitors could represent a potential therapeutic strategy.

In bronchial asthma, elevated levels of MMPs were described and are probably one of the most important inducers of airway remodeling. Certain MMP gene polymorphisms are associated with the risk of asthma development [229]. In BALF and sputum, MMP-9 is increased [206, 303]. Other MMPs (1, 2, 7, 10, 12, 19) were also implicated in asthma [367]. There is strong evidence that MMP-12 is closely associated with bronchial asthma based on animal studies with MMP-12 deficient mice. MMP-12 regulated airway remodeling by its capacity to degrade many extracellular matrix proteins, e.g. elastin, collagen type IV, fibronectin and gelatin [21]. Some viral infections (e.g. respiratory syncytial virus infection) are able to induce MMP-10 [204].

Of the different inhibitors of MMPs, mainly tetracyclines were studied. The results of the studies were inconclusive and contradictory. Tetracyclines are able to maintain MMPs in inactive form. *Doxycycline* in animal models reduced eosinophilic allergen-induced airway inflammation and hyperresponsiveness by reduction of proteolytic activity and expression of MMP-9 [182]. Other MMP inhibitors (e.g. *R94138*) were studied and yielded positive therapeutic effects in animal models of asthma [319]. However, some MMPs – MMP-8 – could also have a protective effect on asthma development [181]. Clinical trials with MMP inhibitors were disappointing, probably due to the broad-spectrum inhibitory effects of currently available compounds.

> Although matrix metalloproteinases seem to be an interesting target for asthma therapy, and despite hopeful animal and *in vitro* results, clinical studies were disappointing and their use in asthma therapy is not recommended.

24. Macrolides

Macrolides (such as *azithromycin, clarithromycin, telithromycin, troleandomycin*) represent an antibiotic class with frequent and long-term use in clinical practice for the treatment of Gram-positive bacteria and atypical microorganisms. They inhibit protein synthesis in the target microorganism. In general, macrolides possess antimicrobial, immunomodulatory and potential antiviral properties [457]. Recently, the possibility of their use in the management of certain asthmatic phenotypes has been explored. In animal models, azithromycin decreased expression of certain cytokines (IL-5, IL-13) and reduced mucus production in the lungs [42].

There are a number of clinical human studies showing that short-term (three weeks) macrolide therapy improved some aspects of lung function, respiratory symptoms and quality of life in asthmatic patients [363]. While the long-term application of macrolides along with corticosteroids did not result in a significant improvement in lung function in the entire cohort, this therapy did yield some beneficial effects in patients with non-eosinophilic asthma. Because corticosteroids inhibit neutrophil apoptosis [305], a cautious steroid taper might be worth considering [68]. New molecules are currently on the horizon [186]. Macrolides have proven value in other neutrophilic airway diseases (chronic obstructive pulmonary disease, cystic fibrosis, panbronchiolitis, bronchiolitis obliterans, bronchiectasis) and there is some evidence of their benefit in adult neutrophilic asthma [10, 65, 186, 394]. Evidence for pediatrics-specific benefit is limited. In one small study with severely asthmatic children, *troleandomycin* showed an ability to reduce the oral methylprednisolone dose by 80%. Despite a dose reduction, an increase of steroid-related side effects was reported [152]. *Troleandomycin* decreased bronchial hyperresponsiveness [22]. *Telithromycin* caused a small but significant reduction in asthma symptoms without changes in lung function compared with the placebo when administered to patients with acute asthmatic exacerbation [230]. Clarithromycin behaves in a similar manner [155], but for both, this does not appear to occur with prednisolone. The studies also described the reduction of inflammatory markers (IL-8 in sputum, neutrophils in sputum) after treatment with macrolides [351, 394]. During pediatric acute wheezing episodes, adjuvant *clarithromycin* therapy decreased epithelial cell cytokine and chemokine production and decreased symptom duration (Table 16) [154, 260].

Another adjuvant benefit is represented by antimicrobial activity of macrolides against *Chlamydophilla pneumonia* and *Mycoplasma pneumonia*, which can be responsible for poor asthma control [368]. Treatment with clarithromycin improved lung function in asthmatics with PCR positivity for these microorganisms [263]. Manipulation with lung microbiome by agents with antibiotic properties may have both beneficial and detrimental effects, which should be taken into consideration. However, our knowledge about these changes and manipulations and their impact on health status is today only superficial and insufficient; further studies are required.

Table 16. Summary of potential clinical effects of macrolides in asthmatic patients

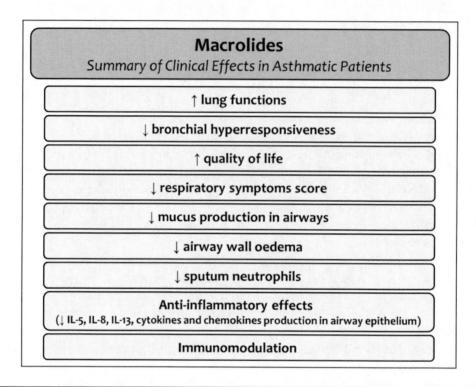

Macrolides have antimicrobial, immunomodulatory and potential antiviral properties, which advocate their potential use in the management of bronchial asthma. Recent evidence suggests improved effectiveness of macrolides in patients with sub-optimally controlled severe neutrophilic asthma and in asthma exacerbations. However, at present, the general use of macrolides in chronic asthma or acute exacerbations cannot be recommended (Wong, 2014). A trial of macrolides could be advocated in patients with a difficult to control disease, particularly in those with neutrophilic inflammation.

25. Statins

Statins are inhibitors of 3-hydroxy-3-methylglutaryl-coenzyme A reductase (HMG-CoA reductase) and are used dominantly as cholesterol-lowering drugs. However, recent studies in animal models and *in vitro* studies revealed their potent anti-inflammatory properties [210, 474]. When statins were added to maintenance corticoid therapy in asthmatics, the results of the studies were contradictory [60, 447]. Recent studies with severe asthmatics showed that the addition of these compounds to the standard controller therapy improved asthma symptoms, decreased the number of exacerbations and reduced corticosteroid use [434, 473]. The combination of corticosteroids with statins leads to the induction of T regulatory cells with subsequent suppression of airway inflammation [295].

Statins possess interesting anti-inflammatory effects. They can be useful as add-on therapy to inhaled corticosteroids in a small subgroup of asthmatic patients. However, their common use in asthma management cannot be recommended based on the current knowledge and evidence. Further studies are needed.

26. Oxidative Stress and Antioxidants

Oxidative stress results from an imbalance between the production of pro-oxidants and antioxidant defense mechanisms in the body. During chronic and acute inflammation, over-production of reactive oxygen species represents the natural protective mechanisms but also the consequences of poorly regulated inflammation with a significant contribution to the post-inflammation consequences (fibrosis, remodeling). The cells formatting airway inflammation infiltrate are an important source of reactive oxygen species in patients with bronchial asthma [12]. Oxidative damage plays an important role in the development, persistence and consequences of bronchial asthma. The oxidative changes of biomacromolecules have many consequences and significantly contribute to the pathogenesis of bronchial asthma. Reactive oxygen species, insufficient function of anti-oxidant defense and oxidation of macromolecules have many consequences: enhanced release of arachidonic acid from cell membranes, hyperreactivity and contraction of airway smooth muscle, increased vascular permeability with airway edema, increased bronchial hyperresponsiveness and mucus secretion, increased synthesis of pro-inflammatory cytokines and chemoattractants, induced release of tachykinins and neurokinins with augmentation of neurogenic inflammation, and impaired response to bronchodilators (Figure 17). The changes are not only the consequence of inflammation, but are also the result of damaged repair mechanisms [16, 17, 223, 228]. On the other hand, it has not been definitely established whether oxidative stress is the reason for or a consequence of chronic inflammation.

It was shown by many authors that *bronchial asthma is significantly associated with increased oxidative stress* expressed by the increased markers of oxidative damage, and the most impressive changes could be observed during acute exacerbation of asthma or in asthma with concomitant allergic rhinitis [16, 17, 25, 223]. The specific selected polymorphisms of antioxidant enzyme genes influencing the final function of the particular enzyme are significantly associated with bronchial asthma and its specific phenotypes [15, 16]. Changes in the levels of oxidants, antioxidants and markers of oxidative damage can be determined in peripheral blood, serum, plasma, bronchoalveolar lavage fluid, lung and bronchial tissues, and even in exhaled breath and its condensate [14, 223]. Due to low concentrations of reactive oxygen species, their extreme reactivity and very short lifetime, their direct measurement is very complicated, as is the estimation of indirect biomarkers of oxidative stress (e.g. markers of lipid peroxidation, decreased content of free thiol groups, total antioxidant capacity of plasma) [17].

Based on the observations from the studies bronchial asthma is associated with decreased antioxidant protection due to (due to changed functions of antioxidant enzymes) or decreased concentrations of non-enzymatic antioxidants, the use of different antioxidants seems to be an interesting mode of supportive anti-asthmatic therapy. Epidemiological data suggest that antioxidants have a significant effect on the incidence and severity of bronchial asthma [153].

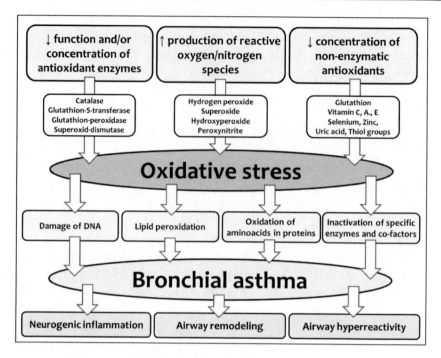

Figure 17. Complex relationship between oxidative stress and bronchial asthma.

Many antioxidants were studied in the treatment of bronchial asthma (e.g. vitamin, A, C, E, β-carotene, co-enzyme Q10, curcumin, flavonoids, and polyphenols); however, the studies brought conflicting and inconclusive results. Therefore, it could be suggested that, in particular, asthmatic subjects with specific polymorphisms of antioxidant enzymes and thus genetically-determined insufficiency or failure of endogenous antioxidant mechanisms could benefit from antioxidant treatment, [17].

> Bronchial asthma is associated with oxidative stress, which participates in different aspects of asthma pathogenesis. However, the therapeutic use of antioxidants was not in general proven in clinical studies for asthma and the appropriate selection of asthmatic patients with the potential to benefit from antioxidant therapy needs further investigation.

27. Beta-glucans

The use of different natural approaches or complementary and alternative medicine (CAM) is very common among patients with bronchial asthma, probably due to the chronic origin of their disease and the long-term application of various synthetic anti-asthmatic therapies [253]. Different approaches of CAM have been the subject of many expert review articles, studies of various designs and systematic reviews. The current form of CAM used in the treatment of asthma includes *natural and synthetic immunomodulators*, *Chinese medicine*, *homeopathy, acupuncture, yoga, aromatherapy, reflexology, relaxation therapy, breathing techniques, massages* and even *prayer* [324]. However, despite the unknown mechanisms of action of some of these approaches, the over-use and preference of different CAM strategies could postpone appropriate anti-asthmatic treatment and worsen the patient's condition. Therefore, in the view of evidence-based medicine, it is only appropriate to use those approaches that can act as complementary support to standard anti-asthmatic treatment, that have a mechanism of action that is at least partially clarified and understood, and that possess some evidence of efficacy based on the results from studies. The use of selected tools of complementary medicine in addition to the conventional treatment is the principle of so-called integrative medicine.

One of the most widely studied groups of natural immunomodulators is β-glucans. β-glucans are a group of biologically active polysaccharides of natural origin with *pleiotropic immunomodulation effects*. Their efficacy has been confirmed in the treatment and prevention of various infectious diseases, oncological disorders, as well as a broad spectrum of immune-mediated conditions (e.g. secondary immunodeficiencies, autoimmune diseases, allergies). The immunomodulation effect is strongly dependent on the β-glucan source, its purity and concentration in the product. The most effective β-glucans are those extracted from mushrooms, e.g. oyster mushroom (*Pleurotus ostreatus*) and shitake. Various *in vitro* experiments and animal studies have confirmed the complex immunomodulatory effect of β-glucans on different components of the immune system. Several of the described effects could be applied in the supportive treatment of allergic diseases (induction of T_H1 response with subsequent suppression of T_H2 cytokine production, increased production of IL-10, TGF-β and IFN-γ, induction of T_H17 lymphocytes, suppression of pro-inflammatory cytokines production, suppression of IgE synthesis) [224, 225, 267]. The anti-allergic effect was also investigated in several human clinical studies. Peroral application of lentinan reduced spontaneous production of specific and total IgE in serum with clinical improvement of symptoms of allergic rhinoconjunctivitis, and the improvement persisted for six months after the end of application [463]. In another placebo-controlled study with allergic rhinitis, application of yeast β-glucan decreased eosinophil content and the production of IL-4 and 5 with an increase of IL-12 in the nasal lavage fluid [248]. In subcutaneous application of β-glucan in 20 children with allergic, partially controlled asthma, the therapy caused a significant increase of IL-10 in serum with a simultaneous decline of daily and nocturnal symptom scores [379]. In two recent placebo-controlled studies, pleuran (β-glucan extracted from *Pleurotus ostreatus*) showed significant complex immunomodulatory effect accompanied by a decline of the respiratory infection rate [226] and the stabilization of IgE production together with a decrease of eosinophils in peripheral blood in atopic children [225].

Complementary medicine is commonly used by asthmatic patients. Integrative medicine uses a conventional therapy with selected effective tools of complementary medicine. β-glucans are one of the most studied natural immunomodulators with pleiotropic immunomodulation effect and with the potential to also be used in the treatment (and even prevention) of allergic diseases. Based on *in vitro* experiments as well as animal and human clinical studies, there is much evidence for the importance of β-glucans in the treatment and prevention of allergic diseases. This opens a new perspective on the use of this widespread and popular group of natural substances.

28. Vitamin D and Bronchial Asthma

Vitamin D is one of the most studied vitamins in recent years. Besides its known role in bone mineralization and calcium homeostasis, there is increasing evidence of its involvement in immune system regulation and the development of various immune mediated diseases, e.g. respiratory disorders, such as bronchial asthma [443]. A deficiency of vitamin D has been suggested as contributing to the worldwide rise of allergy and asthma sufferers. Low levels of vitamin D are associated with adverse asthma outcomes, including worse asthma control, increased corticosteroid use and increased asthma exacerbation rate [61, 62, 94, 360]. Serum vitamin D3 levels were related to subsequent ICS response over 8-12 months of ICS therapy, as assessed by a change in FEV_1, bronchodilator response and airway hyperresponsiveness [458]. These findings are confirmed by an observed inverse relationship between ICS dose and vitamin D levels [183]. However, whether vitamin D plays a causative role or is simple a marker of disease severity remains uncertain [390].

In a recent placebo-controlled childhood study in a small group of children with mild asthma, the supplementation of vitamin D did not cause any significant effect on lung function, symptom score or markers of inflammation [30]. Other interesting results arose from a recent study in Canada. Children in both low and high vitamin D level categories had an increased risk of current wheeze and a reduced rate of change in lung function with age compared to the moderate category. There is a possibility of a U-shaped association between vitamin D levels and respiratory health [328].

The birth cohort studies showed conflicting results. Lower dietary intake of vitamin D by mothers during pregnancy was associated with an increased risk of recurrent wheezing and asthma development in children [137], but a Finnish study has demonstrated that adults receiving vitamin D supplementation in the first year of life had a higher risk of asthma development [221].

In vitro studies with human airway smooth muscle (ASM) cells from asthmatic subjects showed that the active form of vitamin D (1, 25-dihydroxyvitamin D) is able to inhibit ASM proliferation by controlling the cell cycle [119]. On the other hand, vitamin D deficiency has been associated with increased ASM mass in children [183]. Vitamin D deficiency in animal models supports T_H2 differentiation and production of typical cytokine patterns. Vitamin D supplementation reversed this effect and decreased lung infiltration assessed by BALF analysis [428]. Animal model data showed that vitamin D supplementation might be beneficial for the treatment of established diseases; however, the preventative effect of early supplementation was not confirmed [21].

Another possible role of vitamin D is its *adjuvant effects* when used with other therapies. In the mouse model of asthma, supplementation of vitamin D during specific allergen immunotherapy improved final tolerogenic effects [417]. Vitamin D *in vitro* could reverse corticoid resistance and support the production of important anti-inflammatory and regulatory cytokine – interleukin 10.

Oral administration of vitamin D for seven days to corticosteroid-resistant asthmatic patients enhanced *ex vivo* T regulatory cell responses to dexamethasone [462]. Vitamin D3 selectively increases Toll-like receptor 9 expression in IL-10-secreting T regulatory cells. Vitamin D is also able to suppress the T cell proliferation in corticosteroid resistant cells [386].

Current data suggest that vitamin D supplementation may have some anti-inflammatory and immunoregulatory effects and could enhance the anti-inflammatory effects of corticosteroids. It can be supplemented especially in severe asthmatics and in those insensitive to corticotherapy. Screening for vitamin D deficiency could be recommended for severe asthmatics with supplementation for those found to be vitamin D-deficient.

29. Zinc

Zinc (Zn) is an important antioxidant element obtained from food. As an essential micronutrient for more than 100 enzymes involved in human metabolism, it promotes protein folding and helps in the regulation of gene expression. Zinc also plays an important role in modulating the immune system. It is essential for the cellular function of the immune response by acting as an antioxidant microelement. Zinc is an important element in the maintenance of optimal activity of the immune system. Hypozincemia could lead to a variety of defects in growth and the immune system. Low Zn serum levels were frequently found in children with recurrent wheezing and asthma. Zinc deficiency affects the regulation of T-cells and the development of immune hyperreactivity and allergies. Zinc deficiency causes an imbalance of T_H1/T_H2 functions and reduces the production of several cytokines (e.g. IL-2, IFN-γ, TNF-α). The dysbalance between T_H1/T_H2 causes increased inflammation and eosinophilia.

Deficiency of Zn could play a role in airway inflammation. Asthmatics have lower serum zinc levels, hair zinc levels and zinc sputum levels compared to healthy individuals [313, 467]. Low levels of zinc increase the risk of wheezing in small children [123]. A high rate of hypozincemia was described in asthmatic children, and therefore evaluation of serum zinc levels in asthmatics should be performed and a substitution in the diet of those with hypozincemia could be recommended [246]. Zinc supplementation alters NF-κB activity. A recent study provided evidence that zinc supplementation to asthmatics may alter airway reactivity and serum IgE levels. Zinc supplementation in asthmatics is able to reduce symptom score and improve lung function tests [172].

Zinc is an essential micronutrient with an important role in the immune system. Deficiency of zinc is associated with immune dysregulation and development of allergic inflammation. Zinc supplementation could be recommended as a potential treatment for asthmatics, predominantly those with confirmed hypozincemia.

30. Bronchial Thermoplasty

Bronchial thermoplasty (BT) represents a novel, non-pharmacological therapeutic modality for asthma. It involves the application of radiofrequency energy to visible proximal airways to ablate airway smooth muscle selectively. Applied through a flexible bronchoscope, it is the first non-pharmacological interventional therapy approved by the FDA (Food and Drug Administration) for severe asthma. Three randomized clinical trials in patients with moderate-to-severe asthma showed the capacity of BT to improve disease control [85, 112,

343]. The studies demonstrated a significant reduction of severe exacerbation, emergency visits and hospitalizations during 12 months after BT application [85]. The reduction of exacerbation and emergency department visits was maintained for two years after BT [86] and the safety of this therapeutic modality was shown for five years after BT [426]. A recent study showed the durability of BT treatment for a five-year period after BT application with regard to both asthma control and safety. BT has become an important addition to the standard treatment armamentarium and should be considered for patients with severe persistent asthma who remain symptomatic despite therapy with inhaled corticosteroids and LABA [450]. The use of BT and some other treatments for severe asthma (e.g. omalizumab) is able to decrease emergency room visits and hospitalizations, and it generates economic savings in the longer term [308]. According to a recent meta-analysis, bronchial thermoplasty for patients with moderate-to-severe asthma provides a modest clinical benefit in quality of life and lower rates of asthma exacerbations, but no significant difference in asthma control score. This procedure increases the risk of adverse events during treatment but has a reasonable safety profile after completion of the bronchoscopies. Future research should provide a better understanding of the mechanisms of the action of BT and its effects in different asthma phenotypes or in patients with worse lung function [430]. Some authors developed a clinically applicable standardized histologic grading system that identifies structural changes before and after BT in severe asthmatics [176]. However, despite the positive and hopeful results of several studies, the exact utility, efficacy and selection of patients for this therapy is still being discussed and questioned [219].

Bronchial thermoplasty is a novel non-pharmacological bronchoscopically applied therapy for moderate-to-severe asthmatics. Some studies demonstrated its persistent effect and safety. However, further studies are required to better define the role of this option in the treatment of asthma.

---

31. Personalized Therapy of Asthma

Today, the management of asthma is based on many aspects and variables that determine the choice of particular drug(s), their dose, combinations or other non-pharmacological strategies. Based on previous responses to selected therapies, degree of asthma symptoms and their control, the presence of associated comorbidities and atopy, level of inflammatory markers or even the occurrence of unwanted side effects, each physician can "personalize" his approach to particular patients and select the most appropriate and best therapeutic strategy. Despite these already available personalized guides for therapy, side effects occur, disease control fluctuates and symptoms are variably expressed. Therefore, a novel exciting direction for asthma research is that of personalized medicine [445].

Personalized (individualized) medicine is a broad and rapidly advancing field of healthcare that recognizes each person as a unique clinical, genetic, genomic and environmental individual [90]. Personalized medicine uses traditional as well as emerging concepts of the genetic and environmental basis of the disease to individualize prevention, diagnosis and treatment of particular diseases [336]. This approach depends strongly on integrated technologies to utilize a molecular understanding of disease in order to optimize preventive and therapeutic strategies. Personalized medicine is designed to get the right molecules to the right person, at the right time [416]. Several studies showed how the genetic background of a disease could substantially determine the therapeutic response. The carriage of specific gene polymorphism of β_2-receptors modifies the response to the particular bronchodilator [97], the polymorphisms of the genes of leukotriene metabolism pathways could determine the response to antileukotrienes [117], and functional polymorphism of the detoxification gene *NQO1* predicts the need for more intensive anti-inflammatory therapy [175]. At present, a relatively small number of genes have been identified to determine drug treatment, response phenotypes for asthma. As the research in this field is expulsive, personalized medicine becomes more of a reality for asthma patients (Figure 18) [451].

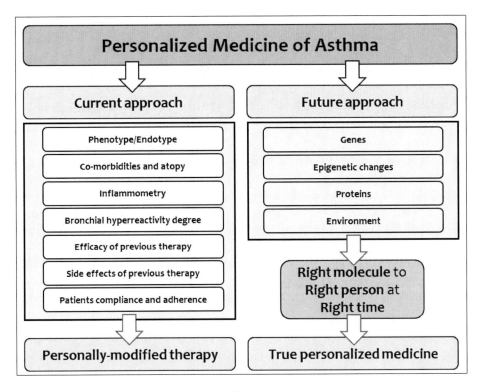

Figure 18. Current and future approach in personalized treatment of asthma.

Conclusion and Perspectives

Bronchial asthma is one of the most important chronic diseases with increasing prevalence worldwide. Understanding the disease pathogenesis, detection of specific subtypes of patients and rational therapy are the crucial cornerstones of current asthma management. Despite the available effective and safe medicaments, a certain proportion of patients require advanced strategies. Research in the field of novel anti-asthmatic therapy is rapidly advancing and several new drugs and compounds for asthma therapy will be available in the near future. However, the future is represented by so-called personalized medicine.

Acknowledgments

This work was supported by project VEGA 1/0252/14 and by projects "Centre of Experimental and Clinical Respirology" (ITMS: 26220120004) and "Martin Biomedical Centre" (ITMS: 26220220187), co-financed from EU sources.

References

[1]   Abraham, S.M., Lawrence, T., Kleiman, A., Warden, P., Medghalchi, M., Tuckermann, J., Saklatvala, J., Clark, A.R., (2006). Antiinflammatory effects of dexamethasone are partly dependent on induction of dual specificity phosphatase 1. *J. Exp. Med.* 203, 1883-1889.

[2]   Abramson, M.J., Puy, R.M., Weiner, J.M., (2003). Allergen immunotherapy for asthma. *Cochrane Database Syst. Rev.* CD001186.

[3]   Abramson, M.J., Puy, R.M., Weiner, J.M., (2010). Injection allergen immunotherapry for asthma. *Cochrane Database Syst. Rev.* CD001186.

[4]   Adcock, I.M., Lane, S.J., (2003). Corticosteroid-insensitive asthma: molecular mechanisms. *J. Endocrinol.* 178, 347-355.

[5]   Adcock, I.M., Chung, F.K., Caramori, G., Ito, K., (2006). Kinase inhibitors and airway inflammation. *Eur. J. Pharmacol.* 533, 118-132.

[6]   Adcock, I.M., Caramori, G., Chung, K.F., (2008). New targets for drug development in asthma. *Lancet.* 372, 1073-1087.

[7]   Akdis, C.A., (2012). Therapies for allergic inflammation: refining strategies to induce tolerance. *Nat. Med.* 18, 736-749.

[8]   Alderton, W.K., Angell, A.D., Craig, C., Dawson, J., Garvey, E., Moncada, S., Monkhouse, J., Rees, D., Russell, L.J., Schwartz, S., Waslidge, N., Knowles, R.G., (2005). GW274150 and GW273629 are potent and highly selective inhibitors of inducible nitric oxide synthase *in vitro* and *in vivo*. *Br. J. Pharmacol.* 145, 301-312.

[9]   Allergic factors associated with the development of asthma and the influence of cetirizine in a double-blind, randomized, placebo-controlled trial: first results of ETAC. Early Treatment of the Atopic Child. *Pediatr. Allergy Immunol.* 1998; 9, 116-124.

[10]   Amayasu, H., Yoshida, S., Ebana, S., Yamamoto, Y., Nishikawa, T., Shoji, T., Nakagawa, H., Hasegawa, H., Nakabayashi, M., Ishizaki, Y., (2000). Clarithromycin suppresses bronchial hyperresponsiveness associated with eosinophilic inflammation in patients with asthma. *Ann. Allergy Asthma Immunol.* 84, 594-598.

[11]   Andersson, F., Kjellman, M., Forsberg, G., Moller, C., Arheden, L., (2001). Comparison of the cost-effectiveness of budesonide and sodium cromoglycate in the management of childhood asthma in everyday clinical practice. *Ann. Allergy Asthma Immunol.* 86, 537-544.

[12]   Andreadis, A.A., Hazen, S.L., Comhair, S.A., Erzurum, S.C., (2003). Oxidative and nitrosative events in asthma. *Free Rad. Biol. Med.* 35, 213-225.

[13]   Arzyan, Z., Holgate, S.T., Radzioch, D., Rezaei, N., (2014). A new era of targeting the ancient gatekeepers of the immune system: toll-like agonists in the treatment of allergic rhinitis and asthma. *Int. Arch. Allergy Immunol.* 164, 46-63.

[14] Babusikova, E., Jesenak, M., Durdik, P., Dobrota, D., Banovcin, P., (2008). Exhaled carbon monoxide as a new marker of respiratory diseases in children. *J. Physiol. Pharmacol.* 59 Suppl 6, 9-17.

[15] Babusikova, E., Jesenak, M., Evinova, A., Banovcin, P., Dobrota, D., (2013). Frequency of polymorphism 262 C/T in catalase gene and oxidant damage in Slovak children with bronchial asthma. *Arch. Bronconeumol.* 49, 507-512.

[16] Babusikova, E., Jesenak, M., Kirschnerova, R., Banovcin, P., Dobrota, D., (2009). Association of oxidative stress and GST-T1 gene with childhood bronchial asthma. *J. Physiol. Pharmacol.* 60 Suppl 5, 27-30.

[17] Babusikova, E., Jurecekova, J., Evinova, A., Jesenak, M., Dobrota, D., (2012). Oxidative damage and bronchial asthma. Respiratory Diseases, Dr. Mostafa Ghanei (Ed.), Rijeka: InTech, 151-176. ISBN 978-953-307-964-6.

[18] Bachert, C., Maspero, J., (2011). Efficacy of second-generation antihistamines in patients with allergic rhinitis and comorbid asthma. *J. Asthma.* 48, 965-973.

[19] Baena-Cagnani, C.E., Berger, W.E., DuBuske, L.M., Gurne, S.E., Stryszak, P., Lorber, R., Danzig, M., (2003). Comparative effects of desloratadine versus montelukast on asthma symptoms and use of beta 2-agonists in patients with seasonal allergic rhinitis and asthma. *Int. Arch. Allergy Immunol.* 130, 307-313.

[20] Baena-Canagnani, C.E., Gomez, R.M., (2014). Current status of therapy with omalizumab in children. *Curr. Opin. Allergy Clin. Immunol.* 14, 149-154.

[21] Baker, K.E., Bonvini, S.J., Donovan, C., Foong, R.E., Han, B., Jha, A., Shaifta, Y., Smit, M., Rohnson, J.R., Moir, L.M., (2014). Novel drug targets for asthma and COPD: Lessons learned from *in vitro* and *in vivo* models. *Pulm. Pharmacol. Ther.* Doi: 10.1016/j.pupt.2014.05.008.

[22] Ball, B.D., Hill, M.R., Brenner, M., Sanks, R., Szefler, S.J., (1990). Effect of low-dose troleandomycin on glucocorticoid pharmacokinetics and airway hyperresponsiveness in severely asthmatic children. *Ann. Allergy.* 65, 37-45.

[23] Ballantyne, S.J., Barlow, J.L., Jolin, H.E., Nath, P., Williams, A.S., Chung, K.F., Sturton, G., Wong, S.H., McKenzie, A.N., (2007). Blocking IL-25 prevents airway hyperresponsiveness in allergic asthma. *J. Allergy Clin. Immunol.* 120, 1324-1331.

[24] Banovcin, P., Buchanec, J., (1989). Mechanisms of bronchial hyperreactivity. *Cesk. Pediatr.* 44, 473-475.

[25] Banovcin, P., Jesenak, M., Michnova, Z., Babusikova, E., Nosal, S., Mikler, J., Fabry, J., Barreto, M., (2009). Factors attributable to the levels of exhaled nitric oxide in asthmatic children. *Eur. J. Med. Res.* 14 Suppl 4, 9-13.

[26] Banovcin, P., Seidenberg, J., von der Hardt, H., (1995). Pressure sensor pletysmography: a method for assessment of respiratory motion in children. *Eur. Respir. J.* 8, 167-171.

[27] Banovcin, P., Seidenberg, J., von der Hardt, H., (1995). Assessment of tidal breathing patterns for monitoring of bronchial obstruction in infants. *Pediatr. Res.* 38, 218-220.

[28] Banovcin, P., Visnovsky, J., (1991). Effect of prostaglandin F2 alpha on the contractile tissue of the respiratory system of the cat in experimental airway inflammation. *Physiol. Res.* 40, 75-79.

[29] Banner, K.H., Igney, F., Poll, C., (2011). TRP channels: emerging targets for respiratory disease. *Pharmacol. Ther.* 130, 371-384.

[30] Bar Yoseph, R., Livnat, G., Schnapp, Z., Hakim, F., Dabbah, H., Goldbart, A., Bentur, L., (2014). The effect of vitamin D on airway reactivity and inflammation in asthmatic children: a double-blind, placebo-controlled trial. *Pediatr. Pulmonol.* Doi: 10.1002/ppul.23076.

[31] Barnes, P.J., (1996). Immunomodulation as asthma therapy: where do we stand? *Eur. Respir. J. Suppl.* 22, 154s-159s.

[32] Barnes, P.J., (2006). How corticosteroids control inflammation: Quintiles Prize Lecture 2005. *Br. J. Pharmacol.* 148, 245-254.

[33] Barnes, P.J., (2006). New therapies for asthma. *Trends Mol. Med.* 12, 515-520.

[34] Barnes, P.J., (2009). Histone deacetylase-2 and airway disease. *Ther. Avd. Respir. Dis.* 3, 235-243.

[35] Barnes, P.J., (2011). Glucocorticosteroids: current and future directions. *Br. J. Pharmacol.* 163, 29-43.

[36] Barnes, P.J., (2011). Triple inhalers for obstructive airways disease: will they be useful? *Expert. Rev. Respir. Med.* 5, 297-300.

[37] Barnes, P.J., (2012). Severe asthma: advances in current management and future therapy. *J. Allergy Clin. Immunol.* 129, 48-59.

[38] Barnes, P.J., (2012). New drugs for asthma. *Semin. Respir. Crit. Care. Med.* 33, 685-694.

[39] Bartho, L., Benko, R., (2013). Should antihistamines be re-considered as antiasthmatic drugs as adjuvants to anti-leukotrienes? *Eur. J. Pharmacol.* 701, 181-184.

[40] Bateman, E.D., Kornmann, O., Ambery, C., Norris, V., (2013). Pharmacodynamics of GSK961081, a bi-functional molecule, in patients with COPD. *Pulm. Pharmacol. Ther.* 26, 581-587.

[41] Beeh, K.M., Meier, J., Meyer, M., Buhl, R., Zahlten, R., Wolff, G., (2006). Bimosiamose, an inhaled small-molecule pan-selectin antagonist, attenuates late asthmatic reactions following allergen challenge in mild asthmatics: a randomized, double-blind, placebo-controlled clinical cross-over-trial. *Pulm. Pharmacol. Ther.* 19, 233-241.

[42] Beigelman, A., Gunsten, S., Mikols, C.L., Vidavsky, I., Cannon, C.L., Brody, S.L., Walter, M.J., (2009). Azithromycin attenuates airway inflammation in a noninfectious mouse model of allergic asthma. *Chest.* 136, 498-506.

[43] Belvisi, M.G., Wicks, S.L., Battram, C.H., Bottoms, S.E., Redford, J.E., Woodman, P., Brown, T.J., Webber, S.E., Foster, M.L., (2001). Therapeutic benefit of a dissociated glucocorticoid and the relevance of in vitro separation of transrepression from transactivation activity. *J. Immunol.* 166, 1975-1982.

[44] Belvisi, M.G., Hele, D.J., (2003). Soft steroids: a new approach to the treatment of inflammatory airways diseases. *Pulm. Pharmacol. Ther.* 16, 321-325.

[45] Belvisi, M.H., Hele, D.J., Birrell, M.A., (2006). Peroxisone proliferator-activated receptor gamma agonists as therapy for chronic airway inflammation. *Eur. J. Pharmacol.* 533, 101-109.

[46] Berry, M.A., Hargadon, B., Shelley, M., Parker, D., Shaw, D.E., Green, R.H., Bradding, P., Brightling, C.E., Wardlaw, A.J., Pavord, I.D., (2006). Evidence of a role of tumor necrosis factor alpha in refractory asthma. *N. Engl. J. Med.* 354, 697-708.

[47] Bhavsar, P., Hew, M., Khorasani, N., Torrego, A., Barnes, P.J., Adcock, I., Chung, K.F., (2008). Relative corticosteroid insensitivity of alveolar macrophages in severe asthma compared to non-severe asthma. *Thorax.* 63, 784-790.

[48] Bhowmick, B., Singh, D., (2008). Novel anti-inflammatory treatments for asthma. *Expert. Rec. Resp. Med.* 2, 617-629.

[49] Biju, P., McCormick, K., Aslanian, R., Berlin, M., Solomon, D., Chapman, R., McLeod, R., Prelusky, D., Eckel, S., Kelly, G., Natiello, M., House, A., Fernandez, X., Bitar, R., Phillips, J., Anthes, J., (2011). Steroidal C-21 mercapto derivatives as dissociated steroids: discovery of an inhaled dissociated steroid. *Bioorgan. Medicinal Chem. Letters.* 21, 6343-6347.

[50] Birrell, M.A., Wong, S., Hardaker, E.L., Catley, M.C., McCluskie, K., Collins, M., Haj-Yahia, S., Belvisi, M.G., (2006). IkappaB kinase-2-independent and –dependent inflammation in airway disease models: relevance of IKK-2 inhibition to the clinicl. *Mol. Pharmacol.* 69, 1791-1800.

[51] Blunt, M.D., Ward, S.G., (2013). Pharmacological targeting of phosphoinositide lipid kinases and phosphatases in the immune system: success, disappointment, and new opportunities. *Front. Immunol.* 3, 1-15.

[52] Blunt, M.D., Ward, S.G., (2013). Targeting PI3K isoforms and SHIP in the immune system: new therapeutics for inflammation and leukemia. *Curr. Opin. Pharmacol.* 12, 444-451.

[53] Boguniewicz, M., Schneider, L.C., Molgrom, H., Newell, D., Kelly, N., Tam, P., Izu, A.E., Jaffe, H.S., Bucalo, L.R., Leung, D.Y., (1993). Treatment of steroid-dependent asthma with recombinant interferon-gamma. *Clin. Exp. Allergy.* 23, 785-790.

[54] Borade, P.S., Ballary, C.C., Currie, G.P., Lee, D.K.C., (2006). Modern H_1-antihistamines in asthma. *Drug Discov. Today Ther. Strat.* 3, 253-259.

[55] Borish, L.C., Nelson, H.S., Corren, J., Bensch, G., Busse, W.W., Whitmore, J.B., Agosti, J.M.; IL-4R Asthma Study Group, (2001). Efficacy of soluble IL-4 receptor for the treatment of adults with asthma. *J. Allergy Clin. Immunol.* 107, 963-970.

[56] Borish, L.C., Nelson, H.S., Lanz, M.J., Claussen, L., Whitmore, J.B., Agosti, J.M., Garrison, L., (1999). Interleukin-4 receptor in moderate atopic asthma. A phase I/II randomized, placebo-controlled trial. *Am. J. Respir. Crit. Care Med.* 160, 1816-1823.

[57] Bousquet, J., Aubier, M., Sastre, J., Izquierdo, J.L., Adler, L.M., Hofbauer, P., Kost, K.D., Harnest, U., Kroemer, B., Albrecht, A., Bredenbroker, D., (2006). Comparison of roflumilast, an oral anti-inflammatory, with beclomethasone dipropionate in the treatment of persistent asthma. *Allergy.* 61, 72-78.

[58] Bousquet, J., Wahn, U., Meltzer, E.O., Fox, H., Hedgecock, S., Thomas, K., Fowler-Taylor, A., (2008). Omalizumab: an anti-immunoglobulin E antibody for the treatment of allergic respiratory diseases. *Eur. Respir. Rev.* 17, 1-9.

[59] Braeckman, R.A., Granneman, G.R., Locke, G.S., Machinist, J.M., Cavanaugh, J.H., Awni, W.M., (1995). The pharmacokinetics of zileuton in healthy and elderly volunteers. *Clin. Pharmacokinet.* 29 Suppl 2, 42-48.

[60] Braganza, G., Chaudhuri, R., McSharry, C., Weir, C.J., Donnelly, I., Jolly, L., Lafferty, J., Lloyd, S.M., Spears, M., Mair, F., Thomson, N.C., (2011). Effects of short-term treatment with atorvastatin in smokers with asthma: a randomized controlled trial. *BMC Pulm. Med.* 11, 16.

[61] Brehm, J.M., Celedon, J.C., Soto-Quiros, M.E., Avila, L., Hunninghake, G.M., Forno, E., Laskey, D., Sylvia, J.S., Hollis, B.W., Weiss, S.T., Litonjua, A.A., (2009). Serum vitamin D levels and markers of severity of childhood asthma in Costa Rica. *Am. J. Respir. Crit. Care Med.* 179, 765-771.

[62] Brehm, J.M., Schuemann, B., Fuhlbrigge, A.L., Hollis, B.W., Strunk, R.C., Zeiger, R.S., Weiss, S.T., Litonjua, A.A., Childhood Asthma Management Program Research Group. *J. Allergy Clin. Immunol.* 126, 52-58.

[63] Brightling, C.E., Bradding, P., Symon, F.A., Holgate, S.T., Wardlaw, A.J., Pavord, I.D., (2002). Mast-cell infiltration of airway smooth muscle in asthma. *N. Engl. J. Med.* 346, 1699-1705.

[64] Brodlie, M., McKean, M.C., Moss, S., Spencer, D.A., (2012). The oral corticosteroid-sparing effect of omalizumab in children with severe asthma. *Arch. Dis. Child.* 97, 604-609.

[65] Brusselle, G.G., Vanderstichele, C., Jordens, P., Deman, R:, Slabbynck, H., RIngoet, V., Verleden, G., Demendts, I.K., Verhamme, K., Delporte, A., Demeyere, B., Claeys, G., Boelens, J., Padalko, E:, Verschakelen, J., Van Maele, G., Deschepper, E., Joos, G.F., (2013). Azithromycin for prevention of exacerbation in severe asthma (AZISAST): a multicenter randomized double-blind placebo-controlled trial. *Thorax.* 68, 322-329.

[66] Bundschih, D.S., Eltze, M., Barsig, J., Wollin, L., Hatzelmann, A., Beume, R., (2001). In vivo efficacy in airway disease models of roflulilast: a novel orally active PDE4 inhibitor. *J. Pharmacol. Exp. Ther.* 297, 280-290.

[67] Burgess, J.K., Oliver, B.G., Poniris, M.H., Ge, Q., Boustany, S., Cox, N., Moir, L.M., Johnson, P.R., Black, J.L., (2006). A phosphodiesterase 4 inhibitor inhibits matrix protein deposition in airways in vitro. *J. Allergy Clin. Immunol.* 118, 649-657.

[68] Bush, A., Saglani, S., (2010). Management of severe asthma in children. *Lancet.* 376, 814-825.

[69] Busse, W.W., Buhl, R., Vidaurre, C.F., Blogg, M., Zhu, J., Eisner, M.D., Canvin, J., (2012). Omalizumab and the risk of malignancy: results from a pooled analysis. *J. Allergy Clin. Immunol.* 129, 983-989.

[70] Busse, W.W., Israel, E., Nelson, H.S., Baker, J.W., Charous, B.L., Young, D.Y., Vexler, V., Shames, R.S.; Daclizumab Asthma Study Group, (2008). Daclizumab improves asthma control in patients with moderate to severe persistent asthma: a randomized, controlled trial. *Am. J. Respir. Crit. Care Med.* 178, 1002-1008.

[71] Busse, W.W., Holgate, S., Kerwin, E., Chon, Y., Feng, J., Lin, J., Lin, S.L., (2013). Randomized, double-blind, placebo-controlled study of brodalumab, a human anti-IL-17 receptor monoclonal antibody, in moderate to severe asthma. *Am. J. Respir. Crit. Care Med.* 188, 1294-1302.

[72] Busse, W.W., Morgan, W.J., Gergen, P.J., Mitchell, H.E., Gern, J.E., Liu, A.H., Gruchalla, R.S., Kattan, M., Teach, S.J., Pongracic, J.A., Chmiel, J.F., Steinbach, S.F., Calatroni, A., Togias, A., Thompson, K.M., Szefler, S.J., Sorkness, C.A., (2011). Randomized trial of omalizumab (anti-IgE) for asthma in inner-city children. *N. Engl. J., Med.* 364, 1005-1015.

[73] Busse, W.W., O'Byrne, P.M., Bleecker, E.R., Lotvall, J., Woodcock, A., Andersen, L., Hicks, W., Crawford, J., Jacques, L., Apoux, L., Bateman, E.D., (2013). Safety and tolerability of the novel inhaled corticosteroid fluticasone furoate in combination with

the β2 agonist vilanterol administered once daily for 52 weeks in patients ≥12 years old with asthma: a randomized trial. *Thorax.* 68, 513-520.

[74] Busse, W.W., Ring, J., Huss-Marp, J., Kahn, J.E., (2010). A review of treatment with mepolizumab, an anti-IL-5 mAb in hypereosinophilic syndrome and asthma. *J. Allergy Clin. Immunol.* 125, 803-813.

[75] Busse, W., Spector, S., Rosen, K., Wang, Y., Alpan, O., (2013). High eosinophil count: a potential biomarker for assessing successful omalizumab treatment effects. *J. Allergy Clin. Immunol.* 132, 485-486e9.

[76] Bustos, G.J., Bustos, D., Bustos, G.J., Romero, O., (1995). Prevention of asthma with ketotifen in preasthmatic children: a three-year follow-up study. *Clin. Exp. Allergy.* 25, 568-573.

[77] Calderon, M.A., Alves, B., Jacobson, M., Hurwitz, B., Sheikh, A., Durham, S., (2007). Allergen injection immunotherapy for seasonal allergic rhinitis. *Cochrane Database Syst. Rev.* 1, CD001936.

[78] Calhoun, W.J., (2001). Anti-leukotrienes for asthma. *Curr. Opin. Pharmacol.* 1, 230-234.

[79] Calignano, A., Katona, I., Desarnaud, F., Giuffrida, A., La Rana, G., Mackle, K., Freund, T.F., Piomelli, D., (2000). Bidirectional control of airway responsiveness by endogenous cannabinoids. *Nature.* 308, 96-101.

[80] Camargo, C.A. Jr., Gurner, D.M., Smithline, H.A., Chapela, R., Fabbri, L.M., Green, S.A., Malice, M.P., Legrand, C., Dass, S.B., Knorr, B.A., Reiss, T.F., (2010). A randomized placebo-controlled study of intravenous montelukast for the treatment of acute asthma. *J. Allergy Clin. Immunol.* 125, 374-380.

[81] Caramori, G., Groneberg, D., Ito, K., Casolari, P., Adcock, I.M., Papi, A., (2008). New drugs targeting Th2 lymphocytes in asthma. *J. Occup. Med. Toxicol.* 3, S6.

[82] Casale, T.B., Busse, W.W., Kline, J.N., Ballas, Z.K., Moss, M.H., Townley, R.G., Mokhtarani, M., Seyfert-Margolis, V., Asare, A., bateman, K., Deniz, Y.; Immune Tolerance Network Group, (2006). Omalizumab pretreatment decreases acute reactions after rush immunotherapy for ragweed-induced seasonal allergic rhinitis. *J. Allergy Clin. Immunol.* 117, 134-140.

[83] Casale, T.B., Stokes, J.R., (2008). Immunomodulators for allergic respiratory disorders. *J. Allergy Clin. Immunol.* 121, 288-296.

[84] Castro, M., Mathur, S., Hargreave, F., Boulet, L.P., Xie, F., Young, J., Wilkins, H.J., Henkel, T., Nair, P., Res-5-0010 Study Group, (2011). Reslizumab for poorly controlled, eosinophilic asthma: a randomized, placebo-controlled study. *Am. J. Respir. Crit. Care Med.* 184, 1125-1132.

[85] Castro, M., Rubin, A., Laviolette, M., Fiterman, J. De Andrade Lima, M., Shah, P.L., Fiss, E., Olivenstein, R., Thomson, N.C., Niven, R.M., Pavord, I.D., Simoff, M., Duhamel, D.R., McEvoy, C., Barbers, R., Ten Hacken, N.H., Wechsler, M.E., Holmes, M., Phillips, M.J., Erzurum, S., Lunn, W., Israel, E., Jarjour, N., Kraft, M., Shargill, N.S., Quiring, J., Berry, S.M., Cox, G.; AIR2 Trial Study Group, (2010). Effectiveness and safety of bronchial thermoplasty in the treatment of severe asthma: a multicenter, randomized, double-blind, sham-controlled clinical trial. *Am. J. Respir. Crit. Care Med.* 182, 116-124.

[86] Castro, M., Rubin, A., Laviolette, M., Hanania, N.A., Armstrong, B., Cox, B.; AIR2 Trial Study Group, (2011). Persistence of effectiveness of bronchial thermoplasty in patients with severe asthma. *Ann. Allergy Asthma Immunol.* 107, 65-70.

[87] Catley, M.C., (2007). Dissociated steroids. *Sci. World. J.* 7, 421-430.

[88] Cates, C.J., Karner, C., (2013). Combination formoterol and budesonide as maintenance and reliever therapy versus current best practice (including inhaled steroid maintenance) for chronic asthma in adults and children. *Cochrane Database Syst. Rev.* 4, CD007313.

[89] Cazzola, M., Page, C.P., Calzetta, L., Matera, M.G., (2012). Pharmacology and therapeutics of bronchodilators. *Pharmacol. Rev.* 64, 450-504.

[90] Chan, I.S., Ginsburg, G.S., (2011). Personalized medicine: progress and promise. *Annu. Rev. Genomics Hum. Genet.* 12, 217-244.

[91] Chatila, T.A., Li, N., Garcia-Lloret, M., Kim, H.J., Nel, A.E., (2008). T-cell effector pathways in allergic diseases: transcriptional mechanisms and therapeutic targets. *J. Allergy Clin. Immunol.* 121, 812-823.

[92] Chen, Y.H., Yao, W.Z., Zhao, M.W., Pang, Y.Z., Tang, C.S., (2005). Cross-talk between calcineurin and protein kinases in airway remodeling in asthma. *Beijing Da. Xue. Xue. Bao.* 37, 599-602.

[93] Chiba, Y., Todoroki, M., Nishida, Y., Tanabe, M., Misawa, M., (2009). A novel STAT6 inhibitor AS1517499 ameliorates antigen-induced bronchial hypercontractility in mice. *Am. J. Respir. Crit. Care Med.* 41, 516-524.

[94] Chinellaro, I., Piazza, M., Sandri, M., Peroni, D., Piacentini, G., Boner, A.L., (2010). Vitamin D serum levels and markers of asthma control in Italian children. *J. Pediatr.* 158, 437-441.

[95] Chrousos, G.P., Kino, T., (2009). Glucocorticoid signaling in the cell. Expanding clinical implications to complex human behavioral and somatic disorders. *Ann. N. Y. Acad. Sci.* 1179, 153-166.

[96] Chung, K.F., Fan, C.K., (2006). Phosphodiesterase inhibitors in airways disease. *Eur. J. Pharmacol.* 533, 110-117.

[97] Chung, L.P., Waterer, G., Thompson, P.J., (2011). Pharmacogenetics of β2 adrenergic receptor gene polymorphisms, long-lasting β agonists and asthma. *Clin. Exp. Allergy.* 41, 312-326.

[98] Ciepiela, O., Zawadzka-Krajewska, A., Kotula, I., van Overveld, F., Kulus, M., Demkow, U., (2014). Sublingual immunotherapy for asthma: affects T-cells but does not impact basophil activation. *Pediatr. Allergy Immunol. Pulmonol.* 27, 17-23.

[99] Ciprandi, G., Cadario, G., Di Gioacchimo, M., Gangemi, S., Minelli, M., RIdolo, E., Valle, C., Verini, M., Boccardo, R., Incorvaia, C., Puccinelli, P., Scurati, S., Frati, F., (2009). Sublingual immunotherapy in polysensitized allergic patients with allergic rhinitis and/or asthma: allergist choices and treatment efficacy. *J. Biol. Regul. Homeostat. Agents.* 23, 165-171.

[100] Ciprandi, G., Cirillo, I., (2006). The lower airway pathology of rhinitis. *J. Allergy Clin. Immunol.* 118, 1105-1109.

[101] Ckless, K., Lampert, A., Reiss, J., Kasahara, D., Poynter, M.E., Irvin, C.G., Lundblad, L.K., Norton, R., van der Vliet, A., Janssen-Heininger, Y.M., (2008). Inhibition of arginase activity enhances inflammation in mice with allergic airway disease, in

association with increases in protein S-nitrosylation and tyrosine nitration. *J. Immunol.* 181, 4255-4264.

[102] Cohen, E.S., Dobson, C.L., Kack, H., Wang, B., Sims, D.A., Lloyd, C.O., England, E., Rees, D.G., Guo, H., Karagiannis, S.N., O'Brien, S., Persdotter, S., Ekdahl, H., Butler, R., Keyes, F., Oakley, S., Carlsson, M., Briend, E., Wilkinson, T., Anderson, I.K., Monk, P.D., von Wachenfeldt, K., Eriksson, P.O., Gould, H.J., Vaughan, T.J., May, R.D., (2014). A novel IgE-neutralizing antibody for the treatment of severe uncontrolled asthma. *MAbs.* 6, 756-764.

[103] Commins, S., Steinke, J.W., Borish, L., (2008). The extended IL-10 superfamily: IL-10, IL-19, IL-20, IL-22, IL-24, IL-26, IL.28, and IL-29. *J. Allergy Clin. Immunol.* 121, 1108-1111.

[104] Corren, J., (2011). Cytokine inhibition in severe asthma: current knowledge and future directions. *Curr. Opin. Pulm. Med.* 17, 29-33.

[105] Corren, J., Lemanske, R.F., Hanania, N.A., Korenblat, P.E., Parsey, M.V., Arron, J.R., Harris, J.M., Scheerens, H., Wu, L.C., Su, Z., Mosesova, S., Eisner, M.D., Bohen, S.P., Matthews, J.G., (2011). Lebrikizumab treatment in adult with asthma. *N. Engl. J. Med.* 365, 1088-1098.

[106] Corrigan, C.J., (1997). Intravenous immunoglobulin therapy for asthma: time for a closer look? *Thorax.* 52, 593-594.

[107] Corrigan, C.J., (2002). Asthma refractory to glucocorticoids: the role of newer immunosuppressants. *Am. J. Respir. Med.* 1, 47-54.

[108] Cosio, B.G., Mann, B., Ito, K., Jazrawi, E., Barnes, P.J., Chung, K.F., Adcock, I.M., (2004). Histone acetylase and deacetylase activity in alveolar macrophages and blood monocytes in asthma. *Am. J. Respir. Crit. Care Med.* 170, 141-147.

[109] Cosio, B.G., Tsaprouni, L., Ito, K., Jazrawi, E., Adcock, I.M., Barnes, P.J., (2004). Theophylline restores histone deacetylase activity and steroid responses in COPD macrophages. *J. Exp. Med.* 200, 689-695.

[110] Costello, P.S., Turner, M., Walters, A.E., Cunningham, C.N., Bauer, P.H., Downward, J., Tybulewicz, V.L., (1996). Critical role of the tyrosine kinase Syk in signaling through the high affinity IgE receptor of mast cells. *Oncogene.* 13, 2595-2605.

[111] Cousins, D.J., McDonald, J., Lee, T.H., (2008). Therapeutic approaches for control of transcription factors in allergic disease. *J. Allergy Clin. Immunol.* 121, 803-309.

[112] Cox, G., Thomson, N.C., Rubin, A.S., Niven, R.M., Corris, P.A., Siersted, H.C., Olivenstein, R., Pavord, I.D., McCormack, D., Chaudhuri, R., Miller, J.D., Laviolette, M.; AIR Trial Study Group, (2007). Asthma control during the year after bronchial thermoplasty. *N. Engl. J. Med.* 356, 1327-1337.

[113] Cox, L., Nelson, H., Lockey, R., Calabria, C., Chacko, T., Finegold, I., Nelson, M., Weber, R., (2011). Allergen immunotherapy: A practice parameter third update. *J. Allergy Clin. Immunol.* 127, S1-S55.

[114] Coyle, T.B., Metersky, M.L., (2013). The effect of the endothelin-1 receptor antagonist, bosentan, on patients with poorly controlled asthma: a 17-week, double-blind, placebo-controlled crossover pilot study. *J. Asthma.* 50, 433-437.

[115] Cruz, A.A., Popov, T., Pawankar, R., Annesi-Maesano, I., Fokkens, W., Kemp, J., Ohta, K., Price, D., Bousquet, J., ARIA Initiative Scientific Committee, (2007). Common characteristics of upper and lower airways in rhinitis and asthma: ARIA update, in collaboration with GA^{2}LEN. *Allergy.* 62 Suppl 84, 1-41.

[116] Cui, Y.Y., D'Agostino, B., Risse, P.A., Marrocco, G., Naline, E., Zhang, Y., Chen, H.Z., Finance, P., Rinaldi-Carmona, M., Rossi, F., Advenier, C., (2007). Cannabinoid CB_2 receptor activation prevents bronchoconstriction and airway edema in a model of gastro-oesophageal reflux. *Eur. J. Pharmacol.* 573, 206-213.

[117] Currie, G.P., Lima, J.J., Sylvester, J.E., Lee, D.K.C., Cockburn, W.J.R., Lipworth, B.J., (2003). Leukotriene C_4 synthase polymorphisms and responsiveness to leukotriene antagonists in asthma. *Br. J. Clin. Pharmacol.* 56, 422-426.

[118] Dal Negro, R.W., Guerriero, M., Micheletto, C., Tognella, S., Visconti, M., (2011). Changes in total IgE plasma concentration measured at the third month during anti-IgE treatment predict future exacerbation rates in difficult-to-treat atopic asthma: a pilot study. *J. Asthma.* 48, 437-441.

[119] Damera, G., Fogle, H.W., Lim, P., Goncharova, E.A., Zhao, H., Banerjee, A., Tliba, O., Krymskaya, V.P., Panettieri, R.A. Jr., (2009). Vitamin D inhibits growth of human airway smooth muscle cells htrough growth factor-induced phosphorylation of retinoblastoma protein and checkpoint kinase 1. *Br. J. Pharmacol.* 158, 1429-1441.

[120] Davies, H., Olson, L., Gibson, P., (2000). Methotrexate as a steroid sparing agent for asthma in adults. *Cochrane Database Syst. Rev.* CD000391.

[121] De Bosscher, K., (2010). Selective glucocorticoid receptor modulators. *J. Steroid. Biochem. Mol. Biol.* 120, 96-104.

[122] De Bosscher, K., Haegeman, G., Elewaut, D., (2010). Targeting inflammation using selective glucocorticoid receptor modulators. *Curr. Opin. Pharmacol.* 10, 497-504.

[123] De Cassia Ribeiro-Silva, R., Fiaccone, R.L., Barretom M.L., da Silva, L.A., Pereira Santos, L.F., Alcantrara-Neves, N.M., (2014). The prevalence of wheezing and its association with serum zinc concentration in children and adolescents in Brazil. *J. Trace Elem. Med. Biol.* 28, 293-297.

[124] De Miguel-Diez, J., Jimenez.Garcia, R., (2014). Considerations for new dual-acting bronchodilator treatments for chronic obstructive pulmonary disease. *Expert. Opin. Investig. Drugs.* 23, 453-456.

[125] Deshpande, D.A., Wang, W.C., McIlmoyle, E.L., Robinett, K.S., Schillinger, R.M., An, S.S., Sham, J.S., Liggett, S.B., (2010). Bitter taste receptors on airway smooth muscle bronchodilate by localized calcium signaling and reverse obstruction. *Nat. Med.* 16, 1299-1304.

[126] Dezitter, Y., Fagart, J., Taront, S., Fay, M., Masselot, B., Hetuin, D., Formstecher, P., Rafestin-Oblin, M.E., Idziorek, T., (2014). A structural explanation of the effects of dissociated glucocorticoids on glucocorticoid receptor transactivation. *Mol. Pharmacol.* 85, 226-236.

[127] Di, C.J., Nelson, C., Bates, G., Parekh, A.B., (2009). Targeting Ca^{2+} release-activated Ca^{2+} channel channels and leukotriene receptors provides a novel combination strategy for treating nasal polyposis. *J. Allergy Clin. Immunol.* 124, 1014-1021.

[128] Domingo, C., Moreno, A., Amengual, M.J., Comet, R., Lujan, M., (2009). Twelve years' experience with methotrexate for GINA treatment step 5 asthma patients. *Curr. Med. Res. Opin.* 25, 367-374.

[129] Drazen, J.M., Yandawa, C.N., Dube, L., Szczerback, N., Hippensteel, R., Pillari, A., Israel, E., Schork, N., Silverman, E.S., Katz, D.A., Drajesk, J., (1999). Pharmacogenetic association between ALOX5 promoter genotype and the response to anti-asthma treatment. *Nat. Genet.* 22, 168-170.

[130] Duan, W., Chan, J.H., Wong, C.H., Leung, B.P., Wong, W.S., (2004). Anti-inflammatory effects of mitogen-activated protein kinase inhibitor U0126 in an asthma mouse model. *J. Immunol.* 172, 7053-7059.

[131] Duan, W., Aguinaldo Datiles, A.M., Leung, B.P., Vlahos, C.J., Wong, W.S., (2005). An anti-inflammatory role for a phosphoinositide 3-kinase inhibitor LY294002 in a mouse asthma model. *Int. Immunopharmacol.* 5, 495-502.

[132] Dykewicz, M.S., (2001). Newer and alternative non-steroidal treatments for asthmatic inflammation. *Allergy Asthma Proc.* 22, 11-15.

[133] Eckstein, J.W., Fung, J. (2003). A new class of cyclosporin analogues for the treatment of asthma. *Expert Opin. Investig. Drugs.* 12, 647-653.

[134] Egan, R.W., Athwal, D., Bodmer, M.W., Carter, J.M., Chapman, R.W., Chou, C.C., Cox, M.A., Emtage, J.S., Fernandez, X., Genatt, N., Indelicato, S.R, Jenh, C.H., Kreutner, W., Kung, T.T., Mauser, P.J., Minnicozzi, M., Murgolo, N.J., Narula, S.K., Petro, M.E., Schilling, A., Sehring, S., Stelts, D., Stephens, S., Taremi, S.S., Zurcher, J., (1999). Effect of Sch 55700, a humanized monoclonal antibody to human interleukin-5, on eosinophilic responses and bronchial hyperreactivity. *Arzneimittelforschung.* 49, 779-790.

[135] Ekoff, M., Nilsson, G., (2011). Mast cell apoptosis and survival. *Adv. Exp. Med. Biol.* 716, 47-60.

[136] Engelbertz, J., Schwenk, T., Kinzinger, U., Schierstedt, D., Verspohl, E.J., (2008). Thyme extract, but not thymol, inhibits endothelin-induced contractions of isolated rat trachea. *Planta Med.* 74, 1436-1440.

[137] Erkkola, M., Kaila, M., Nwaru, B.I., Kronberg-Kippila, C., Ahonen, S., Nevalainen, J., Veijola, R., Pekkanen, J., Ilonen, J., Simell, O., Knip, M., Virtanen, S.M., (2009). Maternal vitamin D intake during pregnancy is inversely associated with asthma and allergic rhinitis in 5-year-old children. *Clin. Exp. Allergy.* 39, 875-882.

[138] Erin, E.M., Leaker, B.R., Nicholson, G.C., Tan, A.J., Green, L.M., Neighbour, H., Zacharasiewicz, A.S., Turner, J., Barnathan, E.S., Kon, O.M., Barnes, P.J., Hansel, T.T., (2006). The effects of a monoclonal antibody directed against. Tumor necrosis factor-alpha in asthma. *Am. J. Respir. Crit. Care Med. 1174, 753-762.*

[139] Evans, D.J., Barnes, P.J., Spaethe, S.M., van Alstyne, E.L., Mitchell, M.I., O'Connor, B.J., (1996). Effect of a leukotriene B4 receptor antagonist, LY293111, on allergen induced responses in asthma. *Thorax.* 51, 1178-1184.

[140] Evans, D.J., Cullinan, P., Geddes, D.M., Walters, E.H., Milan, S.J., Jones, P., (2010). Cyclosporin as an oral corticosteroid sparing agent in stable asthma. *Cochrane Database Syst. Rev.* 4, CD002993.

[141] Eynott, P.R., Nath, P., Leung, S.Y., Adcock, I.M., Bennett, B.L., Chung, K.F., (2003). Allergen-induced inflammation and airway epithelial and smooth muscle cell proliferation: role of Jun N-terminal kinase. *Br. J. Pharmacol.* 140, 1373-1380.

[142] Eynott, P.R., Xu, L., Bennett, B.L., Noble, A., Leung, S.Y., Nath, P., Groneberg, D.A., Adcock, I.M., Chung, K.F., (2004). Effect of an inhibitor of Jun N-terminal protein kinase, SP600125, in single allergen challenge in sensitized rats. *Immunology.* 112, 446-453.

[143] Ezeamuzie, C.I., El-Hashim, A.Z., Renno, W.M., Edafiogho, I.O., (2014). Antiallergic and antiasthmatic effects of a novel enhydratinone ester (CEE-1): Inhibition of activation of both mast cells and eosinophils. *J. Pharmacol. Exp. Ther.* 350, 444-454.

[144] Fahy, J.V., (2006). Anti-IgE: lessons learned from effects on airway inflammation and asthma exacerbation. *J. Allergy Clin. Immunol.* 117, 1230-1232.

[145] Fatemi, F., Sadroddiny, E., Gheibi, A., Mohammadi Farsani, T., Kardar, G.A., (2014). Biomolecular markers in assessment and treatment of asthma. *Respirology.* 19, 514-523.

[146] Finan, P.M., Thomas, M.J., (2004). PI 3-kinase inhibition: a therapeutic target for respiratory disease. *Biochem. Soc. Trans.* 32, 378-382.

[147] Finsnes, F., Lyberg, T., Christensen, G., Skjonsberg, O.H., (2001). Effect of endothelin antagonism on the production of cytokines in eosinophilis airway inflammation. *Am. J., Physiol. Lung. Cell. Mol. Physiol.* 280, L659-L665.

[148] Fiocchi, A., Riva, E., Santini, I., Bernardo, L., Sala, M., Mirri, G.P., (1997). Effect of nedocromil sodium on bronchial hyperreactivity in children with nonatopic asthma. *Ann. Allergy Asthma Immunol.* 79, 503-506.

[149] Fireman, P., Friday, G., (1992). Asthma. A role for IVIG therapy? *Clin. Rev. Allergy.* 10, 135-142.

[150] Flood-Page, P., Menzies-Gow, A.N., Kay, A.B., Robinson, D.S., (2003). Eosinophil's role remains uncertain as anti-interleukin-5 only partially depletes numbers in asthmatic airway. *Am. J. Respir. Crit. Care Med.* 167, 199-204.

[151] Flood-Page, P., Swenson, C., Faiferman, I., Matthews, J., Williams, M., Brannick, L., Robinson, D., Wenzel, S., Busse, W., Hansel, T.T., Barnes, N.C.; International Mepolizumab Study Group. *Am. J. Respir. Crit. Care Med.* 176, 1062-1071.

[152] Flotte, T.R., Loughlin, G.M., (1991). Benefits and complications of troleandomycin (TAO) in young children with steroid-dependent asthma. *Pediatr. Pulmonol.* 10, 178-182.

[153] Fogarty, A., Britton, J., (2000). The role of diet in the etiology of asthma. *Curr. Opin. Pulm. Med.* 30, 615-627.

[154] Fonseca-Aten, M., Okada, P.J., Bowlware, K.L., Chavez-Bueno, S., Mejias, A., Rios, A.M., Katz, K., Olsen, K., Ng, S., Jafri, H.S., McCracken, G.H., Ramilo, O., Hardy, R.D., (2006). Effect of clarithromycin on cytokines and chemokines in children with an acute exacerbation of recurrent wheezing: a double-blind, randomized, placebo-controlled trial. *Ann. Allergy Asthma Immunol.* 97, 457-463.

[155] Fost, D.A., Leung, D.Y., Martin, R.J., Brown, E.E., Szefler, S.J., Spahn, J.D., (1999). Inhibition of methylprednisolone elimination in the presence of clarithromycin therapy. *J. Allergy Clin. Immunol.* 103, 1031-1035.

[156] Franciosi, L.G., Diamant, Z., Banner, K.H., Zuiker, R., Morelli, N., Kamerling, I.M., de Kam, M.L., Burggraaf, J., Cohen, A.F., Cazzola, M., Calzetta, L., Singh, D., Spina, D., Walker, M.J., Page, C.P., (2013). Efficacy and safety of RPL554, a dual PDE3 and PDE4 inhibitor, in healthy volunteers and in patients with asthma or chronic obstructive pulmonary disease: findings from four clinical trials. *Lancet Respir. Med.* 1, 714-727.

[157] Franova, S., Strapkova, S., Mokry, J., Sutovska, M., Joskova, M., Sadlonova, V., Antosova, M., Pavelcikova, D., Fleskova, D., Nosalova, G., (2011). Pharmacologic modulation of experimentally induced allergic asthma. *Interdiscip. Toxicol.* 4, 27-32.

[158] Frew, A.J., (2010). Allergen immunotherapy. *J. Allergy Clin. Immunol.* 125, S306-S313.

[159] Friedman, H.S., Navaratnam, P., McLaughlin, J., (2010). Adherence and asthma control with mometasone furoate versus fluticasone propionate in adolescents and young adults with mild asthma. *J. Asthma.* 47, 994-1000.

[160] Fujitani, Y., Trifilieff, A., Tsuyuki, S., Coyle, A.J., Bertrand, C., (1997). Endothelin receptor antagonists inhibit antigen-induced lung inflammation in mice. *Am. J. Respir. Crit. Care. Med.,* 155, 1890-1894.

[161] Gagliardo, R., Chanez, P., Mathieu, M., Bruno, A., Costanzo, G., Gougat, C., Vachier, I., Bousquet, J., Bonsignore, G., Vignola, A.M., (2003). Persistent activation of nuclear factor-kappaB signaling pathway in severe uncontrolled asthma. *Am. J. Respir. Crit. Care Med.* 168, 1190-1198.

[162] Gajewski, T.F., Fitch, F.W., (1988). Anti-proliferative effect of IFN-γ an immune regulation. I. IFN-γ inhibits the proliferation of Th2 but not Th1 murine helper T lymphocyte clones. *J. Immunol.* 140, 4245-4252.

[163] Galie, N., Hoeper, M.M., Simon, J., Gibbs, R., Simonneau, G., (2011). Liver toxicity of sitaxentan in pulmonary arterial hypertension. *Eur. Heart. J.* 32, 386-387.

[164] Gallelli, L., Busceti, M.T., Vatrella, A., Maselli, R., Pelaia, G., (2013). Update on anticytokine treatment for asthma. *BioMed Res. Int.* 2013, 104315.

[165] Gauvreau, G.M., Boulet, L.P., Schmid-Wirlitsch, C., Cote, J., Duong, M., Killina, K.J., Milot, J., Deschesnes, F., Strinich, T., Watson, R.M., Bredenbroker, D., O'Byrne, P.M., (2011). Roflumilast attenuates allergen-induced inflammation in mild asthmatic subjects. *Respir. Res.* 12, 140.

[166] Gauvreau, G.M., Boulet, L.P., Cockcroft, D.W., Baatjes, A., Cote, J., Deschesnes, F., Davis, B., Strinich, T., Howie, K., Duong, M., Watson, R.M., Renzi, P.M., O'Byrne, P.M., (2008). Antisense therapy against CCR3 and the common beta chain attenuates allergen-induced eosinophilis responses. *Am. J. Respir. Crit. Care Med.* 177, 952-958.

[167] Gauvreau, G.M., Boulet, L.P., Cockcroft, D.W., Fitzgerald, J.M., Carlsten, C., Davis, B.E., Deschesnes, F., Duong, M., Durn, B.L., Howie, K.J., Hui, L., Kasaian, M.T., Killian, K.J., Strinich, T.X., Watson, R.M., Y, N., Zhou, S., Raible, D., O'Byrne, P.M., (2011). Effects of interleukin-13 blockade on allergen-induced airway responses in mild atopic asthma. *Am. J. Respir. Crit. Care Med.* 183, 1007-1014.

[168] Gauvreau, G.M., Boulet, L.P., Cockroft, D.W., Fitzgerald, J.M., Mayers, I., Carlsten, C., Laviolette, M., Killian, K.J., Davis, B.E., Larche, M., Kipling, C., Dua, B., Mosesova, S., Putnam, W., Zheng, Y., Scheerens, H., McClintock, D., Matthews, J.G., O'Byrne, P.M., (2014). OX40L blockade and allergen-induced airway responses in subjects with mild asthma. *Clin. Exp. Allergy.* 44, 29-37.

[169] Gauvreau, G.M., O'Byrne, P.M., Boulet, L.P., Wang, Y., Cockcroft, D., Bigler, J., FitzGerald, J.M., Boedigheimer, M., Davis, B.E., Dias, C., Gorski, K.S., Smith, L., Bautista, E., Comeau, M.R., Leigh, R., Parnes, J.R., (2014). Effects of an anti-TSLP antibody on allergen-induced asthmatic responses. *N. Engl. J. Med.* 370, 2102-2110.

[170] Gelfand, E.W., (2002). Role of histamine in the pathophysiology of asthma: immunomodulatory and anti-inflammatory activities of H1-receptor antagonists. *Am. J. Med.* 113, 2S-7S.

[171] Gernez, Y., Tirouvanziam, R., Yu, G., Ghosn, E.E.B., Reshmwala, N., Nguyen, T., Tsai, M., Galli, S.J., Herzenberg, L.A., Herzenberg, L.A., Nedeau, K.C., (2011). Basophil CD203c levels are increased at baseline and can be used to monitor

omalizumab treatment in subjects with nut allergy. *Int. Arch. Allergy Immunol.* 154, 318-327.

[172] Ghaffari, J., Khalilian, A., Salehifar, E., Khorsani, E., Rezaii, M.S., (2014). Effect of zinc supplementation in children with asthma: a randomized, placebo-controlled trial in northern Islamic Republic of Iran. *East Mediterr. Health J.* 20, 391-396.

[173] Ghosh, S., Erzurum, S.C., (2012). Modulation of asthma pathogenesis by nitric oxide pathways and therapeutic opportunities. *Drug. Discov. Today Dis. Mech.* 9, e89-e94.

[174] Giannini, L., Mastroianni, R., Mariottini, C., Passani, M.B., Nistri, S., Mannaioni, P.F., Masini, E., (2007). Activation of cannabinoid receptors reduces allergen-induced oxidative stress damage during asthma-like reaction in sensitized guinea-pigs. *Inflamm. Res.* 56 Suppl 1, S11-S12.

[175] Goodrich, G.G., Goodman, P.H., Budhecha, S.K., Pritsos, C.A., (2009). Functional polymorphism of detoxification gene NQO1 predicts intensity of empirical treatment of childhood asthma. *Mutat. Res.* 674, 55-61.

[176] Gordon, I.O., Husain, A.N., Charbeneau, J., Krishnan, J.A.? Hogarth, D.K., (2013). Endobronchial biopsy: a guide for asthma therapy selection in the era of bronchial thermoplasty. *J. Asthma.* 50, 634-641.

[177] Gosselin. M., Goulet, S., Wu-Wong, J.R., Wessale, J.L., Opgenorth, T.J., Boulet, L.P., Battistini, B., (2002). Effects of a selective ET(A)-receptor antagonist, atrasentan (ABT-627), in murine mdoels of allergic asthma: demonstration of mouse strain specificity. *Clin. Sci. (Lond.).* 103 Suppl 48, S367-S370.

[178] Gratzl, S., Palca, A., Schmitz, M., Simon, U.H., (2000). Treatment with IFN-alpha in corticoid-unresponsiveness asthma. *J. Allergy Clin. Immunol.* 105, 1035-1036.

[179] Grembiale, R.D., Camporota, L., Naty, S., Tranfa, C.M., Djukanovic, R., Marsico, S.A., (2000). Effects of specific immunotherapy in allergic rhinitis individuals with bronchial hyperresponsiveness. *Am. J. Respir. Crit. Care Med.* 162, 2048-2052.

[180] Grzanka, A., Misiolek, M., Golusinski, W., Jarzab, J., (2011). Molecular mechanisms of glucocorticoids action: implications for treatment of rhinosinusitis and nasal polyposis. *Eur. Arch. Otorhinolaryngol.* 268, 247-253.

[181] Gueders, M.M., Balbin, M., Rocks, N., Foidart, J.M., Gosset, P., Louis, R., Shapiro, S., lopez-Otin, C., Noel, A., Cataldo, D.D., (2005). Matrix metalloproteinase-8 deficiency promotes granulocytic allergen-induced airway inflammation. *J. Immunol.* 175, 2589-2597.

[182] Gueders, M.M., Bertholet, P., Perin, F., Rocks, N., Maree, R., Botta, V., Louis, R., Foidart, M.M., Noel, A., Evrard, B., Cataldo, D.D., (2008). A novel formulation of inhaled doxycycline reduces allergen-induced inflammation, hyperresponsiveness and remodeling by matrix metalloproteinases and cytokines modulation in a mouse model of asthma. *Biochem. Pharmacol.* 75, 514-526.

[183] Gupta, A., Sjoukes, A., Richards, D., Banya, W., Hawrylowicz, C., Bush, A., Saglani, S., (2011). Relationship between serum vitamin D, disease severity, and airway remodeling in children with asthma. *Am. J. Respir. Crit. Care Med.* 184, 1342-1349.

[184] Gupta, S., (2010). Antibodies: Basic mechanisms and emerging concepts. *J. Clin. Immunol.* 30 Suppl 1, S1-S3.

[185] Guyer, B.J., Shimamoto, S.R., Bradhurst, A.L., Grosshard, E.B., Dreskin, S.C., Nelson, H.S., (2006). Mast cell inhibitor R112 is weel tolerated and affects prostaglandin D2

but no other mediators, symptoms, or nasal volumes in a nasal challenge model of allergic rhinitis. *Allergy Asthma Proc.* 27, 208-213.

[186] Haber, V.E., Bosnar, M., Kragol, G., (2014). The design of novel classes of macrolides for neutrophil-dominated inflammatory diseases. *Future Med. Chem.* 6, 657-674.

[187] Hallstrand, T.S., Henderson, W.R., (2010). The evolving role of intravenous leukotriene modifiers in acute asthma. *J. Allergy Clin. Immunol.* 125, 381-382.

[188] Hammad, H., Kool, M., Soullie, T., Narumiya, S., Trottein, F., Hoogsteden, H.C., Lambrecht, B.N., (2007). Activation of the D prostanoid receptor suppresses asthma by modulation of lung dendritic cell function and induction of regulatory T cells. *J. Exp. Med.* 204, 357-367.

[189] Hammad, H., Lambrecht, B.N., (2008). Dendritic cells and epithelial cells: linking innate and adaptive immunity in asthma. *Nat. Rev. Immunol.* 8, 193-204.

[190] Hansbro, N.G., Horvat, J.C., Wark, P.A., Hansbro, P.M., (2008). Understanding the mechanisms of viral induced asthma: new therapeutic directions. *Pharmacol. Ther.* 117, 313-353.

[191] Hansel, T.T., Kharitonov, S.A., Donnelly, L.E., Erin, E.M., Currie, M.G., Moore, W.M., Manning, P.T., Recker, D.P., Barnes, P.J., (2003). A selective inhibitor of inducible nitric oxide synthase inhibits exhaled breath nitric oxide in healthy volunteers and asthmatics. *F.A.S.E.B. J.* 17, 1298-1300.

[192] Haque, S., Boyce, N., Thien, F.C., O'Hehir, R.E., Douglass, J., (2003). Role of intravenous immunoglobulin in severe steroid-dependent asthma. *Intern. Med. J.* 33, 341-344.

[193] Harmanci, K., (2007). Montelukast: its role in the treatment of childhood asthma. *Ther. Clin. Risk Manag.* 3, 885-892.

[194] Hart, T.K., Blackburn, M.N., Brigham-Burke, M., Dede, K., Al-Mahdi, N., Zia-Amirhosseini, P., Cook, R.M., (2002). Preclinical efficacy and safety of pascolizumab (SB 240683): a humanized anti-interleukin-4 antibody with therapeutic potential in asthma. *Clin. Exp. Immunol.* 130, 93-100.

[195] Hart, T.K., Cook, R.M., Zia-Amirhosseini, P., Minthorn, E., Sellers, T.S., Maleeff, B.E., Eustis, S., Schwartz, L.W., Tsui, P., Appelbaum, E.R., Martin, E.C., Bugelski, P.J., Herzyk, D.J., (2001). Preclinical efficacy and safety of mepolizumab (SB-240563), a humanized monoclonal antibody to IL-5, in cynomolgus monkeys. *J. Allergy Clin. Immunol.* 108, 250-257.

[196] Harvima, I.T., Levi-Schaffer, F., Draber, P., Friedman, S., Polakovicova, I., Gibbs, B.F., Blank, U., Nilsson, G., Maurer, M., (2014). Molecular targets on mast cells and basophils for novel therapies. *J. Allergy Clin. Immunol.* Doi: 10.1016/j.jaci.2014.03.007.

[197] Hashimoto, Y., Nakahara, K., (2002). Improvement of asthma after administration of pioglitazone. *Diabetes Care.* 25, 401.

[198] Hasko, G., Szabo, C., (1999). IL-12 as a therapeutic target for pharmacological modulation in immune-mediated and anti-inflammatory diseases: regulation of T helper 1/T helper 2 responses. *Br. J. Pharmacol.* 127, 1295-1304.

[199] Hedman, J., Seideman, P., Albertioni, F., Stenius-Aarniala, B., (1996). Controlled trial of methotrexate in patients with severe chronic asthma. *Eur. J. Clin. Pharmacol.* 49, 347-349.

[200] Henry, P.J., Mann, T.S., Goldie, R.G., (2005). A Rho kinase inhibitor, Y-27632, inhibits pulmonary eosinophilia, bronchoconstriction and airways hyperresponsiveness in allergic mice. *Pulm. Pharmacol. Ther.* 18, 67-74.

[201] Hesslinger, C., Strub, A., Boer, R., Ulrich, W.R., Lehner, M.D., Braun, C., (2009). Inhibition of inducible nitric oxide synthase in respiratory diseases. *Biochem. Soc. Trans.* 37 (Pt 4), 886-891.

[202] Hill, D.A., Siracusa, M.C., Ruymann, K.R., Tait Wojno, E.D., Artis, D., Spergel, J.M., (2014). Omalizumab therapy is associated with reduced circulating basophil populations in asthmatic children. *Allergy.* 69, 674-677.

[203] Himes, B.E., Hunninghake, G.M., Baurley, J.W., Rafaels, N.M., Sleiman, P., Strachan, D.P., Wilk, J.B., Wollis-Owen, S.A., Klanderman, B., Lasky-Su, J., Lazarus, R., Murphy, A.J., Soto-Quiros, M.E., Avila, L., Beaty, T., Mathias, R.A., Ruczinski, I., Barnes, K.C., Celedon, J.C., Cookson, W.O., Gauderman, W.J., Gilliland, F.D., Hakonarson, H., Lange, C., Moffatt, M.F., O'Connor, G.T., Raby, B.A., Silverman, E.K., Weiss, S.T., (2009). Genome-wide association analysis identifies PDE4D as an asthma-susceptibility gene. *Am. J. Hum. Genet.* 84, 581-593.

[204] Hirakawa, S., Kojima, T., Obata, K., Okabayashi, T., Yokota, S., Nomura, K., Obonai, T., Fuchimoto, J., Himi, T., Tsutsumi, H., Sawada, N., (2013). Marked induction of matrix metalloproteinase-10 by respiratory syncytial virus infection in human nasal epithelial cells. *J. Med. Virol.* 85, 2141-2150.

[205] Holz, O., Khalilieh, S., Ludwig-Sengpiel, A., Watz, H., Stryszak, P., Soni, P., Tsai, M., Sadeh, J., Magnussen, H., (2010). SCH527123, a novel CXCR2 antagonist, inhibits ozone-induced neutrophilia in healthy subjects. *Eur. Respir. J.* 35, 564-570.

[206] Hong, Z., Lin, Y.M., Yin, X., Peng, J.L., (2012). Serum MMP-9 is elevated in children with asthma. *Mol. Med. Rep.* 5, 462-464.

[207] Hood, P.P., Cotter, T.P., Costello, J.F., Sampson, A.P., (1999). Effect of intravenous corticosteroid on *ex vivo* leukotriene generation by blood leukocytes of normal and asthmatic patients. *Thorax.* 54, 1075-1082.

[208] Howell, E., McAnulty, R.J., (2006). TGF-β-its role in asthma and therapeutic potential. *Curr. Drug Targets.* 7, 547-565.

[209] Howlett, A.C., Barth, F., Bonner, T.I., Cabral, G., Casellas, P., Devane, W.A., Felder, C.C., Herkenham, M., Mackie, K., Martin, B.R., Mechoulam, R., Pertwee, R.G., (2002). International Union of Pharmacology. XXVII. Classification of Cannabinoid receptors. *Pharmacol. Rev.* 54, 161-202.

[210] Huang, C.F., Peng, H.J., Wu, C.C., Lo, W.T., Shih, Y.L., Wu, T.C., (2013). Effect of oral administration with pravastatin and atorvastatin on airway hyperresponsiveness and allergic reactions in asthmatic mice. *Ann. Allergy Asthma Immunol.* 110, 11-17.

[211] Hypponen, E., Sovio, U., Wjst, M., Patel, S., Pekkanen, J., Hartikainen, A.L., Jarvelinb, M.R., (2004). Infant vitamin D supplementation and allergic conditions in adulthood: northern Finland birth cohort 1966. *Ann. N. Y. Acad. Sci.* 1037, 84-95.

[212] Idzko, M., Hammad, H., van Nimwegen, M., Kool, M., Muller, T., Soullie, T., Willart, M.A., Hijdra, D., Hoogsteden, H.C., Lambrecht, B.N., (2006). Local application of FTY720 to the lung abrogates experimental asthma by altering dendritic cell function. *J. Clin. Invest.* 116, 2935-2944.

[213] Ilmarinen, P., Kankaanranta, H., (2014). Eosinophil apoptosis as a therapeutic target in bronchial asthma. *Bas. Clin. Pharmacol. Toxicol.* 114, 109-117.

[214] Incorvaia, C., Mauro, M., Russelo, M., Formigoni, C., Galeazzo Riario-Sforza, G., Ridolo, E., (2014). Omalizumab, an anti-immunoglobulin E antibody: state of the art. *Drug Design Dev. Ther.* 8, 197-207.

[215] Ito, K., Caramori, G., Adcock, I.M., (2007). Therapeutic potential of phosphatidylinositol 3-kinase inhibitors in inflammatory respiratory disease. *J. Pharmacol. Exp. Ther.* 321, 1-8.

[216] Ito, K., Ito, M., Elliott, W.M., Cosio, B., Caramori, G., Kon, O.M., Barczyk, A., Hayashi, S., Adcock, I.M., Hogg, J.C., Barnes, P.J., (2005). Decreased histone deacetylase activity in chronic obstructive pulmonary disease. *N. Engl. J. Med.* 352, 1967-1976.

[217] Ivanov, S., Linden, A., (2009). Interleukin-17 as a drug target in human disease. *Trends Pharmacol. Sci.* 30, 95-103.

[218] Iyengar, S.R., Hoyte, E.G., Loza, A., Bonaccorso, S., Chiang, D., Umetsu, D.T., Nadeau, K.C., (2013). Immunologic effects of omalizumab in children with severe refractory atopic dermatitis: a randomized, placebo-controlled clinical trial. *Int. Arch. Allergy Immunol.* 162, 89-93.

[219] Iyer, V.N., Lim, K.G., (2014). Bronchial thermoplasty: Reappraising the evidence (or lack thereof). *Chest.* 146, 17-21.

[220] Jakobsson, T., Croner, S., Kjellman, N.I.M., Pettersson, A., Vassella, C., Bjorksten, B., (1994). Slight steroid-sparing effect of intravenous immunoglobulin in children and adolescents with moderately severe bronchial asthma. *Allergy.* 49, 413-420.

[221] Jesenak, M., Babusikova, E., Evinova, A., Banovcin, P., Dobrota, D., (2014). Val66Met polymorphism in the BDNF gene in children with bronchial asthma. *Pediatr. Pulmonol.* Doi: 10.1002/ppul.23065.

[222] Jesenak, M., Babusikova, E., Petrikova, M., Turcan, T., Rennerova, Z., Michnova, Z., Havlicekova, Z., Banovcin, P., (2009). Cough reflex sensitivity in various phenotypes of childhood asthma. *J. Physiol. Pharmacol.* 60 Suppl 5, 61-65.

[223] Jesenak, M., Banovcin, P., Havlicekova, Z., Dobrota, D., Babusikova, E., (2014). Factors influencing the levels of exhaled carbon monoxide in asthmatic children. *J. Asthma.* Jul 3, 1-7.

[224] Jesenak, M., Banovcin, P., Rennerova, Z., Majtan, J., (2014). β-glucans in the treatment and prevention of allergic diseases. *Allergol. Immunopathol. (Madrid).* 42, 149-156.

[225] Jesenak, M., Hrubisko, M., Majtan, J., Rennerova, Z., Banovcin, P., (2014). Antiallergic effect of pleuran (β-glucan from Pleurotus ostreatus) in children with recurrent respiratory tract infections. *Phytother. Res.* 28, 471-474.

[226] Jesenak, M., Majtan, J., Rennerova, Z., Kyselovic, J., Banovcin, P., Hrubisko, M., (2013). Immunomodulatory effect of pleuran (β-glucan from Pleurotus ostreatus) in children with recurrent respiratory tract infections. *Int. Immunopharmacol.* 15, 395-399.

[227] Jesenak, M., Rennerova, Z., Babusikova, E., Havlicekova, Z., Jakusova, L., Villa, M.P., Ronchetti, R., Banovcin, P., (2008). Food allergens and respiratory symptoms. *J. Physiol. Pharmacol.* 59 Suppl 6, 311-320.

[228] Jiang, L., Diaz, P.T., Best, T.M., Stimpfl, J.N., He, F., Zuo, L., (2014). Molecular characterization of redox mechanisms in allergic asthma. *Ann. Allergy Asthma Immunol.* Doi: 10.1016/j.anai.2014.05.030.

[229] Jimenez-Morales, S., Martinez-Aguilar, N., Gamboa-Becerra, R., Jimenez-Ruiz, J.L., Lopez-Ley, D., Lou, H., Saldana-Alvarez, Y., Dean, M., Orozco, L., (2013).

Polymorphisms in metalloproteinase-9 are associated with the risk for asthma in Mexican pediatric patients. *Hum. Immunol.* 74, 998-1002.

[230] Johnston, S.L., Blasi, F., Black, P.N., Martin, R.J., Farrell, D.J., Nieman, R.B., (2006). The effect of telithromycin in acute exacerbations of asthma. *N. Engl. J. Med.* 354, 1589-1600.

[231] Johnstone, D.E., Dutton, A., (1968). The value of hyposensitization therapy for bronchial asthma in children. A 14 year study. *Pediatrics.* 42, 793-802.

[232] Joint Task Force on Practice Parameters, American Academy of Allergy, Asthma and Immunology, American College of Allergy, Asthma and Immunology, Joint Council of Allergy, Asthma and Immunology, (2007). Allergen immunotherapy: A practice parameter, second update. *J. Allergy Clin. Immunol.* 120 (3 Suppl), S25-S85.

[233] Joos, G.F., Gemonpre, P.R., Pauwels, R.A., (2005). Role of tachykinins in asthma. *Allergy.* 55, 321-337.

[234] Joos, G.F., Van, S.J., Kips, J.C., Pauwels, R.A., (1996). The effect of inhaled FK224, a tachykinin NK-1 and NK-2 receptor antagonist, on neurokinin-A-induced bronchoconstriction in asthmatics. *Am. J. Respir. Crit. Care Med.* 153 (6 Pt 1), 1781-1784.

[235] Joos, G.F., Vincken, W., Louis, R., Schelfhout, V.J., Wang, J.H., Shaw, M.J., Cioppa, G.D., Pauwels, R.A., (2004). Dual tachykinin NK1/NK2 antagonist DNK333 inhibits neurokinin A-induced bronchoconstriction in asthma patients. *Eur. Respir. J.* 23, 76-81.

[236] Jutel, M., (2014). Allergen-specific immunotherapy in asthma. *Curr. Treat. Options Allergy.* 1: 213-219.

[237] Kaditis, A.G., Winnie, G., Syrogiannopoulos, G.A., (2007). Anti-inflammatory pharmacotherapy for wheezing in preschool children. *Pediatr. Pulmonol.* 42, 407-420.

[238] Kalish, L.H., Arendts, G., Sack, R., Craig, J.C., (2009). Topical steroids in chronic rhinosinusitis without polyps: a systemic review and meta-analysis. *Otolaryngol. Head Neck Surg.* 141, 674-683.

[239] Kampe, M., Lampinen, M., Stolt, I., Janson, C., Stalenheim, G., Carlson, M., (2012). PI3-kinase regulates eosinophil and neutrophil degranulation in patients with allergic rhinitis and allergic asthma irrespective of allergen challenge model. *Inflammation.* 35, 230-239.

[240] Kannisto, S., Voutilainen, R., Remes, K., Korppi, M., (2002). Efficacy and safety of inhaled steroid and cromone treatment in school-age children: a randomized pragmatic pilot study. *Pediatr. Allergy Immunol.* 13, 24-30.

[241] Kanzov, G., Nowak, D., Magnussen, H., (1995). Short term effect of methotrexate in severe steroid-dependent asthma. *Lung.* 173, 223-231.

[242] Karin, M., Yamamoto, Y., Wang, Q.M., (2004). The IKK NF-kappa B system: a treasure trove for drug development. *Nat. Rev. Drug. Discov.* 3, 17-26.

[243] Kaufman, G.N., Massoud, A.H., Audusseau, S., Benville-Langelier, A.A., Wang, Y., Guay, J., Garellek, J.A., Mourad, W., Piccirillo, C.A., McCusker, C., Mazer, B.D., (2011). Intravenous immunoglobulin attenuates airway hyperresponsiveness in a murine model of allergic asthma. *Clin. Exp. Allergy.* 41, 718-728.

[244] Kawaguchi, M., Kokubu, F., Fujita, J., Huang, S.K., Kizawa, N., (2009). Role of interleukin-17F in asthma. *Inflamm. Allergy Drug Targ.* 8, 383-389.

[245] Kenyon, N.J., Bratt, J.M., Lee, J., Luo, J., Franzi, L.M., Zeki, A.A., Lam, K.S., (2013). Self-assembling nanoparticles containing dexamethasone as a novel therapy in allergic airways inflammation. *PLoS. One.* 8, e7773.

[246] Khanbabaee, G., Omidian, A., Imanzadeh, F., Adibeshgh, F., Ashayeripanah, M., Rezaei, N., (2014). Serum level of zinc in asthmatic patients: a case-control study. *Allergol. Immunopathol. (Madrid).* 42, 19-21.

[247] Kim, M.S., Cho, K.A., Cho, Y.J., Woo, S.Y., (2013). Effects of interleukin-9 blockade on chronic airway inflammation in murine asthma models. *Allergy Asthma Immunol. Res.* 5, 197-206.

[248] Kirmaz, C., Bayrak, P., Yilmaz, O., Yuksel, H., (2005). Effects of glucan treatmend on the Th1/Th2 balance in patients with allergic rhinitis: a double-blind placebo-controlled study. *Eur. Cytokine Netw.* 16, 128-134.

[249] Kirsten, A., Watz, H., Kretschmar, G., Pedersen, F., Bock, D., Meyer-Sabellek, W., Magnussen, H., (2011). Efficacy of the pan-selectin antagonist Bimosiamose on ozone-induced airway inflammation in healthy subjects: a double blind, randomized, placebo-controlled, cross-over clinical trial. *Pulm. Pharmacol. Ther.* 24, 555-558.

[250] Kishiyama, J.L., Valacer, D., Cunningham-Rundles, C., Sperber, K., Richmond, G.W., Abramson, S., Glovsky, M., Stiehm, R., Stocks, J., Rosenberg, L., Shames, R.S., Corn, B., Shearer, W.T., Bacot, B., DiMaio, M., Tonetta, S., Adelman, D.C., (1999). A multicenter, randomized, double-blind, placebo-controlled trial of high-dose intravenous immunoglobulin for oral corticosteroid-dependent asthma. *Clin. Immunol.* 91, 126-133.

[251] Kline, J.N., (2007). Eat dirt: CpG DNA and immunomodulation of asthma. *Proc. Am. Thorac. Soc.* 4, 283-288.

[252] Kling, J., (2014). Benralizumab improves asthma symptoms. *Medscape.* May 28.

[253] Klinger, B., McKee, M.D., Sackett, E., Levenson, H., Kenney, J., Karasz, A., (2012). An integrative medicine approach to asthma: who responds? *J. Altern. Complem. Med.* 18, 939-945.

[254] Klos, K., Kruszewski, J., (2001). Preliminary estimation of results of high-dose intravenous immunoglobulin in severe steroid-dependent adult asthma. *Pol. Merkur. Lekarski.* 11, 379-383.

[255] Kon, O.M., Sihra, B.S., Compton, C.H., Leonard, T.B., Kay, A.B., Barnes, N.C., (1998). Randomised, dose-ranging, placebo-controlled study of chimeric antibody to CD4 (keliximab) in chronic severe asthma. *Lancet.* 352, 1109-1113.

[256] Kon, O.M., Sihra, B.S., Loh, L.C., Barkans, J., Compton, C.H., Barnes, N.C., Larche, M., Kay, A.B., (2001). The effects of an anti-CD4 monoclonal antibody, keliximab, on peripheral blood CD4+ T-cells in asthma. *Eur Respir. J.* 18, 45-52.

[257] Kondo, N., Katsunuma, T., Odajima, Y., Morikawa, A., (2006). A randomized open-label comparative study of montelukast versus theophylline added to inhaled corticosteroid in asthmatic children. *Allergol. Int.* 55, 287-293.

[258] Kopriva, F., Janostakova, A., Jarmila, S., Zapalka, M., Hajduch, M., (2006). Montelukast decreases plasma endothelin-1 and serum eosinophil cationic protein levels in paediatric atopic asthma. *Clin. Drug Investig.* 26, 351-356.

[259] Korhonen, K., Dunder, T., Klaukka, T., Reijonen, T.M., Issakoff, K., Kiviharju, M., Linna, O., Remes, K., Korppi, M., (2004). Do inhaled steroids differ from cromones in terms of hospital admission rates for asthma in children? *Acta Paediatr.* 93, 1612-1618.

[260] Koutsoubari, I., Papaevangelou, V., Konstantinou, G.N., Makrinioti, H., Xepapadaki, P., Kafetzis, D., Papadopoulos, N.G., (2012). Effect of clarithromycin on acute asthma exacerbations in children: an open randomized study. *Pediatr. Allergy Immunol.* 23, 385-390.

[261] Kovalev, I.E., Kovaleva, V.L., Rumiantseva, E.I., (2008). Mechanisms of the therapeutic effect of immunoglobulins in the treatment of bronchial asthma. *Eksp. Klin. Farmakol.* 71, 48-51.

[262] Kotlyarov, A., Neininger, A., Schubert, C., Eckert, R., Birchmeier, C., Volk, H.D., Gaestel, M., (1999). MAPKAP kinase 2 is essential for LPS-induced TNF-alpha biosynthesis. *Nat. Cell. Biol.* 1, 94-97.

[263] Kraft, M., Cassell, G.H., Pak, J., Martin, R.J., (2002). *Mycoplasma pneumonia* and *Chlamydia pneumonia* in asthma: effect of clarithromycin. *Chest.* 121, 1782-1788.

[264] Krause, K., Spohr, A., Zuberbier, T., Church, M.K., Maurer, M., (2013). Up-dosing with bilastine results in improved effectiveness in cold contact urticarial. *Allergy.* 68, 921-928.

[265] Krinner, E.M., Raum, T., Petsch, S., Bruckmaier, S., Schuster, I., Petersen, L., Cierpka, R., Abebe, D., Molhoj, M., Wolf, A., Sorensen, P., Locher, M., Baeuerle, P.A., Hepp, J., (2007). A human monoclonal IgG1 potently neutralizing the pro-inflammatory cytokine GM-CSF. *Mol. Immunol.* 44, 916-925.

[266] Krystofova, J., Jesenak, M., Banovcin, P., (2011). Bronchial asthma and obesity in childhood. *Acta Medica (Hradec Kralove).* 54, 102-106.

[267] Ku, S.K., Kim, J.W., Cho, H.R., Kim, K.Y., Min, Y.H., Park, J.H., Kim, J.S., Park, J.H., Seo, B.I., Roh, S.S., (2012). Effect of β-glucan originated from *Aureobasidium pullulans* on asthma induced by ovalbumin in mouse. *Arch. Pharm. Res.* 35, 1073-1081.

[268] Kubavat, A.H., Khippal, N., Tak, S., Rijhwani, P., Bhargava, S., Patel, T., Shah, N., Kshatriya, R.R., Mittal, R., (2013). A randomized, comparative, multicentric clinical trial to assess the efficacy and safety of zileuton extended-release tablets with montelukast sodium tablets in patients suffering from chronic persistent asthma. *Am. J. Ther.* 20, 154-162.

[269] Kume, H., (2008). RhoA/Rho-kinase as a therapeutic target in asthma. *Curr. Med. Chem.* 15, 2876-2885.

[270] Lagente, V., Advenier, C., /2004). New nitric oxide-donating drugs for the treatment of airway diseases. *Curr. Opin. Investig. Drugs.* 5, 537-541.

[271] Landgraf, R.G., Jancar, S., (2008). Endothelin A receptor antagonist modulates lymphocyte and eosinophil infiltration, hyperreactivity and mucus in murine asthma. *Int. Immunopharmacol.* 8, 1748-1753.

[272] Lazarus, S.C., Chinchilli, V.M., Rollings, N.J., Boushey, H.A., Cherniack, R., Craig, T.J., Deykin, A., DiMango, E., Fish, J.E., Ford, J.G., Israel, E., Kiley, J., Kraft M., Lemanske, R.F. Jr., Leone, F.T., Martin, R.J., Pesola, G.R., Peters, S.P., Sorkness, C.A., Szefler, S.J., Wechsler, M.E., Fahy, J.V., National Heart Lung and Blood Institute's Asthma Clinical Research Network, (2007). Smoking affects response to inhaled corticosteroids or leukotriene receptor antagonists in asthma. *Am. J. Respir. Crit. Care Med.* 175, 783-790.

[273] Leckie, M.J., Ten Brinke, A., Khan, J., Diamant, Z., O'Connor, B.J., Walls, C.M., Mathur, A.K., Cowley, H.C., Chung, K.F:, Djukanovic, R., Hansel, T.T., Holgate, S.T.,

Sterk, P.J., Barnes, P.J., (2000). Effects of an interleukin-5 blocking monoclonal antibody on eosinophils, airway hyper-responsiveness, and the late asthmatic response. *Lancet.* 356, 2144-2148.

[274] Lee, J.H., Sohn, J.H., Ryu, S.Y., Hong, C.S., Moon, K.D., Park, J.W., (2013). A novel human anti-VCAM-1 monoclonal antibody ameliorates airway inflammation and remodelling. *J. Cell. Mol. Med.* 17, 1271-1281.

[275] Lee, K.S., Lee, H.K., Hayflick, J.S., Lee, Y.C., Puri, K.D., (2006). Inhibition of phosphoinositide 3-kinase δ attenuates allergic airway inflammation and hyperresponsiveness in murine asthma model. *F.A.S.E.B. J.* 20, 455-465.

[276] Lee, H., Lee, K., Yoon, J., Lee, M., Kim, H., Lee, J., Uijeongbu, I., (2008). Therapeutic comparison between low-dose sustained-release theophylline dry syrup and capsule in children with mild persistent asthma. *Ann. Allergy Asthma Immunol.* 100, A33-A34.

[277] Lee-Fowler, T.M., Guntur, V., Dodam, J., Cohn, L.A., DeClue, A.E., Reinero, C.R., (2012). The tyrosine kinase inhibitor masitinib blunts airway inflammation and improves associated lung mechanics in a feline model of chronic allergic asthma. *Int. Arch. Allergy Immunol.* 158, 369-374.

[278] Leff, A.R., (2000). Role of leukotrienes in bronchial hyperresponsiveness and cellular responses in the airways. *Am. J. Respir. Crit. Care Med.* 161, S125-S132.

[279] Leung, D.Y.M., Bloom, J.W., (2003). Update on glucocorticoid action and resistance. *J. Allergy Clin. Immunol.* 111, 3-22.

[280] Leung, D.Y.M., Sampson, H.A., Yunginger, J.W., Burks, A.W. Jr., Schneider, L.C., Wortel, C.H., Davis, F.M., Hyun, J.D., Shanahan, W.R. Jr.; Avon Longitudinal Study of Parents and Children Study Team, (2003). Effect of anti-IgE therapy in patients with peanut allergy. *N. Engl. J. Med.* 348, 986-993.

[281] Lever, R., Page, C.P., (2002). Novel drug development opportunities for heparin. *Nat. Rev. Drug. Discov.* 1, 140-148.

[282] Levi-Schaffer, F., Eliashar, R., (2009). Mast cell stabilizing properties of antihistamines. *J. Investig. Dermatol.* 129, 2549-2551.

[283] Levy, B.D., Lukacs, N.W., Berlin, A.A., Schmidt, B., Guilford, W.J., Serhan, C.N., Parkinson, J.F., (2007). Lipoxin A4 stable analogs reduce allergic airway responses via mechanisms distinct from CysLT1 receptor antagonism. *F.A.S.E.B. J.* 21, 3877-3884.

[284] Li, L.B., Goleva, E., Hall, C.F., Ou, L.S., Leung, D.Y., (2004). Superantigen-induced corticosteroid resistance of human T cells occurs through activation of the mitogen-activated protein kinase (extracellular signal-regulated kinase (MEK-ERK) pathway. *J. Allergy Clin. Immunol.* 114, 1059-1069.

[285] Li, J.J., Wang, W., Baines, K.J., Bowden, N.A., Hansbro, P.M., Gibson, P.G., Kumar, R.K., Foster, P.S., Yang, M., (2010). IL-27/IFN-γ induce MyD88-dependent steroid-resistant airway hyperresponsiveness by inhibiting glucocorticoid signaling in macrophages. *J. Immunol.* 185, 4401-4409.

[286] Lin, H., Boesel, K.M., Griffith, D.T., Prussin, C., Foster, B., Romero, F.A., Townley, R., Casale, T.B., (2004). Omalizumab rapidly decreases nasal allergic response and FcεRI on basophils. *J. Allergy Clin. Immunol.* 113, 297-302.

[287] Liu, X., Li, M., Wu, Y., Zhou, Y., Zeng, L., Huang, T., (2009). Anti-IL-33 antibody treatment inhibits airway inflammation in murine model of allergic asthma. *Biochem. Biophys. Res. Commun.* 386, 181-185.

[288] Long, A.A., (2009). Monoclonal antibodies and other biologic agents in the treatment of asthma. *Landes Biosci.* 1, 237-246.

[289] MacGlashan, D. Jr., Honigberg, L.A., Smith, A., Buggy, J., Schroeder, J.T., (2011). Inhibition of IgE-mediated secretion from human basophils with a highly selective Bruton's tyrosine kinase, Btk, inhibitor. *Int. Immunopharmacol.* 11, 475-479.

[290] Maddur, M.S., Othy, S., Hedge, P., Vani, J., Lacroix-Desmazes, S., Bayry, J., Kaveri, S.V., (2010). Immunomodulation by intravenous immunoglobulin: role of regulatory T cells. *J. Clin. Immunol.* 30 Suppl 1, S4-S8.

[291] Magrioti, V., Kokotos, G., (2010). Phospholipase A2 inhibitors as potential therapeutic agents for the treatment of inflammatory diseases. *Expert Opin. Ther. Pat.* 20, 1-18.

[292] Makatani, M., Fujitani, Y., Takimoto, M., Oda, K., Sasaki, Y., Hori, S., Inui, T., Sakaki, J., Okada, T., Hoshiko K., Yamamura, T., (2000). Effect of a novel bifunctional endothelin receptor antagonist, IRL 3630A, on guinea pig respiratory mechanics. *Eur. J. Pharmacol.* 406, 139-147.

[293] Mancel, E., Drouet, M., Sabbah, A., (1999). Membrane stabilizers (cromones and ketotifen). *Allerg. Immunol. (Paris).* 31, 103-105.

[294] Maneechotesuwan, K., Xin, Y., Ito, K., Jazrawi, E., Lee, K.Y., Usmani, O.S., Barnes, P.J., Adcock, I.M., (2009). Suppression of GATA-3 nuclear import and phosphorylation: a novel mechanism of corticosteroid action in allergic disease. *PLoS Med.* 6, e1000076.

[295] Maneechotesuwan, K., Kasetsinsombat, K., Wamanuttajinda, V., Wongkajornsilp, A., Barnes, P.J., (2013). Statins enhance the effects of corticosteroids on the balance between regulatory T cells and Th17 cells. *Clin. Exp. Allergy.* 43, 212-222.

[296] Mastalerz, L., Kumik, J., (2010). Antileukotriene drugs in the treatment of asthma. *Polskie Archiwum Medycyny Wewnetrznej.* 120, 103-108.

[297] Masuda, E.S., Schmitz, J., (2008). Inhibitors as treatment for allergic rhinitis. *Pulm. Pharmacol. Ther.* 21, 461-467.

[298] Mata, M., Martinez, I., Melero, J.A., Tenor, H., Cortijo, J., (2013). Roflumilast inhibits respiratory syncytial virus infection in human differentiated bronchial epithelial cells. *PLoS One.* 8, e69670.

[299] Matera, M.G., Cazzola, M., (2007). Ultra-long-acting beta2-adrenoreceptor agnoists: an emerging therapeutic option for asthma and COPD? *Drugs.* 67, 503-515.

[300] Mathioudakis, A.G., Chatzimavridou-Grigoriadou, V., Evangelopoulou, E., Mathioudakis, G.A., (2013). Vasoactive intestinal peptide inhaled agonists: potential role in respiratory therapeutics. *Hippokratia.* 17, 12-16.

[301] Matsumuto, H., (2014). Serum periostin: a novel biomarker for asthma management. *Allergol. Int.* 63, 153-160.

[302] Matsuno, O., Komori, C., Hang, Y., Matsumoto, T., Minamoto, S., (2012). Effectiveness of omalizumab in a patient with severe asthma, low serum IgE level, and lack of sensitized allergens induced by oral steroid therapy: the usefulness of impulse oscillation for assessment of omalizumab therapy. *J. Asthma.* 49, 839-842.

[303] Mattos, W., Lim, S., Russell, R., Jatakanon, A., Chung, K.F., Barnes, P.J., (2002). Matrix metalloproteinase-9 expression in asthma: effect of asthma severity, allergen challenge, and inhaled corticosteroids. *Chest.* 122, 1543-1552.

[304] Mazer, B.D., Gelfand, E.W., (1991). An open-label study of high-dose intravenous immunoglobulin in severe childhood asthma. *J. Allergy Clin. Immunol.* 87, 976-983.

[305] Meagher, L.C., Cousin, J.M., Seckl, J.R., Haslett, C., (1996). Opposing effects of glucocorticoticoids on the rate of apoptosis in neutrophilic and eosinophilic granulocytes. *J. Immunol.* 156, 4422-4428.

[306] Medina-Tato, D.A., Watson, M.L., Ward, S.G., (2006). Leukocyte navigation mechanisms as targets in airway diseases. *Drug Discov. Today.* 11, 866-879.

[307] Meja, K.K., Rajendrasozhan, S., Adenuga, D., Biswas, S.K., Sundar, I.K., Spooner, G., Marwick, J.A., Chakravarty, P., Fletcher, D., Whittaker, P., Megson, I.L., Kirkham, P.A., Rahman, I., (2008). Curcumin restores corticosteroid function in monocytes exposed to oxidants by maintaining HDAC2. *Am. J. Respir. Crit. Care Med.* 39, 312-323.

[308] Menzella, F., Zucchi, L., Piro, R., Galeone, C., Castagnetti, C., Facciolongo, N., (2014). A budget impact analysis of bronchial thermoplasty for severe asthma in clinical practice. *Adv. Ther.* Ahead of print.

[309] Mercado, N., To, Y., Ito, K., Barnes, P.J., (2011). Nortriptyline reverses corticosteroid insensitivity by inhibition of PI3Kδ. *J. Pharmacol. Exp. Ther.* 337, 465-470.

[310] Meltzer, E.O., Berkowitz, R.B., Grossbard, E.B., (2005). An intranasal Syk-kinase inhibitor (R112) improves the symptoms of seasonal allergic rhinitis in a park environment. *J. Allergy Clin. Immunol.* 115, 791-796.

[311] Mokry, J., Joskova, M., Mokra, D., Christensen, I., Nosalova, G., (2013). Effects of selective inhibition of PDE4 and PDE7 on airway reactivity and cough in healthy and ovalbumin-sensitized guinea pigs. *Adv. Exp. Med. Biol.* 756, 57-64.

[312] Mokry, J., Mokra, D., (2013). Immunological aspects of phosphodiesterase inhibition in the respiratory system. *Respir. Physiol. Neurobiol.* 187, 11-17.

[313] Morgan, C.I., Ledford, J.R., Zhou, P., Page, K., (2011). Zinc supplementation alters airway inflammation and airway hyperresponsiveness to a common allergen. *J. Inflamm.* 8, 36.

[314] Montuschi, P., Peters-Golden, M.L., (2010). Leukotriene modifiers for asthma treatment. *Clin. Exp. Allergy.* 40, 1732-1741.

[315] Moote, W., Kim, H., (2011). Allergen-specific immunotherapy. *Allergy Asthma Clin. Immunol.* 7 (Suppl 1), S5.

[316] Mori, T., Saito, K., Ohki, Y., Arakawa, H., Tominaga, M., Tokuyama, K., (2011). Lack of transient receptor potential vanilloid-1 enhances Th2-biased immune response on airways in mice receiving intranasal, but not intraperitoneal sensitization. *Int. Arch. Allergy Immunol.* 156, 305-312.

[317] Morley, J., (1992). Cyclosporin A in asthma therapy: a pharmacological rationale. *J. Autoimmun.* 5 Suppl A, 265-269.

[318] Mukhopadhyay, S., Hoidal, J.R., Mukherjee, T.K., (2006). Role of TNF-α in pulmonary pathophysiology. *Respir. Res.* 7, 125.

[319] Mukhopadhyay, S., Sypek, J., Tavendale, R., Gartner, U., Winter, J., Li, W., Page, K., Fleming, M., Brady, J., O'Toole, M., Macgregor, D.F., Goldman, S., Tam, S., Abraham, W., Williams, C., Miller, D.K., Palmer, C.N., (2010). Matrix metalloproteinase-12 is a therapeutic target for asthma in children and young adults. *J. Allergy Clin. Immunol.* 126, 70-76.

[320] Mungan, D., Misirligil, Z., Sin, B., Kaya, A., Demirel, Y., Gurbuz, L., (1995). Cyclosporin in steroid dependent asthma. *Allergol. Immunopathol (Madr).* 23, 202-206.

[321] Nakamura, Y., Ghaffar, O., Olivenstein, R., Taha, R.A., Soussi-Gounni, A., Zhang, D.H., Ray, A., Hamid, Q., (1999). Gene expression of the GATA-3 transcription factor is increased in atopic asthma. *J. Allergy Clin. Immunol.* 103 (2 Pt 1), 215-222.

[322] Nath, P., Eynott, P., Leung, S.Y.? Adcock, I.M., Bennerr, B.L., Chung, K.F., (2005). Potential role of c-Jun NH2-terminal kinase in allergic airway inflammation and remodeling: effects of SP600125. *Eur. J. Pharmacol.* 506, 273-283.

[323] Nevin, B.J., Broadley, K.J., (2004). Comparative effects of inhaled budesonide and the NO-donating budesonide derivative, NCX1020, against leucocyte influx and airway hyperreactivity following lipopolysaccharide challenge. *Pulm. Pharmacol. Ther.* 17, 219-232.

[324] Ng, T.P., Wong, M.L., Hong, C.Y., Koh, K.T.C., Goh, L.G., (2003). The use of complementary and alternative medicine by asthma patients. *Q. J. Med.* 96, 747/754.

[325] Niggemann, B., Jacobsen, L., Dreborg, S., Ferdousi, H.A., Halken, S., Host, A., Koivikko, A., Koller, D., Norberg, L.A., Urbanek, R., Valovirta, E., Wahn, U., Moller, C., PAT Investigator Group, (2006). Five-year follow-up on the PAT study: specific immunotherapy and long-term prevention of asthma in children. *Allergy.* 61, 855-859.

[326] Niggemann, B., Leupold, W., Schuster, A., Schuster, R. van Berg, A., Grubl, A., von der Hardt, H., Eibl, M.M., Wahn, U., (1998). Prospective, double-blind, placebo-controlled, multicenter study on the effect of high-dose, intravenous immunoglobulin in children and adolescents with severe bronchial asthma. *Clin. Exp. Allergy.* 28, 205-210.

[327] Niimi, K., Ge, Q., Moir, L.M., Ammit, A.J., Trian, T., Burgess, J.K., Black, J.L., Oliver, B.G., (2012). β_2-agonists upregulate PDE4 mRNA but not protein or activity in human airway smooth muscle cells from asthmatic and nonasthmatic volunteers. *Am. J. Physiol. Lung Cell Mol. Physiol.* 302, L334-342.

[328] Niruban, S.J., Alagiakrishnan, K., Beach, J., Senthilselvan, A., (2014). Association of vitamin D with respiratory outcomes in Canadian children. *Eur. J. Clin. Nutr.* Doi: 10.1038/ejcn.2014.121.

[329] Noga, O., Hanf, G., Kunkel, G., (2003). Immunological and clinical changes in allergic asthma following treatment with omalizumab. *Int. Arch. Allergy Immunol.* 131, 46-52.

[330] Norman, G., Faria, R., Paton, F., Llewellyn, A., Fox, D., Palmer, S., Clifton, I., Paton, J., Woolacott, N., McKenna, C., (2013). Omalizumab for the treatment of severe persistent allergic asthma: a systematic review and economic evaluation. *Health Technol. Assess.* 17, 1-161.

[331] Norman, P., (2011). Selective PI3Kδ inhibitors, a review of the patent literature. *Expert Opin. Ther. Pat.* 21, 1773-1790.

[332] Normansell, R., Walker, S., Milan, S.J., Walters, E.H., Nair, P., (2014). Omalizumab for asthma in adults and children (Review). *Cochrane Database Syst. Rev.* CD003559.

[333] Nosal, S., Sutovska, M., Nosalova, G., Banovcin, P., Sutovsky, J., Franova, S., (2007). Age-dependent changes of airway obstruction parameters. *J. Physiol. Pharmacol.* 58 Suppl 5 Pt 2, 493-500.

[334] O'Byrne, P.M., (2000). Why does airway inflammation persist? *Am. J. Respir. Crit. Care Med.* 161, S186-S187.

[335] O'Byrne, P.M., Bleecker, E.R., Bateman, E.D., Busse, W.W., Woodcock, A., Forth, R., Toler, W.T., Jacques, L., Lotvall, J., (2014). Once-daily fluticasone furoate alone or combined with vilanterol in persistent asthma. *Eur. Respir. J.* 43, 773-782.

[336] Offit, K., (2011). Personalized medicine: new genomics, old lessons. *Hum. Genet.* 130, 3-14.

[337] Ogawa, S., Lozach, J., Benner, C., Pascual, G., Tangirala, R.K., Westin, S., Hoffmann, A., Subramaniam, S., David, M., Rosenfeld, M.G., Glass, C.K., (2005). Molecular determinants of crosstalk between nuclear receptors and toll-like receptors. *Cell.* 122, 707-721.

[338] Oh, C.K., Leigh, R., McLaurin, K.K., Kim, K., Hutquist, M., Molfino, N., (2013). A randomized, controlled trial to evaluate the effect of an anti-interleukin-9 monoclonal antibody in adults with uncontrolled asthma. *Respir. Res.* 14, 93.

[339] Oliver, A., Bjermer, L., Quinn, D., Saggu, P., Thomas, P., Yarnall, K., Lotvall, J., (2013). Modulation of allergen-induced bronchoconstriction by fluticasone furoate and vilanterol alone or in combination. *Allergy.* 68, 1136-1142.

[340] Park, S.J., Lee, Y.C., (2010). Interleukin-17 regulation: an attractive therapeutic approach for asthma. *Respir. Res.* 11, 78.

[341] Park, H.W., Yang, M.S., Park, C.S., Kim, T.B., Moon, H.B., Min, K.U., Kim, Y.Y., Cho, S.H., (2009). Additive role of tiotropium in severe asthmatics and Arg16Gly in ADRB2 as a potential marker to predict response. *Allergy.* 64, 778-783.

[342] Paul-Clark, M.J., Roviezzo, F., Flower, R.J., Cirino, G., Soldato, P.D., Adcock, I.M., Perretti, M., (2003). Glucocorticoid receptor nitration leads to enhanced anti-inflammatory effects of novel steroid ligands. *J. Immunol.* 171, 3245-3252.

[343] Pavord, I.D., Cox, G., Thomson, N.C.m Rubin, A.S., Corris, P.A., Niven, R.M., Chung, K.F., Laviolette, M.; RISA Trial Study Group, (2007). Safety and efficacy of bronchial thermoplasty in symptomatic, severe asthma. *Am. J. Respir. Crit. Care Med.* 176, 1185-1191.

[344] Pelaia, G., Vatrella, L., Gallelli, L., Renda, T., Cazzola, M., Maselli, R., Marsico, S.A., (2006). Respiratory infections and asthma. *Respir. Med.* 100, 775-784.

[345] Pelaia, G., Vatrella, A., Maselli, R., (2012). The potential of biologics for the treatment of asthma. *Nature Rev. Drug. Disc.* 11, 958-972.

[346] Peters, S.P., Kunselman, S.J., Icitovic, N., Moore, W.C., Pascual, R., Ameredes, B.T., Boushey, H.A., Calhoun, W.J., Castro, M., Cherniack, R.M., Craig, T., Denlinger, L., Engle, L.L., DiMango, E.A., Fahy, J.V., Israel, E., Jarjour, N., Kazani, S.D., Kraft, M., Lazarus, S.C., Lemanske, R.F. Jr., Lugogo, N., Martin, R.J., Meyers, D.A., Ramsdell, J., Sorkness, C.A., Sutherland, E.R., Szefler, S.J., Wasserman, S.I., Walter, M.J., Wechsler, M.E., Chinchilli, V.M., Bleecker, E.R., National Heart, Lung, and Blood Institute Asthma Clinical Research Network. Tiotropium bromide step-up therapy for adults with uncontrolled asthma. *N. Engl. J. Med.* 364, 1715-1726.

[347] Peters-Golden, P., Henderson, W.R. Jr., (2007). Mechanisms of disease: leukotrienes. *N. Engl. J. Med.* 357, 1841-1954.

[348] Petersen, B.C., Lukacs, N.W., (2012). IL-17A and IL-25: therapeutic targets for allergic and exacerbated asthmatic disease. *Future. Med. Chem.* 4, 833-836.

[349] Petru, V., Carbolova, A., Matulka, M., Stejskal, J., (1991). Sodium nedocromil (Tilade) in the treatment of severe forms of asthma in children. *Cs. Pediat.* 46, 349-351.

[350] Pettpher, R., Hansel, T.T., Ramer, R., (2007). Antagonism of the prostaglandin D2 receptors DP1 and CRTH2 as an approach to treat allergic diseases. *Nat. Rev. Drug Discov.* 6, 313-325.

[351] Piacentini, G.L., Peroni, D.G., Bodini, A., Pigozzi, R., Costella, S., Loiacono, A., Boner, A.L., (2007). Azithromycin reduces bronchial hyperresponsiveness and neutrophilic airway inflammation in asthmatic children: a preliminary report. *Allergy Asthma Proc.* 28, 194-198.

[352] Pite, H., Gaspar, A., Paiva, M., Leiria-Pinto, P., (2013). Omalizumab under 12 years old: real-life practice. *Allergol. Immunopathol. (Madrid).* 41, 133-136.

[353] Plewako, H., Arvidsson, M., Petruson, K., Oancea, I., Holmberg, K., Adelroth, E., Gustafsson, H., Sandstrom, T., Rak, S., (2002). The effect of omalizumab on nasal allergic inflammation. *J. Allergy Clin. Immunol.* 110, 68-71.

[354] Popescu, F.D., (2003). New asthma drugs acting on gene expression. *J. Cell. Mol. Med.* 7, 475-486.

[355] Putney, J.W. Jr., (2001). Pharmacology of capacitative calcium entry. *Mol. Interv.* 1, 84-94.

[356] Quarcoo, D., Weixler, S., Groneberg, D., Joachim, R., Ahrens, B., Wagner, A.H., Hecker, M., Hamelmann, E., (2004). Inhibition of signal transducer and activator of transcription 1 attenuates allergen-induced airway inflammation and hyperreactivity. *J. Allergy Clin. Immunol.* 114, 288-295.

[357] Rabe, K.F., Tenor, H., Dent, G., Schudt, C., Liebig, S., Magnussen, H., (1993). Phosphodiesterase isozymes modulating inherent tone in human airways: identification and characterizations. *Am. J. Physiol.* 264, L458-464.

[358] Rabinovitch, N., Gelfand, E.W., Leung, D.Y.M., (1999). The role of immunoglobulin therapy in allergic diseases. *Allergy.* 54, 662-668.

[359] Raemdonck, K., De Alba J., Birrell, M.A., Grace, M., Maher, S.A., Irvin, C.G., Fozard, J.R., O'Byrne, P.M., Belvisi, M.G., (2012). A role for sensory nerves in the late asthmatic response. *Thorax.* 67, 19-25.

[360] Rajabbik, M.H., Lotfi, T., Alkhaled, L., Fares, M., El-Hajj Fuleihan, G., Mroueh, S., Akl, E.A., (2014). Association between low vitamin D levels and the diagnosis of asthma in children: a systematic review of cohort studies. *Allergy Asthma Clin. Immunol.* 10, 31.

[361] Rajesh, M., Pan, H., Mukhopadhyay, P., Batkai, S., Osei-Hyiaman, D., Hasko, G., Liaudet, L., Gao, B., Pacher, P., (2007). Pivotal advance: Cannabinoid 2 receptor agonist HU-308 protects against hepatic ischemia/reperfusion injury by attenuating oxidative stress inflammatory response, and apoptosis. *J. Leucocyt. Biol.* 82, 1382-1389.

[362] Ravichand, D.M., Laxmipathi, K., Sheshayamma, V., Abhay, A.P., (2006). Cytokine and chemokine modulators as novel targets for asthma. *Indian J. Allergy Asthma Immunol.* 20, 53-65.

[363] Reiter, J., Demirel, N., Mendy, A., Gasana, J., Vieira, E.R., Colin, A.A., Quizon, A., Forno, E., (2013). Macrolides for the long.term management of asthma: a meta-analysis of randomized clinical trials. *Allergy.* 68, 1040-1049.

[364] Richards, M.L., Lio, S.C., Sinha, A., Tieu, K.K., Sircar, J.C., (2004). Novel 2-(substituted pnenyl) benzimidazole derivatives with potent activity against IgE, cytokines, and CD23 for the treatment of allergy and asthma. *J. Med. Chem.* 47, 6451-6454.

[365] Robinson, P.D., Van Asperen, P., (2009). Asthma in childhood. *Pediatr. Clin. North. Am.* 56, 191-226.

[366] Robinson, P.D., Van Asperen, P., (2013). Newer treatments in the management of pediatric asthma. *Pediatr. Drugs.* 15, 291-302.

[367] Rogers, N.K., Clements, D., Dongre, A., Harrison, T.W., Shaw, D., Johnson, S.R., (2014). Extra-cellular matrix protein induce matrix metalloproteinase-1 (MMP-1) activity and increase airway smooth muscle contraction in asthma. *PLoS One.* 9, e90565.

[368] Ronchetti, R., Biscione, G.L., ROnchetti, F., Ronchetti, M.P., Martella, S., Falasca, C., Casini, C., Barreto, M., Villa, M.P., (2005). Why Chlamydia pneumonia is associated with asthma and other chronic conditions? Suggestions from a survey in unselected 9 yr old schoolchildren. *Pediatr. Allergy Immunol.* 16, 145-150.

[369] Ronchetti, R., Jesenak, M., Rennerova, Z., Barreto, M., Ronchetti, F., Villa, M.P., (2009). Relationship between atopic asthma and the population prevalence rates for asthma or atopy in children: atopic and nonatopic asthma in epidemiology. *Allergy Asthma Proc.* 30, 55-63.

[370] Ronchetti, R., Jesenak, M., Ronchetti, F., Rennerova, Z., (2010). Is asthma caused by atopy (positive skin prick tests)? Epidemiologic evidence suggests a negative answer. *Inflamm. Allergy Drug Targets.* 9, 91-96.

[371] Rosenwasser, L.J., (1998). Biological activities of IL-1 and itrs role in human diseae. *J. Allergy Clin. Immunol.* 102, 344-350.

[372] Rosenwasser, L.J., Busse, W.W., Lizambri, R.G., Olejnik, T.A., Totoritis, M.C., (2003). Allergic asthma and an anti-CD23 mAb (IDEC-152): results of a Phase I, single-dose, dose-escalating clinical trial. *J. Allergy Clin. Immunol.* 112, 563-570.

[373] Ross, R.N., Nelson, H.S., Finegold, I., (2000). Effectiveness of specific immunotherapy in the treatment of allergic rhinitis: an analysis. *Clin. Ther.* 22, 342-350.

[374] Rovati, G.E., Capra, V., (2007). Cysteinyl-leukotriene receptors and cellular signals. *Sci. World J.* 7, 1375-1392.

[375] Ruhl, R., Halpern, G.M., Gerschwin, M.E., (1993). Unconventional approaches to drug therapy in severe asthma. *Allergol. Immunopathol (Madr).* 21, 53-60.

[376] Salmun, L.M., Barlan, I., Wolf, H.M., Eibl, M., Twarog, F.J., Geha, R.S., Schneider, L.C., (1999). Effect of intravenous immunoglobulin on steroid consumption in patients with severe asthma: a double-blind, placebo-controlled, randomized trial. *J. Allergy Clin. Immunol.* 103, 810-815.

[377] Sampson, A.P., Siddiqui, S., Buchanan, D., Howarth, P.H., Holgate, S.T., Holloway, J.W., Sayers, I., (2000). Variant LTC4 synthase allele modifies cysteinyl leukotriene synthesis in eosinophils and predicts clinical response to zafirlukast. *Thorax.* 55, S28-S31.

[378] Sankar, J., Lodha, R., Kabra, S.K., (2008). Doxofylline: The next generation methylxanthine. *Indian J. Pediatr.* 75, 251-254.

[379] Sarinho, E., Medeiros, D., Schor, D., Rego Silva, A., Sales, V., Motta, M.E., Costa, A., Azoubel, A., Rizzo, J.A., (2009). Production of ointerleukin-10 in asthmatic children after beta-1,3-glucan. *Allergol. Immunopathol. (Madrid).* 37, 188-192.

[380] Schaafsma, D., Bos, I.S., Zuidhof, A.B., Zaagsma, J., Meurs, H., (2008). The inhaled Rho kinase inhibitor Y-27632 protects against allergen-induced acute bronchoconstriction, airway hyperresponsiveness, and inflammation. *Am. J. Physiol. Lung. Cell Mol. Physiol.* 295, L214-L219.

[381] Schelfhout, V., Louis, R., Lenz, W., Heyrman, R., Pauwels, R., Joos, G.R., (2006). The triple neurokinin-receptor antagonist CS-003 inhibits neurokinin A-induced bronchoconstriction in patients with asthma. *Pulm. Pharmacol. Ther.* 19, 413-418.

[382] Schmidt, D.T., Watson, N., Dent, G., Ruhlmann, E., Brandscheid, D., Magnussen, H., Rabe, K.F., (2000). The effect of selective and non-selective phosphodiesterase inhibitors on allergen- and leukotriene C_4-induced contractions in passively sensitized human airways. *Br. J. Pharmacol.* 131, 1607-1618.

[383] Schuster, A., Wahn, V., (1993). Intravenous immunoglobulins in bronchial asthma: a therapeutic alternative? *Infusionsther. Transfusionsmed.* 20 Suppl 1, 141-144.

[384] Schwartz, H.J., Hostoffer, R.W., McFadden, E.R. Jr., Berger, M., (2006). The response to intravenous immunoglobulin replacement therapy in patients with asthma with specific antibody deficiency. *Allergy Asthma Proc.* 27, 53-58.

[385] Sedlak, V., Koblizek, V., (2010). Future treatment of asthma. *Klin. Farmakol. Famr.* 24, 71-74.

[386] Searing, D.A., Zhang, Y., Murphy, J.R., Hauk, P.J., Goleva, E., Leung, D.Y., (2010). Decreased serum vitamin D levels in children with asthma are associated with increased corticosteroid use. *J. Allergy Clin. Immunol.* 125, 995-1000.

[387] Seddon, P., Bara, A., Ducharme, F.M., Lasserson, T.J., (2006). Oral xanthines as maintenance treatment for asthma in children. *Cochrane Database Syst. Rev.* CD002885.

[388] Seitz, M., Kamgang, R.K., Simon, H.U., Villiger, P.M., (2005). Therapeutic interleukin (IL) 1 blockade normalizes increased IL1β and decreased tumour necrosis factor α and IL10 production in blood mononuclear cells of a patient with CINCA syndrome. *Ann. Rheum. Dis.* 64, 1802-1803.

[389] Shapiro, D., Deering-Rice, C.E., Romero, E.G., Hughen, R.W., Light, A.R., Veranth, J.M., Reilly, C.S., (2013). Activation of transient receptor potential ankyrin-1 (TRPA1) in lung cells by wood smoke particulate material. *Chem. Res. Toxicol.* 26, 750-758.

[390] Shee, C., (2013). Is hypovitaminosis D a consequence rather than a cause of disease? *Thorax.* 68, 679.

[391] Sigman, K., Ghibu, F., Sommerville, W., Toledano, B.J., Bastein, Y., Cameron, L., Hamid, Q.A., Mazer, B., (1998). Intravenous immunoglobulin inhibits IgE production in human B lymphocytes. *J. Allergy Clin. Immunol.* 102, 421-427.

[392] Simon, H.U., (2006). Cytokine and anti-cytokine therapy for asthma. *Curr. Allergy Asthma Rep.* 6, 117-121.

[393] Simon, H.U., Seelbach, H., Ehmann, R., Schmitz, M., (2003). Clinical and immunological effects of low-dose IFN-α treatment in patients with corticosteroid-resistant asthma. *Allergy.* 58, 1250-1255.

[394] Simpson, J.L., Powell, H., Boyle, M.J., Scott, R.J., Gibson, P.G., (2008). Clarithromycin targets neutrophilic airway inflammation in refractory asthma. *Am. J. Respir. Crit. Care Med.* 177, 148-155.

[395] Singh, D., Kane, B., Molfino, N.A., Faggioni, R., Roskos, L., Woodcock, A., (2010). A phase I study evaluating the pharmacokinetics, safety and tolerability of repeat dosing with a human IL-33 antibody (CAT-354) in subject with asthma. *BMC Pulm. Med.* 10, 3.

[396] Singh, D., Richards, D., Knowles, R.G., Schwartz, S., Woodcock, A., Langley, S., O'Connor, B.J., (2007). Selective inducible nitric oxide synthase inhibition has not effect on allergen challenge in asthma. *Am. J. Respir. Crit. Care Me.* 176, 988-993.

[397] Singh, J., Adams, S., Carter, M.B., Cuervo, H., Lee, W.C., Lobb, R.R., Pepinsky, R.B., Petter, R., Scott, D., (2004). Rational design of potent and selective VLA-4 inhibitors and their utility in the treatment of asthma. *Curr. Top Med. Chem.* 4, 1497-1507.

[398] Skoner, D.P., Meltzer, E.O., Milgrom, H., Stryszak, P., Teper, A., Staudinger, H., (2011). Effects of inhaled mometasone furoate on growth velicity and adrenal function: a placebo-controlled trial in children 4 – 9 years old with mild persistent asthma. *J. Asthma.* 48, 848-859.

[399] Slavin, R.G., Ferioli, C., Tannenbaum, S.J., Martin, C., Blogg, M., (2009). Asthma symptom re-emergence after omalizumab withdrawal correlates well with increasing IgE and decreasing pharmacokinetic concentrations. *J. Allergy Clin. Immunol.* 123, 107-113.

[400] Sole, D., Costa-Carvalho, B.T., Soares, F.J., Rullo, V.V., Naspitz, C.K., (1996). Methotrexate in the treatment of corticodependent asthmatic children. *J. Investig. Allergol. Clin. Immunol.* 6, 126-130.

[401] Soler, M., Matz, J., Townley, R., Buhl, R., O'Brien, J., Fox, H., Thirlwell, J., Gupta, N., Della Cioppa, G., (2001). The anti-IgE antibody omalizumab reduces exacerbations and steroid requirement in allergic asthmatics. *Eur. Respir. J.* 18, 254-261.

[402] Sorkness, C.A., Wildfire, J.J., Calatroni, A., Mitchell, H.E., Bussee, W.W., O'Connor, G.T., Pongracic, J.A., Ross, K., Gill, M.A., Kattan, M., Morgan, W.J., Teach, S.J., Gergen, P.J., Liu, A.H., Szefles, S.J., (2013). Reassessment of omalizumab-dosing strategies and pharmacodynamics in inner-city children and adolescents. *J. Allergy Clin. Immunol. Pract.* 1, 163-171.

[403] Soucek, L., Buggy, J.J., Kortlever, R., Adimoolam, S., Monclus, H.A., Allende, M.T., Swigart, L.B., Evan, G.I., (2011). Modelling pharmacological inhibition of mast cell degranulation as a therapy for insulinoma. *Neoplasia.* 13, 1093-1100.

[404] Spears, M., Donnelly, I., Jolly, L., Brannigan, M., Ito, K., McSharry, C., Lafferty, J., Chaudhuri, R., Braganza, G., Bareille, P., Sweeney, L., Adcock, I.M., Barnes, P.J., Wood, S., Thomson, N.C., (2009). Bronchodilatory effect of the PPAR-gamma agonist rosiglitazone in smokers with asthma. *Clin. Pharmacol. Ther.* 86, 49-53.

[405] Spector, S.L., (1997). Alternative treatment in the patient with intractable asthma. *Curr. Opin. Pulm. Med.* 3, 23-29.

[406] Spooner, C.H., Saunders, L.D., Rowe, B.H., (2000). Nedocromil sodium for preventing exercise-induced bronchoconstriction. *Cochrane Database Syst. Rev.* CD001183.

[407] Steinhilber, D., Hofmann, B., (2014). Recent advances in the search for novel 5-lipoxygenase inhibitors. *Bas. Clin. Pharmacol. Toxicol.* 114, 70-77.

[408] Steiss, J.O., Schmidt, A., Nahrlich, L., Zimmer, K.P., Rudloff, S., (2012). Immunoglobulin E monitoring and reduction of omalizumab therapy in children and adolescents. *Allergy Asthma Proc.* 33, 77-81.

[409] Stengel, P.W., Rippy, M.K., Cockerham, S.L., Devane, W.A., Silbaugh, S.A., (1998). Pulmonary actions of anandamide, an endogenous cannabinoid receptor agonist, in guinea pigs. *Eur. J. Pharmacol.* 355, 57-66.

[410] Stengel, P.W., Cockerham, S.L., Silbaugh, S.A., (2007). Inhaled anandamide reduces leukotriene D4-induced airway obstruction in guinea pigs. *Eur. J. Pharmacol.* 557, 66-68.

[411] Stenton, G.R., Mackenzie, L.F., Tam, P., Cross, J.L., Harwig, C., Raymond, J., Toews, J., Wu, J., Ogden, N., MacRury, T., Szabo, C., (2013). Characterization of AQX-1125, a small molecule SHIP-1 activator: Part 1. Effects on inflammatory cell activation and chemotaxis in vitro and pharmacokinetic characterization in vivo. *Br. J. Pharmacol.* 168, 1506-1518.

[412] Stenton, G.R., Mackenzie, L.F., Tam, P., Cross, J.L., Harwig, C., Raymond, J., Toews, J., Chernoff, D., MacRury, T., Szabo, C., (2013). Characterization of AQX-1125, a small molecule SHIP-1 activator: Part 1. Efficacy studies in allergic and pulmonary inflammation models in vivo. *Br. J. Pharmacol.* 168, 1519-1529.

[413] Suessmuth, S., Freihorst, J., Gappa, M., (2003). Low-dose theophylline in childhood asthma: a placebo-controlled, double-blind study. *Pediatr. Allergy Immunol.* 14, 394-400.

[414] Sutovska, M., Adamkov, M., Kocmalova, M., Mesarosova, L., Oravec, M., Franova, S., (2013). CRAC ion channels and airway defense reflexes in experimental allergic inflammation. *Adv. Exp. Med. Biol.* 756, 39-48.

[415] Sutovska, M., Kocmalova, M., Adamkov, M., Vybohova, D., Mikolka, P., Mokra, D., Hatok, J., Antosova, M., Franova, S., (2013). The long-term administration of Orai 1 antagonist possesses antitussive, bronchodilatory and anti-inflammatory effects in experimental asthma model. *Gen. Physiol. Biophys.* 32, 251-259.

[416] Szefler, S.J., (2011). Personalised medicine for asthma management in pregnancy. *Lancet.* 378, 963-964.

[417] Taher, Y.A., van Esch, B.C.A.M., Hofman, G.A., Henricks, P.A.J., van Oosterhour, A.J.M., (2008). 1α,25-Dihydroxyvitamin D3 potentiates the benefitial effects of allergen immunotherapy in a mouse model of allergic asthma: role for IL-10 and TGF-beta. *J. Immunol.* 180, 5211-5221.

[418] Takahashi, N., Ogino, K., Takemoto, K., Hamanishi, S., Wang, D.H., Takigawa, T., Shibamori, M., Ishiyama, H., Fujikura, Y., (2010). Direct inhibition of arginase attenuated airway allergic reactions and inflammation in a Dermatophagoides farina-induced NC/Nga mouse model. *Am. J., Physiol. Lung Cell Mol Physiol.* 299, L17-L24.

[419] Taki, F., Kume, H., Kobayashi, T., Ohta, H., Aratake, H., Shimokata, K., (2007). Effects of Rho-kinase inactivation on eosinophilia and hyper-reactivity in murine airways by allergen challenges. *Clin. Exp. Allergy.* 37, 599-607.

[420] Tamachi, T., Maezawa, Y., Ikeda, K., Kagami, S., Hatano, M., Seto, Y., Suto, A., Suzuki, K., Watanabe, N., Saito, Y., Tokuhisa, T., Iwamoto, I., Nakajima, H., (2006). IL-25 enhances allergic airway inflammation by amplifying a T_H2 cell-dependent pathway in mice. *J. Allergy Clin. Immunol.* 118, 606-614.

[421] Tantisira, K.G., Drazen, J.M., (2009). Genetics and pharmacogenetics of the leukotriene pathway. *J. Allergy Clin. Immunol.* 124, 422-427.

[422] Taylor, D.A., McGrath, J.L., O'Connor, B., Barnes, P.J., (1998). Allergen-induced early and late asthmatic responses are not affected by inhibition of endogenous nitric oxide. *Am. J. Respir. Crit. Care Med.* 158, 1298-1300.

[423] Taylor, D.A., McGrath, J.L., Orr, L.M., Barnes, P.J., O'Connor, B.J., (1998). Effect of endogenous nitric oxide inhibition on airway responsiveness to histamine and adenosine-5'-monophosphate in asthma. *Thorax.* 53, 483-489.

[424] Tha-In, T., Bayry, J., Metselaar, H.J., Kaveri, S.V., Kwekkeboom, J., (2008). Modulation of the cellular immune system by intravenous immunoglobulin. *Trends Immunol.* 29, 608-615.

[425] Thomson, N.C., Patel, M., Smith, A.D., (2012). Lebrikizumab in the personalized management of asthma. *Biologics.* 6, 329-335.

[426] Thomson, N.C., Rubin, A.S., Niven, R.M., Corris, P.A., Siersted, H.C., Olivenstein, R., Pavord, I.D., McCormack, D., Laviolette, M., Shagill, N.S., Cox, G.; AIR Trial Study Group, (2011). Long-term (5 year) safety of bronchial thermoplasty: Asthma Intervention Research (AIR) Trial. *BMC Pulm. Med.* 11, 8.

[427] Tintinger, G.R., Feldman, C., Theron, A.J., Anderson, R., (2010). Montelukast: More than a cysteinyl leukotriene receptor antagonists? *Sci. World J.* 10, 2403-2413.

[428] Topilski, I., Flaishon, L., Naveh, Y., Harmelin, A., Levo, Y., Shachar, I., (2004). The anti-inflammatory effects of 1,25-dihydroxyvitamin D3 on Th2 cells in vivo are due in part to control of integrin-mediated T lymphocyte homing. *Eur. J. Immunol.* 34, 1068-1076.

[429] Torphy, T.J., Undem, B.J., Cieslinski, L.B., Luttmann, M.A., Reeves, M.L., Hay, D.W., (1993). Identification, characterization, and functional role of phosphodiesterase isozymes in human airway smooth muscle. *J. Pharmacol. Exp. Ther.* 165, 1213-1223.

[430] Torrego, A., Sola, I., Munoz, A.M., Roque, I., Figuls, M., Yepes-Nunez, J.J., Alonso-Coello, P., Plaza, V., (2014). Bronchial thermoplasty for moderate to severe persistent asthma in adults. *Cochrane Database Syst. Rev.* 3, CD009910.

[431] Torres, T., Vilaca, S., Velho, G., Selores, M., (2012). Etanercept-induced asthma in a psoriatic patient resolving with transition to ustekinumab. *Eur. J. Dermatol.* 22, 696-697.

[432] Trevor, J.L., Deshane, J.S., (2014). Refractory asthma: mechanisms, targets, and therapy. *Allergy.* 69, 817-827.

[433] Trian, T., Burgess, J.K., Niimi, K., Moir, L.M., Ge, Q., Berger, P., Liggett, S.B., Black, J.L., Oliver, B.G., (2011). β_2-agonist induced cAMP is decreased in asthmatic airway smooth muscle due to increased PDE4D. *PLoS One.* 6, e20000.

[434] Tse, S.M., Li, L., Butler, M.G., Fung, V., Kharbanda, E.O., Larkin, E.K., Vollmer, W.M., Miroshnik, I., Rusinak, D., Weiss, S.T., Lieu, T., Wu, A.C., (2013). Statin exposure is associated with decreased asthma-related emergency department visits and oral corticosteroid use. *Am. J. Respir. Crit. Care Med.* 188, 1076-1082.

[435] Tsitoura, D.C., Rothman, P.B., (2004). Enhancement of MEK/ERK signaling promotes glucocorticoid resistance in CD4$^+$ T cells. *J. Clin. Invest.* 113, 619-627.

[436] Tudhope, S.J., Catley, M.C., Fenwick, P.S., Russell, R.E., Rumsey, W.L., Newton, R., Barnes, P.J., Donnelly, L.E., (2007). The role of IkappaB kinase 2, but not activation of NF-kappaB, in the release of CXCR3 ligands from IFN-gamma-stimulated human bronchial epithelial cells. *J. Immunol.* 179, 6237-6245.

[437] Underwood, D.C., Osborn, R.R., Kotzer, C.J., Adams, J.L., Lee, J.C., Webb, E.F., Carpenter, D.C., Bochnowicz, S., Thomas, H.C., Hay, D.W., Griswold, D.E., (2000). SB-239063, a potent p38 MAPK kinase inhibitor, reduces inflammatory cytokine

production, airways eosinophil infiltration, and persistence. *J. Pharmacol. Exp. Ther.* 293, 281-288.

[438] Usami, A., Ueki, S., Ito, W., Kobayashi, Y., Chiba, T., Mahemuti, G., Oyamada, H., Kamada, Y., Fujita, M., Kato, H., Saito, N., Kayaba, H., Chihara, J., (2006). Theophylline and dexamethasone induce peroxisome proliferator-activated receptor-gamma expression in human eosinophils. *Pharmacology.* 77, 33-37.

[439] Van Schoor, J., Joos, G.F., Chasson, B.L., Brouard, R.J., Pauwels, R.A., (1998). The effect of the NK2 tachykinin receptor antagonist SR 48968 (saredutant) on neurokinin A-induced bronchoconstriction in asthmatics. *Eur. Respir. J.* 12, 17-23.

[440] Valovirta, E., (2011). Effect of AIT in children including potential to prevent the development of asthma. *Allergy.* 66 (Suppl 95), 53-54.

[441] Vayssiere, B.M., Dupont, S., Choquart, A., Petit, F., Garcia, T., Marchandeau, C., Gronemeyer, H., Resche-Rigon, M., (1997). Synthetic glucocorticoids that dissociate transactivation and AP-1 transrepression exhibit anti-inflammatory activity in vivo. *Mol. Endocrinol.* 11, 1245-1255.

[442] Vichyanond, P., (2011). Omalizumab in allergic diseases, a recent review. *Asian Pac. J. Allergy Immunol.* 29, 209-219.

[443] Vojtkova, J., Ciljakova, M., Vojarova, L., Janikova, K., Michnova, Z., Sagiova, V., (2012). Hypovitaminosis D in children with type 1 diabetes mellitus and its influence on biochemical and densitometric parameters. *Acta Medica (Hradec Kralove).* 55, 18-22.

[444] Vrugt, B., Wilson, S., van Velzen, E., Bron, A., Shute, J.K., Holgate, S.T., Djukanovic, R., Aalbers, R., (1997). Effects of high dose intravenous immunoglobulin in two severe corticosteroid insensitive asthmatic patients. *Thorax.* 52, 662-664.

[445] Wadsworth, S.J., Sandford, A.J., (2013). Personalised medicine and asthma diagnosis/management. *Curr. Allergy Asthma Rep.* 13, 118-129.

[446] Wahn, V., Orange, J., Alexis, A., Ballow, M., Belohradsky, B.H., Berger, M., Bonagura, V., Bonilla, F.A., Borte, M., Bussel, J.B., Chinen, J., Christiansen, O.B., Coski, C.L., Ebell, W., Gold, R., Goldman, F., Harville, T., Hoffmann, F., Horneff, G., Jordan, S.C., Korinthenberg, R., Meyer, C.U., Nadal, D., Niggemann, B., Roos, R., Sacher, R.A., Schulze, I., Siegel, J., Spaeth, P., Sundel, R.P., Van Holten, R.W., Wallington, T., Wehmeier, A., Zepp, F., (2008). Bremen: UNI-MED Verlag, 1. edition, 207 pp. ISBN 978-3-8374-1011-2.

[447] Walker, D.Y., Edwards, K.L., (2013). Statins in the treatment of asthma. *Am. J. Health. Sys. Pharm.* 70, 1661-1669.

[448] Wang, Y.H., Angkasekwinai, P., Lu, N., Voo, K.S., Arima, K., Hanabuchi, S., Hippe, A., Corrigan, C.J., Dong, C., Homey, B., Yao, Z., Ying, S., Huston, D.P., Liu, Y.J., (2007). IL-25 augments type 2 immune responses by enhancing the expansion and functions of TSLP-DC-activated Th2 memory cells. *J. Exp. Med.* 204, 1837-1847.

[449] Wechsler, M.E., (2013). Inhibiting interleukin-4 and interleukin-13 in difficult-to-control asthma. *N. Engl. J. Med.* 368, 2511-2513.

[450] Wechsler, M.E:, Laviolette, M., Rubin, A.S., Fiterman, J., Lapa, J.R., Shah, P.L., Fiss, E., Olivenstein, R., Thomson, N.C., Nives, R.M., Pavord, I.A., Simoff, M., Hales, J.B., McEvoy, C., Slebos, D.J., Holmes, M., Phillips, M.J., Erzurum, S.C., Hanania, N.A., Sumino, K., Kraft, M., Cox, G., Sterman, D.H., Hogart, K., Austin, J.H.M., Shargill, N.S., Quiring, J., Armstrong, B., Castro, M.; Asthma Intervention Research 2 Trial

Study Group, (2013). Bronchial thermoplasty: Long-term safety and effectiveness in patients with severe asthma. *J. Allergy Clin. Immunol.* 132, 1295-1302.

[451] Weiss, S.T., (2012). New approaches to personalized medicine for asthma: Where are we? *J. Allergy Clin. Immunol.* 129, 327-334.

[452] Wenzel, S.E., Barnes, P.J., Bleecker, E.R., Bousquet, J., Busse, W., Dahlen, S.E., Holgate, S.T., Meyers, D.A., Rabe, K.F., Antczak, A., Baker, J., Horvath, I., Mark, Z., Bernstein, D., Kerwin, E., Schlenker-Herceg, R., Lo, K.H., Watt, R., Barnathan, E.S., Chanez, P.; T03 Asthma Investigators, (2009). A randomized, boulde-blind, placebo-controlled study of tumor necrosis factor-alpha blockade in severe persistent asthma. *Expert. Opin. Investig. Drugs.* 18, 1421-1423.

[453] Wenzel, S., Ford, L., Pearlman, D., Spector, S., Sher, L., Skobieranda, F., Wang, L., Kirkesseli, S., Rocklin, R., Bock, B., Hamilton, J., Ming, J.E., Radin, A., Stahl, N., Yancopoulos, G.D., Graham, N., Pirozzi, G., (2013). Dupilumab in persistent asthma with elevated eosinophil levels. *N. Engl. J. Med.* 368, 2455-2466.

[454] Wenzel, S., Wilbraham, D., Fuller, R., Getz, E.B., Longphre, M., (2007). Effect of an interleukin-4 variant on late phase asthmatic response to allergen challenge in asthmatic patients: results of two Phase 2a studies. *Lancet.* 370, 1422-1431.

[455] Williams, J., Johnson, S., Mascali, J.J., Smith, H., Rosenwasser, L.J., Borish, L., (1992). Regulation of low affinity IgE receptor (CD23) expression on mononuclear phagocytes in normal and asthmatic subjects. *J. Immunol.* 149, 2823-2829.

[456] Wilson, A., (2002). Are antihistamines useful in managing asthma? *Curr. Opin. Allergy Clin. Immunol.* 2, 53-59.

[457] Wong, E.H., Porter, J.D., Edwards, M.R., Johnston, S.L., (2014). The role of macrolides in asthma: current evidence and future directions. *Lancet Respir. Med.* Doi: 10.1016/S2213-2600(14)70107-9.

[458] Wu, A.C., Tantisira, K., Li, L., Fuhlbrigge, A.L., Weiss, S.T., Litonjua, A., (2012). Effect of vitamin D and inhaled corticosteroid treatment on lung function in children. *Am. J. Respir. Crit. Care Med.* 186, 508-513.

[459] Wu, F.Q., Zhu, S.Y., He, C.X., Gu, M.X., (2009). Effects of fasudil on the expression of Rho-kinase-1 and airway inflammation in a mouse model of asthma. *Chin. J. Tuberc. Respir. Dis.* 32, 847-849.

[460] Wulff, H., Castle, N.A., (2010). Therapeutic potential of KCa3.1 blockers: recent advances and promising trends. *Expert Rev. Clin. Pharmacol.* 3, 385-396.

[461] Xiang, Z., Moller, C., Nilsson, G., (2006). IgE-receptor activation induces survival and Bfl-1 expression in human mast cells but not basophils. *Allergy.* 61, 1040-1046.

[462] Xystrakis, E., Kusumakar, S., Boswell, S., Peek, E., Urry, Z., Richards, D.F., Adikibi, T., Pridgeon, C., Dallman, M., Loke, T.K., Robinson, D.S., Barrat, F.J., O'Garra, A., Lavender, P., Lee, T.H., Corrigan, C., Hawrylowicz, C.M., (2006). Reversing the defective induction of IL-10-secreting regulatory T cells in glucocorticoid-resistant asthma patients. *J. Clin. Invest.* 116, 146-155.

[463] Yamada, J., Hamuro, J., Natanaka, H., Hamabata, K., Kinoshita, S., (2007). Alleviation of seasonal allergic symptoms with superfine beta-1,3-glucan: a randomized study. *J. Allergy Clin. Immunol.* 119, 1119-1126.

[464] Yamamoto, N., Takeshita, K., Shichijo, M., Kokubo, T., Sato, M., Nakashima, K., Ishimori, M., Nagai, H., Li, Y.F., Yura, T., Bacon, K.B., (2003). The orally available spleen tyrosine kinase inhibitor 2-[7-(3,4-dimethoxyphenyl)-imidazo[1,2-c]pyrimidin-

5-ylamino]nicotinamide dihydrochloride (BAY 61-3606) blocks antigen-induced airway inflammation in rodents. *J. Pharmacol. Exp. Ther.* 306, 1174-1181.

[465] Yamashita, N., Tashimo, H., Ishida, H., Kaneko, F., Nakano, J., Kato, H., Hirai, K., Horiuchi, T., Ohta, K., (2002). Attenuation of airway hyperresponsiveness in a murine asthma model by neutralization of granulocyte-macrophage colony-stimulating factor (GM-CSF). *Cell. Immunol.* 219, 92-97.

[466] Yazid, S., Sinniah, A., Solito, E., Calder, V., Flower, R.J., (2013). Anti-allergic cromones inhibit histamine and eicosanoid release from activated human and murine mast cells by releasing Annexin A1. *PLoS One.* 8, e58963.

[467] Yilmaz, E.A., Ozmen, S., Bostanci, I., DIbek Misirlioglu, E., Ertan, U., (2011). Erythrocyte zinc levels in children with bronchial asthma. *Pediatr. Pulmonol.* 46, 1189-1193.

[468] Yoshihara, S., Morimoto, H., Yamada, Y., Abe, T., Arisaka, O., (2004). Cannabinoid receptor agonists inhibit sensory nerve activation in guinea pigs. *Am. J. Respir. Crit. Care Med.* 170, 941-946.

[469] Yoshihara, S., Morimoto, H., Ohori, M., Yamada, Y., Abe, T., Arisaka, O., (2005). The cannabinoid receptor agonist WIN 55212-2 inhibits neurogenic inflammation in airway tissues. *J. Pharmacol. Sci.* 98, 77-82.

[470] Yoshii, A., Iizuka, K., Dobashi, K., Horie, T., Harada, T., Nakazawa, T., Mori, M., (1999). Relaxation of contracted rabbit tracheal and human bronchial smooth muscle by Y-27632 through inhibition of Ca^{2+} sensitization. *Am. J. Respir. Cell Mol. Biol.* 20, 1190-1200.

[471] Yoshino, T., Ishikawa, J., Ohga, K., Morokata, T., Takezawa, R., Morio, H., Okada, Y., Honda, K., Yamada, T., (2007). YM-58483, a selective CRAC channel inhibitor, prevents antigen-induced airway eosinophilia and late phase asthmatic responses via Th2 cytokine inhibition in animal model. *Eur. J. Pharmacol.* 560, 225-233.

[472] Youngchaiyund, P., Lee, T.B., (1986). Effect of nedocromil sodium in the immediate response to antigen challenge in asthmatic patients. *Clin. Allergy.* 16, 129-134.

[473] Zeki, A.A., Oldham, J., Wilson, M., Fortenko, O., Goyal, V., Last, M., Last, A., Patel, A., Last, J.A., Kenyon, N.J., (2013). Statin use and asthma control in patients with severe asthma. *BMJ Open.* 3, e003314.

[474] Zeki, A.A., Thai, P., Kenyon, N.J., Wu, R., (2012). Differential effects of simvastatin on IL-13-induced cytokine gene expression in primary mouse tracheal epithelial cells. *Respir. Res.* 13, 38.

[475] Zielen, S., Kardos, P., Madonini, E., (2010). Steroid-sparing effects with allergen-specific immunotherapy in children with asthma: A randomized controlled trial. *J. Allergy Clin. Immunol.* 126, 942-949.

Reviewed by:

Prof. Peter Banovcin, M.D., Ph.D. – Department of Pediatrics, Comenius University in Bratislava, Jessenius Faculty of Medicine in Martin, Slovakia

Assoc. Prof. Vladimír Pohanka, M.D., Ph.D., MPH, FCCP – 4th Department of Pediatrics, Slovak Medical University in Bratislava, Poprad, Slovakia

In: Advances in Respiratory Therapy Research
Editor: Miloš Jeseňák

Chapter 2

Therapeutic Use of Nitric Oxide Synthase Inhibitors in Respiratory Diseases with Bronchial Hyperreactivity

Martina Antosova[1]* and Juraj Mokry[2]
[1]Department of Physiology,
[2]Department of Pharmacology,
Comenius University Jessenius Faculty of Medicine, Martin, Slovakia

Abstract

Chronic inflammatory diseases of the respiratory tract represent a serious global problem. The continuous updates and advances in knowledge about their pathogenesis and incidences evoke many questions. One question is the position of nitric oxide (NO) in the respiratory system. Nitric oxide is a small mediator/messenger important for both the physiology and pathophysiology of airways. This dual position is changed in accordance to many factors e.g. age, gender, hormonal activity, the influence of exogenous irritants etc. Nitric oxide is produced in relatively small amounts in a healthy organism. Chronic inflammation during respiratory diseases is often associated with an increase of NO production through the action of nitric oxide synthases, predominantly inducible nitric oxide synthase (iNOS). The role of other enzymes participating in formation of NO (e.g. arginase – competition for NO production substrate L-Arginine) in the pathogenesis of respiratory diseases is also important. Therefore, modulation of this enzymatic activity is very interesting for many researchers focused on the identification of new markers and trends in the therapy of chronic inflammatory airways disease.

* Corresponding Author address: Martina Antosova, MSc., Ph.D., MBA, Department of Physiology, Jessenius Faculty of Medicine in Martin, Comenius University in Bratislava, Mala Hora 4, 036 01, Martin, Slovak Republic, e-mail: Martina.Antosova@jfmed.uniba.sk

Enzyme inhibitors have positive effects in experiments. These substances modulate bronchial hyperreactivity, the number of inflammatory cells, specific airway resistance and the level of nitric oxide in exhaled air. There are many experimental and clinical studies (Phase II) regarding the use of these substances in respiratory diseases. However, their results are controversial. Is it possible to use the inhibitor of nitric oxide synthase in the treatment of chronic airway inflammation e.g. in bronchial asthma? Which effect of the inhibitors might be particularly effective in the treatment of cases related to overproduction of nitric oxide?

This chapter focuses on the possibilities of treatment with nitric oxide synthase inhibitors and the potential benefit of those inhibitors in the treatment of respiratory diseases with bronchial hyperreactivity. The information is supported by the results with non-selective and selective NO-synthase inhibitors, which were tested in an animal model of allergic inflammation/hyperreactivity.

Keywords: Bronchial Hyperreactivity, Enzyme Inhibitors, Nitric oxide, Nitric Oxide Synthase, Therapy

1. Introduction

There are two types of nitric oxide—exogenous and endogenous. Exogenous NO is a free radical, highly reactive gas, one of the ten most unstable molecules in nature. A relatively stable amount (10 to 100 ppb) is present in the atmospheric air. A lethal dose for humans is considered to be a concentration of 5000 ppb [34]. The respiratory system in healthy humans produces NO both in the upper and lower respiratory tracts (approximately 20 ppb), with very high levels of NO in the nose and sinuses (approximately 900 ppb) [48]. These amounts of NO are involved in the regulation of many physiological processes in the airways as well as in pathogenesis of a number of airways diseases, both acute and chronic.

The basic substrate for nitric oxide biosynthesis is L-arginine. This semi-essential amino acid is also a precursor for the synthesis of other molecules e.g. urea, creatine, polyamines etc. The synthesis and catabolism of L-arginine is affected by several enzymes, such as arginine-succinate synthase, arginase isoenzymes, *NO-synthase* and arginine decarboxylase in human cells. Nitric oxide is produced through the process of NO-synthases. The knowledge of their structures, functions and possibilities of their modulation significantly contributes to understanding the effects of nitric oxide and is important for the planning of potential therapeutic strategies as well. In the human body, NO-synthases are present as three major isoforms, which require several cofactors and prosthetic groups to function properly. For each of these isoforms there are many specific differences at the level of structural, transcriptional and post-translational regulations of their catalytic activity. Differences in the cell and tissue localization of NO-synthases in airways, differences in activity and some other specific characteristics (e.g. expression after specific stimulus affection, chromosome localization etc.) are already recognized in the respiratory tract [4]. The basic characteristic of NO-synthase is associated with their location. *Neuronal nitric oxide synthase - nNOS* is expressed *in* all levels of the respiratory tract - in the cytosol of the epithelial cells, in the smooth muscle cells and in the nerve fibers of the respiratory and vascular system [69]. The density of the nerve fibers decreases from the trachea toward the small bronchi. nNOS-containing nerve fibers were also detected around the submucosal glands, but their impact on the regulation of secretion is at the present unknown [21]. *It is assumed that this isoform can be involved in the development of bronchial hyperreactivity* [12, 18]. *Inducible nitric oxide synthase - iNOS,* is sometimes referred to as immune or inflammatory type NOS [78]. The expression of this isoform in the airways is increased mainly by the action of proinflammatory cytokines. iNOS is a cytoplasmic enzyme detected in the epithelium of the proximal and terminal bronchioles [1, 64], alveolar cells II type [82], lung fibroblasts [67], in bronchial smooth muscle and blood vessels [29], mast cells [27], endothelial cells [63], neutrophils, [8] etc.

Nitric oxide produced by iNOS has anti-microbial, anti-tumor, cytostatic and cytotoxic effects associated predominantly with the production of free radicals [74]. It has a protective role in a variety of bacterial and parasitic infections and in response to inflammation. On the other hand, the increase of iNOS activity is associated with various infectious and inflammatory diseases. *This isoform plays a major role in the pathogenesis of inflammatory diseases of the airways such as bronchial asthma* [6; 69]. Increased activity of iNOS causes relaxation of vascular smooth muscle, increases vascular permeability, increases mucus secretion, inflammatory cell infiltration, damages the epithelium layer, modulates the function of immune cells and mediates respiratory inflammation [52]. *Endothelial NO synthase - eNOS* is located in the epithelium of the trachea, bronchi and alveoli [64]. It has also been detected in the endothelial cells of large pulmonary blood vessels, in the nasal mucosa and in the basal membrane of the ciliary microtubules [40]. *It is assumed that NO produced by eNOS reduces the bronchial hyperreactivity* [18]. Currently there is a fourth isoform - *mitochondrial* (mtNOS, [45]. This isoform has not been identified satisfactorily yet and its participation in physiological and pathological processes in the airways can be only hypothesized.

The isoforms of NO-synthase can be divided according to expression pattern and the relationship between the levels of intracellular calcium to dependent and independent intracellular calcium levels. Some results show that the constitutive isoforms can be induced under similar conditions as the iNOS and it may be expressed constitutively in some cells like airway epithelium [23]. This relationship is important in bronchial hyperreactivity too.

Based on the information, it is evident that all of these three isoforms are involved in the regulation of physiological functions in airways. The changes in NO-synthases activities and the subsequent change in the levels of NO are important for the pathogenesis of various airway diseases.

Several articles describe "the optimal level of NO," which is primarily associated with the activity of the constitutive NO synthase (cNOS). The theory of "the optimal level" points out that under physiological conditions cNOS produces relatively small, stable amounts of NO involved in the regulation of physiological processes. Because these amounts are formed almost continuously, their blockade should have a negative effect on the regulation of the fundamental physiological processes occurring in the airways. On the other hand, in inflammatory conditions, inductive isoform (iNOS) is activated, which is able to produce abnormally high amounts of NO with a pathogenic effect in a relatively short time. Its blockade in these conditions would be beneficial and reduce the symptoms induced by overproduction of NO (e.g. edema, improved ventilation, etc.).

2. The Main Effects of Nitric Oxide in Airways

The most important effect of NO in the airways is a regulation of bronchomotor tone. Nitric oxide is a major neurotransmitter/mediator of the inhibitory nonadrenergic noncholinergic (NANC) system and the regulation of bronchial tone is provided along with cholinergic and adrenergic systems. In addition, it is involved in the regulation of blood flow and modulates the onset and progression of inflammatory processes. Nitric oxide also has an important role in the regulation of mucociliary transport and the production of surfactant. Its importance has been described in the process of the development of lung tissue. The basic effects of NO in the respiratory system are summarized in Table 1.

Table 1. Basic effects of NO in airways and association with NO-synthase

Target	Physiology	Pathophysiology	NOS
Bronchial smooth muscle	relaxation	changes of reactivity/ hyperreactivity	nNOS
Vessel smooth muscle	vasodilatation	plasma exudation/ edema	eNOS
Immune system	anti-inflammatory effect, antiviral, antiparasital, antibacterial effect	proinflammatory effect	iNOS
Epithelium	mucocilial clearance regulation	mucus hypersecretion	nNOS/eNOS /iNOS

2.1. Nitric Oxide and Regulation of Bronchomotor Tone

One of the basic effects of NO is the regulation of bronchomotor tone. The nonadrenergic noncholinergic system was identified in the tracheal smooth muscle of animals and humans. This system is classified as an excitatory (contractile) system (eNANC) or inhibitory (relaxation) system (iNANC) [79]. Several studies indicate that the major neurotransmitter of the iNANC system is nitric oxide. This neurotransmitter predominantly mediates the bronchodilation. The importance of NO as a neurotransmitter of the iNANC system has been demonstrated by studies in isolated guinea pig trachea and later in human tissue isolated from the airways. The importance of this neurotransmission is supported by the fact that application of NO-synthase inhibitors in *in vitro* conditions has significantly increased the cholinergic contraction stimulated pharmacologically [13]. Nitric oxide works as a functional antagonist in the smooth muscles found in airways. It reacts against the bronchoconstriction induced by acetylcholine and other bronchoconstriction mediators such as bradykinin, histamine and methacholine [73]. This effect was also observed in asthmatic patients after inhalation of NO or after administration of NO donors [77]. iNANC neurons are located mostly in the deeper layers of the airways. In the airways, the iNANC system was also detected in the parasympathetic, sympathetic and sensory ganglia (jugular more than nodose), in bronchial blood vessels and submucosal glands [13, 68]. It is assumed that NO is released together with acetylcholine and other NANC neurotransmitters for the modulation of cholinergic responses.

The bronchodilation mediated by the iNANC system is associated with increased levels of cGMP in smooth muscle, indicating a modulation of bronchomotor tone via the NO / cGMP cascade. This mechanism is mediated by the soluble guanylyl cyclase (GC-S). The literature presents that NO released mainly by cNOS binds to the Fe^{2+} in heme of GC-S with changes in the activity of this enzyme. The result is a transformation of guanosine triphosphate (GTP) to cyclic guanosine monophosphate, which in turn activates cGMP-dependent protein kinase. This process catalyzes the phosphorylation of various proteins, activates or inhibits certain types of ion channels (calcium, potassium), or regulates the activity of phosphodiesterase [35; 55]. The result is a variety of cellular processes, such as the relaxation of smooth muscle cells in bronchi [32; 78]. It is known that cGMP causes the relaxation of smooth muscle by reducing the intracellular calcium or by reducing the sensitivity of the contractile system to calcium [69]. The effect of NO on the smooth muscle in airways is secured solely by this mechanism. A second messenger, cGMP, mediates the majority of the NO effects in the airways. Therefore, the changes in the NO / cGMP pathway may be also one of the causes of respiratory diseases associated with obstruction and hyperreactivity [70].

The bronchomotor tone is not only under the control of NO formed and released in smooth muscle cells, but also under the control of the epithelium involved in this process. After removing the epithelium, contractile responses to a variety of spasmogens was increased [68]. This result confirms that endogenous NO released by epithelium acts as a relaxing factor. In the respiratory system of guinea pigs NO did not cause a direct effect on basal bronchial tone, but reduced the contractile response to parasympathomimetic, histamine, bradykinin etc. [19]. Removing the epithelium along with direct effects of exogenous stimuli on smooth muscle may also contribute to bronchial hyperreactivity [13].

2.2. Nitric Oxide and Regulation of Vascular Tone

Nitric oxide is an important regulator of vascular tone. It is an effective vasodilator and plays an important role in the regulation of blood flow through the lungs. Release of NO in endothelial cells of the pulmonary circulation regulates basal vascular tone and prevents vasoconstriction [68]. Deficiency and overproduction of NO are both unfavorable for pulmonary circulation. Reduced NO production promotes vasoconstriction and pulmonary hypertension; overproduction causes hypotension and is often associated with sepsis [15]. The opinions about the effect of NO on the microvasculature and vascular permeability are unclear. NOS inhibitors blocked plasma leakage in the microvasculature after exposure to some mediators – e.g. leukotriene D4, demonstrating the significant effect of NO in plasma extravasation. Increased levels of NO may cause increased blood flow in the lungs, increased vascular permeability, and exudation of plasma into the interstitium and formation of an edema [25]. This process is primarily caused by activation of the neurokinin receptor (NK1), and by activation of the leukotriene or histamine receptors [39]. This process is affected and worsened by the formation of free radicals [62].

2.3. Nitric Oxide and Mucociliary Transport

The production and characteristics of mucus significantly affects mucociliary transport. Nitric oxide stimulates submucosal glands in the airways, resulting in increased mucus production [59]. These findings were confirmed by the application of NO donors leading to a significant increase of mucus secretion. Conversely, the application of NOS inhibitors suppresses the mucus secretion. These results indicate that the secretion of mucus in the airways is mediated by mechanisms depending on the intracellular production of NO [2]. Nitric oxide also contributes to the control of mucociliary transport. Ciliary motility is an important defense mechanism and it is enhanced e.g. by the effects of proinflammatory cytokines. The participation of NO in this process was confirmed with NOS inhibitors, which suppressed ciliary motility and with L-arginine, which stimulated ciliary motility [68]. Decreased production of NO has been observed in primary ciliary dyskinesia, Kartageners syndrome and cystic fibrosis (accompanied by impaired ciliary clearance). The effect of NO on the mucociliary transport mechanism may be associated with the modulation of phosphodiesterases or by modulating the activity of ion channels [14, 20]. The question that remains is which type of channels is the most important for the signal transmission in NO signaling. The interactions of calcium channels are not yet completely elucidated. From existing information, it is obvious that these types of channels provide the support of Ca^{2+} dependent constitutive NOS isoforms. A different model works in the chloride ion channels (activated by the NO). An increase in chloride ion conductivity is involved in the regulation of the balance between Na^+ and Cl^-, thus influencing secretion and mucociliary transport in the airways. Potassium channels are mainly in smooth muscle cells and are responsible for the relaxation of smooth muscle. Based on the available information we can assume that NO is a physiological regulator of mucociliary clearance and changes in the production and activity may be important in the pathophysiology of respiratory diseases associated with changes in mucus secretion and mucociliary transport.

2.4. Nitric Oxide and Inflammation

Nitric oxide acts as an important mediator of inflammation in the respiratory system. iNOS expression and subsequent NO production in the cells of the respiratory epithelium and in inflammatory and immune cells is significantly increased in acute and chronic inflammation. Is overproduction of NO a protective or negative factor? The data presents antiviral, antibacterial, antiparasitic and other protective effects of NO produced by iNOS. Many of these effects are associated with the production of free radicals. A key mechanism in this process is the interaction of NO with free radicals, mainly with the superoxide radical with subsequent production of the peroxynitrite [3]. Peroxynitrite as a powerful oxidant can cause significant cell damage. The damage flows directly by the nitration of tyrosine, resulting in irreversible dysfunction of critical proteins or by the formation of other toxic substrates harmful to primary cells [10, 71]. The final substances can be deleterious for primary etiology but can also increase the production of pro-inflammatory cytokines, prostaglandins or other pro-inflammatory mediators [30, 74]. An increase of NO production is also typical for eosinophilic inflammation in bronchial asthma. Significant proof of NO participation in inflammatory airway diseases is an increased level of NO and oxidation products in exhaled breath [42, 49].

3. Inhibitors of NO-Synthases

Currently we cannot say which isoform is most important for the pathogenetic process of bronchial hyperreactivity. The results of experimental work and the clinical trials remain quite controversial. In spite of this fact, development of the specific inhibitors of NO-synthases is a very interesting field of research. The level of nitric oxide can be reduced by inhibition of membrane transport of L-arginine into the cell or by directly blocking enzymes synthesizing NO. The effect of inhibition of NO was observed in models of acute arthritis, inflammatory nephritis, chronic ileitis, diabetes, etc. There is available data about bronchial asthma, too. The topical application of an inhibitor of NO-synthase in the experiment slowed the progression of these diseases and therefore, the development of similar substances is currently of high interest. In addition, these substances are important for recent understanding and detailed description of physiological and pathological processes with participation of NO. Although we observe progress in the molecular modeling and activity of NO-synthase inhibitors in experimental studies, these substances are still not used in clinical practice and their application into clinical practice is currently complicated. Animal models do not correlate completely with the primate experiments or diseases in humans. They are also expensive and ethically questionable. A number of tested substances also exhibit a certain degree of toxicity, lack of selectivity or loss of activity by the changes of conditions *in vitro* to *in vivo* or vice versa. Most of these substances also do not have pharmacokinetic properties suitable for oral use. One of the most important factors of NO-inhibitors is their selectivity. Based on the selectivity we can classify the NO-synthase inhibitors as:

- non-selective,
- partially selective,
- selective,
- modulators of NOS (e.g. cofactors).

Non-selective NO-synthase inhibitors are classified as endogenous or synthetic analogs of L-arginine, for example NG-monomethyl-L-arginine (L-NMMA), NG-nitro-L-arginine methyl ester (L-NAME), NG-nitro-L-arginine (L-NA), N-iminoethyl-L-ornithine (L-NIO), L-NIL [N^6-(1-iminoethyl)-L-lysine hydrochloride and NG -amino-L-arginine (L-NAA). They block activity of both the constitutive and inductive isoforms of NO synthases. One of the mechanisms of the process of non-selective NO-synthase inhibitors is the blockade of the L-arginine delivery system, which is responsible for substrate transport into the cell [56]. The blockade may be reversible or irreversible. Despite of the lack of selectivity and some non-specific effects, analogue-based inhibitors of L-arginine are fully used in the experiments to clarify the pathophysiological significance of NO and to clarify the protective effects of reducing NO levels in various inflammatory conditions. Some of these analogs have shown selectivity for one of the isoforms of NO synthase in *in vitro* conditions and a different efficacy may be reflected in *in vivo* conditions [26, 54]. Administration of NO-synthase inhibitors reduced the degree of inflammation and tissue damage in animal models of acute inflammation [36] and reduced immune complex-induced vascular injury in rat lungs [57]. Most used non-selective NOS-inhibitor is L-NAME, which has predominantly cNOS selectivity (Table 2). Many of the arginine-based inhibitors of NOS provide potent inhibition of NOS; have low toxicity, and predictable pharmacokinetics. The major problem is low selectivity among NOS isoforms [80].

Therapeutic potential is associated with specific selective inhibitors. The most important for research activity is *inductive NO-synthase* because this isoform is active in many of pathological processes including airway inflammation, and may contribute to chronic inflammatory diseases such as bronchial asthma. Induction of NO synthase in *in vivo* conditions is a complex process resulting from the activation of a wide range of cells. The induction occurs simultaneously in different parts of the body, and therefore complete inhibition is not possible. However, the development of selective inhibitors of iNOS has rapid progress and a wide spectrum of partially selective or selective iNOS inhibitors is used in experimental and clinical studies. The literature describes studies in the field of pain, hypotension, inflammation, stroke, asthma, arthritis, neuropathy, etc. Generally, the inhibitors of inducible isoform could be effective in the treatment of these diseases. Currently we know of many structurally different iNOS-selective inhibitors such as 1400W, GW273629, AR-C102222, BYK191023, the recently presented BYK402750, ONO1714, SC-51, BBS-1, aminoguanidine, and some derivates of L-arginine [33]. All of these inhibitors have high iNOS selectivity and efficacy in *in vivo* conditions (Table 2). GW274150 has an excellent selectivity to iNOS. This compound shows favorable pharmacokinetics, negligible toxicity and can be administered orally. Among all known inhibitors of NO synthases, GW274150 currently has the highest chance to be approved for medical use [80]. In patients with asthma, GW274150 in a dose of 90 mg once daily for 14 days was administered for at least 6 months before the trial was evaluated. The treatment with this selective inhibitor reduced the exhaled NO level but had no effects on airway hyperreactivity or on airway inflammatory cell count after an allergen challenge [75].

Table 2. Enzymatic potency of human NOS-isoforms and efficacy in in vivo conditions of standards NOS inhibitors (LPS induces increase in plasma NO_x levels in rat) (n.d. – not defined) [33]

Inhibitor	IC50(uM) iNOS	IC50(uM) nNOS	IC50(uM) eNOS	EC50 (uM/kg/hod) *in vivo*
L-NMMA	1.3	1.3	0.66	11.1
L-NAME	44	3.4	2.8	n.d.
L-NIL	0.5	3.4	12	1
1400 W	0.13	3.4	66	2.3
GW274150	0.58	11	41	1.6
AR-C102222	0.25	0.48	>100	0.75
BYK191023	0.09	17	160	16.3
BYK402750	0.09	5.2	74	7

Historically, one of the specific iNOS inhibitors is glucocorticosteroids (GCS), as they inhibit iNOS directly via down regulation of its expression [65]. GCS inhibit also cytokine release and have many other anti-inflammatory effects. The difference between GCS and selective NOS inhibitors is in the duration of the inhibition. GCS prevent the expression and induction of the enzyme whereas iNOS inhibitors inhibit the action of the enzyme at any time after its induction [56]. In fact, none of the tested inhibitors reached the desired effect, and therefore they have not yet been approved for clinical use.

One of the most representative compounds from the group of selective inhibitors of iNOS is *aminoguanidine*. Currently, there are numerous studies about the positive effects of aminoguanidine in different types of inflammation and shock. The disadvantage of its use is the relatively high doses required to achieve its effects. The desired effect of aminoguanidine in *in vivo* conditions was achieved after administration of 1545 mg of inhibitors per kg of body weight. The positive/beneficial effects of aminoguanidine were also observed in the experiments with diabetes mellitus, shock, autoimmune encephalomyelitis or pulmonary edema (prevention of plasma exudation). These effects were primarily associated with the inhibition of iNOS activity, as well as other iron-containing enzymes (e.g. catalase). The mechanism also involves inhibition of the metabolism of histamine and inhibition of polyamine catabolism. Aminoguanidine hydrolysis leads to the formation of toxic products - semicarbazide and hydrazine.

Activity of constitutive NO-synthases isoforms, like most of the Ca^{2+} calmodulin dependent enzyme can be inhibited, for example, through calmodulin antagonists (calmidazolium, chlorpromazine). Some of substances such as S-methyl-L-thiocitrulline and S-ethyl-L-thiocitrulline [24], exhibit a degree of selectivity in *in vitro* conditions for nNOS. cNOS inhibitors can be grouped based on their selectivity to cNOS, nNOS and eNOS inhibitors. Selective inhibitors of eNOS do not currently exist. Nitric oxide produced by endothelial NO synthase is a key signal molecule of vascular homeostasis, including the regulation of vascular tone and blood pressure. In addition it has anti-atherogenic function, anti-inflammatory, antithrombotic and antiproliferative effects. Inhibition of NO synthesis in the endothelium could induce the endothelial dysfunction, which is a pre-condition for numerous cardiovascular diseases. Therefore, the effort to develop selective inhibitors of iNOS and nNOS is of higher significance. Selective nNOS inhibitors have been tested primarily in relation to neurodegenerative diseases, such as Parkinson's, Alzheimer's and Huntington's disease. Because nNOS is important for the formation of NO in neurons, it is considered to participate in the process of neuroprotection. Experimental inhibitors of nNOS include 7-NI, L-NNA, TRIM, ARL17477 but their selectivity is problematic.

7-NI (7-nitro-indazole) was described as another specific nNOS inhibitor. It inhibits cerebellar nNOS *in vitro,* exhibits antinociceptive activity *in vivo* in mice, affecting neuronal death induced by toxicity and motoric and cognitive functions. The mechanism that triggers 7-NI processes is complex; it binds to the enzyme prosthetic groups, and subsequently affects the binding sites for L-arginine.

In conclusion, we can say that achieving selective inhibition of specific NO synthase is a realistic target and may have future therapeutic and commercial value, but at this time still requires more experimental and clinical data.

4. Inhibitors of NO-synthases and Therapy of Respiratory Diseases with Bronchial Hyperreactivity

Nitric oxide is a basic physiological mediator and regulation of NO release is associated with various inflammatory diseases, including respiratory diseases. Bronchial hyperreactivity (BHR) is defined as an abnormal response of the airways to a variety of stimuli (e.g. allergens, chemical irritants, cold air, hypoxia, viral infection, pharmacological stimuli etc.). The other definitions describe an excessive bronchial narrowing and an exaggerated bronchoconstriction response of the airways to various inhaled stimuli [68]. It is an important symptom present in asthma, upper respiratory tract infections, but also in gastro esophageal reflux. Its development is influenced by several risk factors including atrophy, gender, age, smoking, and the change in status of a pulmonary function [31]. Various cell types including epithelial, inflammatory, neuronal and vascular smooth muscle cells and airway cells, release mediators that participate in the pathogenesis of hyperreactivity. The most important are histamine, leukotrienes, prostaglandins, adenosine, acetylcholine, substance P, neurokinin A and NO [38]. In the case of bronchial hyperreactivity induced by these mediators, nitric oxide has a protective role. NO can affect experimentally induced contraction of bronchial smooth muscle by a negative feedback system and act as a single bronchodilator mediator. Increase of airways reactivity is usually reversible after administration of anticholinergic agents [50]. The rise of cholinergic activity can be a basic mechanism causing the hyperreactivity, and can significantly illustrate the dysfunction of NANC, too [28, 9, 50]. NO as a major mediator of the iNANC system has the most important role in the process of onset and development of bronchial hyperreactivity. It is significantly involved in the regulation of bronchomotoric tone, and therefore changes in the level, activity, and mechanism of action of NO may cause changes in the airway reactivity [5].

There is a presumption that inhibition of nitric oxide synthesis increases airway reactivity in lab animals and in humans [41; 73]. On the other hand, substitution of L-arginine as a precursor of NO synthesis and an increasing level of NO, may have a positive effect on the response induced by various bronchoconstriction stimuli or can completely block the hyperreactivity [23]. At this point, we can return to the theory of "optimal level" and focus on the participation of isoforms in the development of bronchial hyperreactivity. The most important isoform in this aspect is the inductive isoform, which exhibits significant activity in the development of BHR induced for example by allergens. Increased iNOS expression and activity correlates with increased levels of NO in exhaled air. Increased expression of iNOS in both inflammatory cells and airway epithelium, results in the formation of large amounts of NO. These quantities reduced the expression and activity of constitutive NOS and desensitized GC-S, indicating that iNOS is one of important factors in the development of bronchial hyperreactivity [52, 53].

We have carried out several experiments using non-selective and selective inhibitors of NO synthase in a model of allergen-induced hyperreactivity. Repeated allergen sensitization (ovalbumin) at specific time intervals in our experiments caused an increase of smooth muscle reactivity to histamine and acetylcholine *in vivo* and *in vitro*. Data from the literature indicate a different use of the allergen as a factor of inducing airway hyperreactivity. The result of sensitization depends on the type of allergen, doses and methods of allergen application, and on the different types of sensitizing modes. Ovalbumin, the main chicken egg protein, was used to induce an allergic reaction in sensitized animals. The dose of ovalbumin was optimized according to the work of Koarai et al. [44] and Jain et al. [37] to 100μg/ml and it was applied at certain times during the 14-day sensitization process. The animals were given the allergen subcutaneously and intraperitoneally on the first day, intraperitoneally on the third day and by inhalation at the fourteenth day. The changes of reactivity were observed in *in vivo* (30 minutes and 4 hours after allergen application) and *in vitro* conditions. Healthy adult guinea pigs (TRIK) of both genders were used for the experiment we conducted. Changes in the respiratory system in guinea pigs caused by sensitization of allergens are similar to the changes in the human airway. The airway reactivity was recorded in *in vitro* conditions in response to cumulative doses ($10^{-8} - 10^{-3}$ mol.l^{-1}) of histamine and acetylcholine (Sigma Aldrich®). The animals were euthanized 24 hours after the last allergen exposure. The trachea and lung were removed and small thin strips from these organs were prepared and placed into organ bath with Krebs-Henseleit solution. The solution was continuously aerated with mixture of 95% O_2 and 5% CO_2 at pH 7.4 ± 0.1 and temperature $37.0 \pm 0.5°C$. The tissue strips were exposed at the first to the tension of 4.0 g (30 minutes - loading phase). Thereafter, the tension was reduced to a baseline of 2.0 g (30 minutes - adaptation phase). Krebs-Henseleit solution was changed every 10 minutes. The changes of trachea and lung tissue strips reactivity to cumulative doses of both bronchoconstrictors after one hour of tissue incubation were recorded.

We must admit that any animal model of airway hyperreactivity or asthma does not simulate the full symptoms of human disease and many results in experimental work are controversial. Eynot et al. [16] demonstrated in ovalbumin sensitized rats induced iNOS and increased level of exhaled NO shortly after ovalbumin challenge. After administration of selective iNOS inhibitor SC-51 both BHR and number of neutrophils in lungs were reduced. After repeated sensitization, SC-51 reduced also number of eosinophils and CD4-positive T-cells [17]. Studies with NOS knockout animals are also interesting. Methacholine-mediated bronchial hyperreactivity was reduced only in nNOS- and in nNOS/eNOS double deficient mice, but was not significantly different in iNOS-knockout animals [11]. Decreased BHR was demonstrated also after L-NAME and aminoguanidine treatment in identic knockout animals [46]. One of the preferred examinations of respiratory inflammation is a detection of nitric oxide in exhaled air and nasal nitric oxide. It has been confirmed that levels of exhaled NO correlate with levels of eosinophilic inflammation in the lungs, and therefore this non-invasive measurement is very popular. It is recommended for repeated measurements of treatment efficacy in subjects with corticosteroid treatment. Some data indicate advantages and possibilities in self-monitoring of diseases such as bronchial asthma. However, measurement of exhaled condensate is used in the clinical practice for detailed analysis, e.g. prostaglandins, free radicals, etc. It has already been mentioned that iNOS is active in the inflammatory processes. Despite the fact that its inhibitors have beneficial effects in animal models, several clinical studies describe very low efficacy. For example, a Phase II study in mildly asthmatic humans using highly selective iNOS inhibitor GW274150 showed only low efficacy on early and late asthmatic response despite potent inhibition of exhaled NO [75].

In our recent study, aminoguanidine hydrochloride (hydrazinecarboximidamide monohydrochloride, CH6N4.HCl, substance Sigma Aldrich®) was used as a selective inhibitor of inducible NO synthase in a constant dose of 50mg/1ml solvent/ kg of body weight in guinea pigs. The inhibitor was administered to healthy animals and those with allergic hyperreactivity induced by ovalbumin in two therapeutic regimens – acute and chronic. The acute administration in healthy animals was performed through three days of intraperitoneal administration. In sensitized animals, the inhibitor was administered 30 minutes before the last sensitization (inhalation). We have found that acute administration of selective iNOS inhibitor aminoguanidine significantly increased reactivity of tracheal smooth muscle to histamine in *in vitro* conditions. A similar effect was observed in ovalbumin-sensitized animals. The chronic therapeutic regimen was performed in healthy animals through 14 days of intraperitoneal administration of the inhibitor. The same intervals, doses and route of administration were used in sensitized animals. Long-term administration provided opposite, however non-significant, results in healthy animals. Contrary to this, the results obtained in sensitized animals were similar to that obtained after acute administration of the inhibitor.

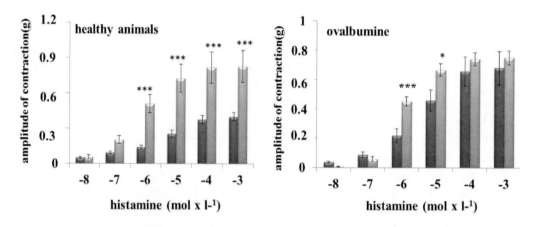

Figure 1. The changes of tracheal smooth muscle reactivity to histamine after acute administration of specific iNOS inhibitor aminoguanidine (grey columns) in healthy animals (left panel) and ovalbumin sensitized animals (right panel) in comparison to the control groups (healthy animals or OVA sensitized animals – black columns). * p<0.05, *** p<0.001.

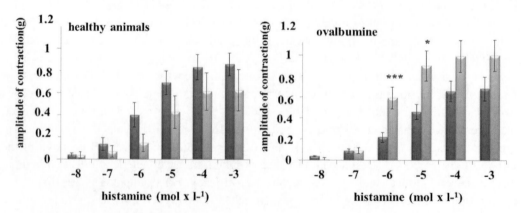

Figure 2. The changes of tracheal smooth muscle reactivity to histamine after chronic administration of specific iNOS inhibitor aminoguanidine (grey columns) in healthy animals (left panel) and ovalbumin sensitized animals (right panel) in comparison to the control groups (healthy animals or OVA sensitized animals – black columns). * p<0.05, *** p<0.001.

These results may support a theory of inducible NO synthase participation in the regulation of bronchomotoric tone and airway reactivity and during physiological conditions. It is known that allergic inflammation is characterized by increased activity of iNOS, but its role in the process of bronchial hyperreactivity remains unclear. The main factors involved in the increase of iNOS activity are primarily cytokines (IFN-γ, IL-1β, TNF-α), as well as an increase of the nuclear transcription factor NF-κB [1]. On the other side, the activity of iNOS, for example, is reduced by epidermal growth factor (EGF) or cytokines produced by Th2 lymphocytes (IL-4, 8, 10) etc. These data indicate that the inductive NO-synthase is under the control of stimulatory and inhibitory cytokines controlling and regulating its activity during allergic inflammation. Based on published data we suppose that the high production of nitric oxide by iNOS has predominantly prohyperreactive effects, which depend on damage of the epithelia in airways, deregulation and desensitization of guanylyl cyclase and on significant transformation to free radicals. iNOS expression was increased for several hours after exposure to allergens, which subsequently elevated levels of NO in exhaled air [58; 66]. The expression of this enzyme was increased mainly in the epithelium and inflammatory cells. It is known that both IFN-γ and the induction of an inducible isoform inhibit the expression of constitutive NO synthase [81]. After the application of the selective iNOS inhibitor SC-51, the allergen-induced hyperreactivity was reduced, but allergic (mainly eosinophilic) inflammation of the respiratory tract was not affected [16]. The selective iNOS inhibitor (aminoguanidine) used under our conditions demonstrated the opposite effect. It increased airway hyperreactivity induced by allergen. It is possible that this effect could be caused by an insufficient dose of aminoguanidine or other factors could be involved in the regulation of the bronchomotor tone in our model of hyperreactivity. Literature describing the use of aminoguanidine under the same conditions showed that the small doses of the inhibitor administered before ovalbumin potentiated acute bronchial hyperreactivity, while high doses of aminoguanidine administered prophylactically reduce the allergen-induced hyperreactivity. Is iNOS responsible for production of prohyperreactive nitric oxide or not? Selective inhibitors of iNOS have anti-inflammatory and tissue protective effects in the majority of animal experiments. However, caution must be used in cases of translation of the results to clinical conditions, as the enzymatic regulation in animals and humans is probably different. Many studies show conflicting evidence. Instead of some positive results for the roles of iNOS in pathogenesis of BHR, our results showed that the effect of inhibitors could also be negative.

Another question is how much contributes to the constitutive isoform on the total NO production. Many non-selective inhibitors have been used in experimental and clinical studies but the most frequently used is NG-nitro-L-arginine methyl ester (L-NAME). Inhalation of L-NAME in humans with mild allergy induced asthma had no significant effects on early and late asthmatic response or on lung function measured as FEV1 [76]. The other non-selective inhibitor L-NMMA was detrimental because of increased pulmonary pressure due to the eNOS inhibition and excessive pulmonary vessel vasoconstriction [7]. In our study with guinea pigs, we have used a non-selective NO-synthase inhibitor L-NAME (substance Sigma Aldrich®) at a dose of 40mg/1ml solvent/kg of the body weight. L-NAME is chemically N-omega-Nitro-L-arginine methyl ester hydrochloride ($C_7H_{16}CIN_5O_4$). In addition to NOS inhibition, it inhibits cGMP production in endothelial cells. Similarly, to aminoguanidine, the inhibitor was administered to healthy animals and animals with allergic hyperreactivity induced by ovalbumin in two therapeutic regimens – acute and chronic. The therapeutic regimens were designed as in the aminoguanidine studies. We found that acute administration of a non-selective NOS inhibitor L-NAME significantly increased the reactivity of tracheal smooth muscle to histamine in *in vitro* conditions. These results confirmed that a deficit in endogenous NO produced by cNOS may contribute to airway hyperreactivity.

Similar effects were observed in ovalbumin-sensitized animals. The chronic administration of L-NAME evoked a significant increase of tracheal smooth muscle reactivity to histamine in healthy and sensitized animals.

Comparable results were observed in other experimental work, where it was possible to suppress the increase of reactivity by the application of NO donors, or by direct inhalation of NO [43]. Mehta et al. [51] noticed that L-NAME increased bronchial reactivity to histamine in the control group of healthy guinea pigs, but not in the group of animals sensitized to the allergen.

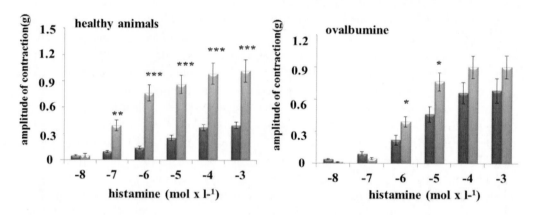

Figure 3. The changes of tracheal smooth muscle reactivity to histamine after acute administration of non-selective NOS inhibitor L-NAME (grey columns) in healthy animals (left panel) and ovalbumin sensitized animals (right panel) in comparison to the control groups (healthy animals or OVA sensitized animals – black columns). * $p<0.05$, ** $p<0.01$, *** $p<0.001$.

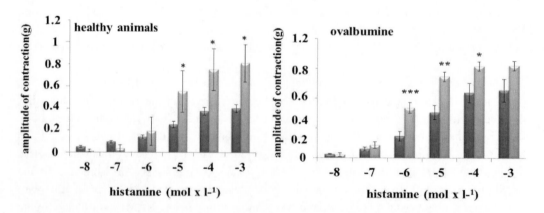

Figure 4. The changes of tracheal smooth muscle reactivity to histamine after chronic administration of non-selective NOS inhibitor L-NAME (grey columns) in healthy animals (left panel) and ovalbumin sensitized animals (right panel) in comparison to with the control groups (healthy animals or OVA sensitized animals – black columns). * $p<0.05$, ** $p<0.01$, *** $p<0.001$.

Nogami et al. [61] observed that the application of L-NAME potentiated the allergen-induced hyperreactivity, suggesting protective effects of NO produced mostly by cNOS.

The question of which cNOS participates in the regulation of airway tone is still open. The method of administration is important for results. The inhalation of L-NAME before sensitization induced an increase of reactivity to histamine. In hyperreactive animals, the effect of the inhibitor was more significant. In our experiments we administered inhibitors in different ways – by inhalation, directly to the tissue strips (incubation in the organ baths) and intraperitoneally. We have observed small differences, which may be important for interpretation and for translation of results. Based on our results we can say that the effects of NO-synthase inhibitions depend on both the mode of administration and the duration of application of the inhibitor.

Based on the available data we can suggest which of the isoforms is important in the regulation process of airway bronchomotor tone. Neuronal NOS is located mainly in the iNANC airways system and together with the others, NANC mediator and cholinergic and adrenergic system regulates bronchodilation. Nitric oxide released by eNOS localized in the epithelium at different levels of the respiratory system also participates in the control of smooth muscle tone [18]. Lee et al. [47] found that the distribution of the eNOS genotype was significantly higher in patients with asthma compared to the control group. This supports the theory of eNOS participation in BHR pathogenesis. Another theory assumes that the reduction of nNOS activity and subsequent NO deficiency has a prohyperreactive effect. NO released by this isoform in physiological conditions acts as a functional antagonist of excitatory cholinergic neurotransmission and its inhibition, evoked bronchoconstriction [12, 18]. The other theory suggests the normal function of the two cNOS (eNOS, nNOS) in bronchial hyperreactivity, with increased expression and activity of iNOS [60; 72]

Despite the fact that the pathogenesis of many chronic inflammatory diseases of the airways is relatively well understood, the question of the participation of the various isoforms of NO synthase in the pathogenesis of some symptoms remains open. More reliable responses could be obtained from experiments with strict selective inhibitors of constitutive isoforms or inductive NO-synthase. Another important aspect is the participation of other isoforms of NOS in inflammatory process, e.g. mitochondrial. Based on our results we assume that all three isoforms cooperate and are involved in the pathogenesis of bronchial hyperreactivity. It is possible that there are some inter-specie differences, since the studies have only been performed in various animals (guinea pig, rat). Another possible explanation is the activation of different cell types depending on the means of sensitization, duration of the repeated allergen administration, negative feedback via the overproduction of NO and subsequent reduction of NOS activity and other mechanisms.

Conclusion

The development of new drugs for the treatment of respiratory diseases is of great interest. These diseases are accompanied by a significant deterioration of the patient's quality of life. A drug discovery, which would improve symptomatology and can be applied not only in acute cases, but also as a preventive and therapeutic tool, may be of great benefit for even patients without chronic respiratory airways diseases. In our research with L-NAME we have demonstrated very positive and promising effects of this non-specific inhibitor in influencing BHR. Decreased levels of exhaled nitric oxide in experimental animals, decreased numbers of inflammatory cells in bronchoalveolare lavage, and decreased values of the selected markers of oxidative stress in the peripheral blood (e.g. 3-nitrotyrosine, TBARS) add to these assumptions. A comprehensive approach in further phases of experiments must be applied to selective inhibitors as well. Our results indicate that the use of an inhibitor of NO-synthase in the treatment of respiratory diseases associated with bronchial hyperreactivity is possible. It is very important to continue the discussion about the theory of "optimal level" of NO and about the involvement and participation of the various isoforms of NO synthase in the physiology and pathology of the processes occurring in the airways.

Acknowledgments

This work was supported by the project "The increasing of opportunities for career growth in research and development in the medical sciences," co-financed from EU sources.

References

[1]   Adcock, I.M.; Brown, C.R.; Kwon, O.; Barnes, P.J. 1994. Oxidative stress NF kappa B DNA binding and inducible NOS mRNA in human epithelial cells. *Biochem Biophys Res Commun. 199*, 1518-1524.

[2]   Adler, K.B.; Fischer B.M.; Li H.; Choe N.H.; Wright, D.T. 1995. Hypersecretion of mucin is response to inflammatory mediators by guinea pig tracheal epithelial cells in vitro is blocked by inhibition of nitric oxide synthase. *Am J Respir Cell Mol Biol. 13*, 526-530.

[3]   Aizawa, H. 1999. Role of nitric oxide in airway inflammation and hyperresponsiveness in bronchial asthma. *Allergy Inter. 48*, 25-30.

[4]   Alderton, W.K.; Cooper, CH.E.; Knowles, R.G. 2001. Nitric oxide synthases: structure, function and inhibition. *Biochem J. 357*, 593-615.

[5]   Antosova, M.; Strapkova, A.; Plevkova, J. 2011. Bronchial hyperreactivity: pathogenesis and treatment options. *Op J of Mol Integ Physiol. 1*, 43-51.

[6]   Barnes, P.J. 1999. NO or no NO in asthma? *Thorax. 51*, 218-220.

[7]   Bekes, C.E.; Dellinger, R.P.; Brooks, D.; Edmondson, R.; Olivia, C.T.; Parrillo, J.E. 2004. Critical care medicine as a distinct product line with substantial financial profitability: the role of business planning. *Crit. Care Med. 32*, 1207–1214.

[8]   Blackford, J.A.; Antonini, J.M.J.; Castranova, V.; Dey, R.D.; 1994. Intratracheal instillation of silica up-regulates inducible nitric oxide synthase gene expression and increases nitric oxide production in alveolar macrophages and neutrophils. *Am J Respir Crit Care Med. 11*, 426-431.

[9]   Canning, B.J.; Fischer, A. 2001. Neural regulation of airway smooth muscle tone. *Respir Physiol. 125*, 113-127.

[10] Cucchiaro, G.; Tatum, A.H.; Brown, M.C.; Camporesi, E.M.; Daucher, J.W.; Hakim, T.S. 1999. Inducible nitric oxide synthase in the lung and exhaled nitric oxide after hyperoxia. *Am J Physiol Lung Cell Mol Physiol. 277(3)*, L636-L644.

[11] de Sanctis, G.T.; MacLean, J.A.; Hamada, K.; Mehta, S.; Scott, J.A.; Jiao, A.; Yandava, C.N.; Kobzik, L.; Wolyniec, W.W;, Fabian, A.J.; Venugopal, C.S.; Grasemann, H.; Huang, P.L.; Drazen, J.M. 1999. Contribution of nitric oxide synthases 1, 2, and 3 to airway hyperresponsiveness and inflammation in a murine model of asthma. *J Exp Med. 189*, 1621 -1630.

[12] de Sanctis, G.T.; Metha, S.; Kobzik, L.; Yandava, C.; Jiao, A.; Huang, P.L.; Drazen, J.M. 1997. Contribution of type I NOS to expired gas NO and bronchial responsiveness in mice. *Am J Physiol Lung Cell Mol Physiol. 273*, L883-L888.

[13] di Maria, G.U.; Spicuzza, L.; Mistretta, A.; Mazzarella, G. 2000. Role of endogenous nitric oxide in asthma. *Allergy. 55*, 31-35.

[14] Duszyk, M. 2001. Regulation of anion secretion by nitric oxide in human airway epithelial cells. *Am J Physiol. 281*, L450-L457.

[15] Dweik, R.A. 2001. The promise and reality of nitric oxide in the diagnosis and treatment of lung disease. *Cleveland Clin J Med. 68(6)*, 486-490.

[16] Eynott, P.R.; Groneberg, D.A.; Caramori, G.; Adcock, I.M.; Donnelly, L.E.; Kharitonov, S.A.; Barnes, P.J.; Chung, K.F. 2002. Role of nitric oxide in allergic inflammation and bronchial hyperresponsiveness. *Eur. J. Pharmacol. 452*, 123–133.

[17] Eynott, P.R.; Paavolainen, N.; Groneberg, D.A.; Noble, A.; Salmon, M.; Nath, P.; Leung, S.Y.; Chung, K.F. 2003. Role of nitric oxide in chronic allergen-induced airway cell proliferation and inflammation. *J. Pharmacol Exp Ther. 304*, 22–29.

[18] Feletou, M.; Lonchampt, M.; Coge, F.; Galizzi, J.P.; Bassoullet, C.; Merial, C.; Robineau, P.; Boutin, J.A.; Huang, P.L.; Vanhoutte, P.M.; Canet, E. 2001. Regulation of murine airway responsiveness by endothelial nitric oxide syntase. *Am J Physiol Lung Cell Mol Physiol. 281*, 258-267.

[19] Figini, M.; Ricciardolo, F.L.M.; Javdan, P.; Nijkamp, F.P.; Emanueli, C.; Pradelles, P.; Folkerts, G.; Geppetti, P. 1996. Evidence that epithelium-derived relaxing factor released by bradykinin in guinea-pig trachea is nitric oxide. *Am J Respir Crit Care Med. 153*, 918–23.

[20] Fischer, B.M.; Rochelle, L.G.; Voynow, J.A.; Akley, N.J.; Adler, K.B. 1999. Tumor necrosis factor − α stimulates mucin secretion and cyclic GMP production by guinea pig tracheal epithelial cells in vitro. *Am J Respir Cell Mol Biol. 20*, 413-422.

[21] Fischer, A.; Hoffman, B. 1996. Nitric oxide synthase in neurons and nerve fibers of lower airways and in vagal sensory ganglia of man. Correlation with neuropeptides. *Am J Respir Crit Care Med. 154(1)*, 209-216.

[22] Folkerts, G.; Nijkamp, F.P. 1998. Airway epithelium: more than just a barrier! *TIPS. 19*, 334-341.

[23] Folkerts, G.; van der Linde, H.J.; Nijkamp, F.P. 1995. Virus-induced airway hyperresponsiveness in guinea pigs is related to a deficiency in nitric oxide. *J Clin Invest. 95*, 26-30.

[24] Furfine, E.S.; Harman, M.F.; Paith, J.E.; Knowles, K.C.; Salter, M.; Kiff, R.J.; Duffy, C.; Hazeiwood, K.; Oplinger, J.A.; Garvey, E.P. 1994. Potent and selective inhibition of human nitric oxide synthases. *Biol Chem. 269*, 26677-26683.

[25] Gabazza, E.C.; Taguchi, O.; Tamaki, S.; Murashima, S.; Kobayashi, H.; Yasui, H.; Kobayiashi, T.; Hataji, O.; Adachi, Y. 2000. Role of nitric oxide in airway remodelling. *Clin Sci. 98,* 291-294.

[26] Garvey, E.P.; Oplinger, J.A.; Tanouty, C.J.; Sherman, P.A.; Fowler, M.; Marshall, S.; Harmon, M.F.; Paith, J.E.; Furfine, E. S. 1994. Potent and selective inhibition of human nitric oxide synthases. *Biol Chem. 269,* 26669-26676.

[27] Gilchrist, M.; Savoie, M.; Nohara, O.; Wills, F.L.; Wallace, J.L.; Befus, A.D. 2002. Nitric oxide synthase and nitric oxide production in in vivo-derived mast-cell. *J Leukoc Biol. 71,* 618-624.

[28] Grasseman, H.; Yandava, C.N.; Storm van's Gravesande, K.; Deykin, A.; Pilari, A.; Ma, J.; Sonna, L.A.; Lilly, C.; Stampfer, M.J.; Israel, E.; Silverman, E.K.; Drazen, J.M. 2000. A neuronal NO synthase (NOS1) gene polymorphism in associated with asthma. *Biochem Biophys Res Commun. 272(2),* 391-394.

[29] Griffith, M.J.; Liu, S.; Curzen, N.P.; Messent, M.; Evans, T.W. 1995. In vivo treatment with endotoxin induces nitric oxide synthase in rat main pulmonary artery. *Am J Physiol Lung Cell Mol Physiol. 268,* L509-L518.

[30] Grisham, M.B.; Jourd'Heuil, D.; Wink, D.A. 1999. Nitric oxide. I. Physiological chemistry of nitric oxide and its metabolites: implications in inflammation. *Am J Physiol. 276,* G315-G321.

[31] Grootendorst, D.C.; Rabe, K.F. 2004. Mechanisms of bronchial hyperreactivity in asthma and chronic obstructive pulmonary disease. *Proc Am Thorac Soc. 1,* 77-87.

[32] Hamad, A.S.M.; Clayton, A.; Islam, B.; Knox, A.J. 2003. Guanylyl cyclases, nitric oxide, natriuretic peptides, and airway smooth muscle function. *Am J Physiol Lung Cell Mol Physiol. 285,* L973-L983.

[33] Hesslinger, Ch.; Strub, A.; Boer, R.; Wolf-Rudiger, U.; Lehner, M.D.; Braun, C. 2009. Inhibition of inducible nitric oxide synthase in respiratory diseases. *Biocheml Soc Trans.37(4),* 886-91.

[34] Himashree, G.; Dass, D.; Banerjee, P.K.; Selvamurthy, W. 2003. Nitric oxide and the respiratory system. *Curr Sci. 85(5),* 607-614.

[35] Charles, A. 1999. Nitric oxide pumps up calcium signalling. *Nature Cell Biol. 1(8),* E193-E195.

[36] Ialenti, A.; Ianaro, A.; Moncada, S.; Di Rosa, M. 1992. Modulation of acute inflammation by endogenous nitric oxide. *Eur Pharmacol. 21 (1),* 177-182.

[37] Jain, D.; Chhabra, S.K.; Raj, H.G. 2004. Effect of sensitization on membrane ion fluxes and intracellular calcium in guinea pigs. *Ind J Med Res. 120,* 534-541.

[38] Joos, G.F. 2003. Bronchial hyperresponsiveness: too complex to be useful? *Curr Opin Pharmacol. 3(3),* 233-238.

[39] Kageyama, N.; Miura, M.; Ichinose, M.; Tomaki, M.; Ishikawa, J.; Ohuchi, Y.; Endoh, N.; Shirato, K. 1997. Role of endogenous nitric oxide in airway microvascular leakage induced by inflammatory mediators. *Eur Respir J. 10,* 13-19.

[40] Kawamoto, H.; Takumida, M.; Takeno, S.; Wantabe, H.; Fukushima, N.; Yajin, K. 1998. Localization of nitric oxide synthase in human nasal mucosa with nasal allergy. *Acta Otolaryngol. 539,* 65-70.

[41] Kesler, B.S.; Mazzone, S.B.; Canning, B.J. 2002. Nitric oxide-dependent modulation of smooth muscle tone by airway parasympatethic nerves. *Am J Respir Crit Care Med. 165,* 481-488.

[42] Kharitonov, S.A. 2005. Influence of different therapeutic strategies on exhaled NO and lung inflammation in asthma and COPD. *Vasc Pharmacol. 43,* 371-378.

[43] Khassawneh, M.Y.; Dreshaj, I.A.; Liu S.; Chang, C.H.H.; Haxhiu, M.A.; Martin, R.J. 2002. Endogenous nitric oxide modulates responses of tissue and airway resistance to vagal stimulation in piglets. *J Appl Physiol. 93,* 450-456.

[44] Koarai, A.; Ichinose, M.; Sugiura, H.; Tomaki, M.; Watanabe, M.; Yamagata, S.; Komaki, Y.; Shirato, K.; Hattori, T.; 2002. iNOS depletion completely diminished reactive nitrogen species formation after an allergic response. *Eur Respir J. 20,* 609-616.

[45] Lacza, Snipes J.A.; Yhang, J.; Horvath, E.M.; Figueroa, J.P.; Szabo, C.; Busija, D.W. 2003. Mitochondrial nitric oxide synthase is nor eNOS, nNOS or iNOS. *Free Radic Biol Med. 35,* 1217-1228.

[46] Landgraf, R.G.; Russo, M.; Jancar, S. 2005. Acute inhibition of inducible nitric oxide synthase but not its absence suppresses asthma-like responses. *Eur J Pharmacol. 518,* 212–220.

[47] Lee, Y.C.; Cheon, K.T.; Lee, H.B.; Kim, W.; Rhee, Y.K.; Kim, D.S. 2000. Gene polymorphisms of endothelial nitric oxide synthase and angiotensin-converting enzyme in patients with asthma. *Allergy. 55,* 959–63.

[48] Lundberg, J.O.; Weitzberg, E. 1999. Nasal nitric oxide in man. *Thorax. 54,* 946–952.

[49] Marshall, H.E.; Stamler, J.S. 2000. NO waiting to exhale in asthma. *Am J Respir Crit Care Med. 161,* 685-687.

[50] Mazzone, S.B.; Canning, B.J. 2002. Evidence for differential reflex regulation of cholinergic and noncholinergic parasympathetic nerves innervating the airways. *Am J Respir Crit Care Med. 165,* 1076-1083.

[51] Mehta, S.; Drazen, J.M.; Lilly, C.M. 1997. Endogenous nitric oxide and allergic bronchial hyperresponsiveness in guinea pigs. *Am J Physiol. 273(3),* L656-662.

[52] Meurs, H.; Maarsingh, H.; Zaagsma, J. 2003. Arginase and asthma: novel insights into nitric oxide homeostasis and airway hyperresponsiveness. *TIPS. 24(9),* 450-455.

[53] Meurs, H.; McKay, S.; Maaarshing, H.; Haamer, M.A.M.; Macie, L.; Molendijk, N.; Zaagsma, J. 2002. Increased arginase activity underlies allergen-induced deficiency of cNOS-derived nitric oxide and airway hyperresponsiveness. *Br J Pharmacol. 136,* 391-398.

[54] Misko, P.; Moore, W.M.; Kasten, P.; Nickols, C.A.; Corhett, J.A.; Tilton, K.C.; McDaniel, M.L.; Williamson, J.K.; Currie, M.C. 1993. Selective inhibition of the inducible nitric oxide synthasc by aminoguanidine. *Eur Pharmacol. 233,* 119-125.

[55] Morgan, L. 2000. Nitric oxide: a challenge to chiropractic. *J Can Chiropr Assoc. 44(1),* 40-48.

[56] Moncada, S.; Higgs, E.A. 1995. Molecular mechanisms and therapeutic strategies related to nitric oxide. *FASEB J. 9,* 1319-1330.

[57] Mulligan, M.S.; Warren, J.S.; Smith, C.W.; Anderson, D.C.; Yeh, C.G.; Rudolph, A.R.; Ward, P.A. 1992. Lung injury after deposition of IgA immune complexes: requirements for CD18 and L-arginine. *J Immunol. 148,* 3086-3092.

[58] Mulligan, M.S.; Hevel, J.M.; Marletta, M.A.; Ward, P.A. 1991. Tissue injury caused by deposition of immune complexes is L-arginine dependent. *Proc Nat Acad Sci USA. 88,* 6338-6342.

[59] Nagaki, M.; Shimura, M.N.; Irokawa, T.; Sasaki, T.; Shirato, K. 1995. Nitric oxide regulation of glycoconjugate secretion from feline and human airways in vitro. *Respir Physiol. 102,* 89-95.

[60] Nevin, B.J.; Broadley, K.J. 2002. Nitric oxide in respiratory diseases. *Pharmacol Ther. 95,* 259-293.

[61] Nogami, H.; Umeno, E.; Kano, S.; Hirose, T.; Nishima, S. 1998 Effect of nitric oxide synthase inhibitor on allergen- and hyperventilation-induced bronchokonstriction in guinea-pigs. *Eur Respir J. 12,* 1318-1321.

[62] Ohuchi, Y.; Ichinose, M.; Miura, M.; Kageyama, N.; Tomaki, M.; Endoh, N.; Mashito, Y.; Sugiura, H.; Shirato, K. 1998. Induction of nitric oxide synthase by lipopolysaccharide inhalation enhances substance P-induced microvascular leakage in guinea-pigs. *Eur Respir J. 12,* 831-836.

[63] Palmer, R.M.; Ferrige, A.G.; Moncada, S. 1987. Nitric oxide release accounts for the biological activity of endothelium derived relaxing factor. *Nature. 327(6122),* 524-526.

[64] Pechkovsky, D.V.; Zissel, G.; Goldmann, T.; Einhaus, M.; Taube, C.; Magnussen, H.; Schlaak, M.; Muller-Quernheim, J. 2002. Pattern of NOS2 and NOS3 mRNA expression in human A549 cells and primary cultured AECII. *Am J Physiol Lung Cell Mol Physiol. 282,* L684-L692.

[65] Radomski, M.W.; Palmer, K.M.J.; Moncada, S. 1990. Glucocorticoids inhibit the expression of an inducible, but not the constitutive, nitric oxide synthase in vascular endothelial cells. *Proc Nat Acad Sci USA. 87,*10043-10047.

[66] Renzi, P.M.; Sebastiao, N.; Al Assaad, A.S.; Giaid, A.; Hamid, Q. 1997. Inducible nitric oxide synthase mRNA and immunoreactivity in the lungs of rats eight hours after antigen challenge. *Am J Respir Cell Mol Biol. 17,* 36-40.

[67] Romanska, H.M.; Polak, J.M.; Coleman, R.A.; James, R.S.; Harmer, D.W.; Allen, J.C.; Bishop, A.E. 2002. iNOS gene upregulation is associated with the early proliferative response of human lung fibroblasts to cytokine stimulation. *J Pathol. 197,* 372-379.

[68] Ricciardolo, F.L.M. 2003. Multiple role of nitric oxide in the airways. *Thorax. 58,* 175-182.

[69] Ricciardolo, F.L.M.; Sterk, P.J.; Gaston, B.; Folkerts, G. 2004. Nitric oxide in health and disease of the respiratory system. *Physiol Res. 84,* 731-765.

[70] Sadeghi-Hashjin, G.; Folkerts, G.; Henricks, P.A.J.; van de Loo, P.G.F.; van der Linde, H.J.; Dik, I.E.M.; Nijkamp, F.P. 1996a. Induction of guinea pig airway hyperresponsiveness by inactivation of guanylate cyclase. *Eur J Pharmacol. 302(1-3),* 109-115.

[71] Sadeghi-Hashjin, G.; Folkerts, G.; Henricks, P.A.; Verheyen, A.K.; van der Linde, H.J.; Ark, I.; Coene, A.; Nijkamp, F.P. 1996b. Peroxynitrite induces airway hyperresponsiveness in guinea pigs in vitro and in vivo. *Am J Respir Crit Care Med. 153,* 1697-1701.

[72] Samb, A.; Pretolani, M.; Dinh-Xuan, A-T.; Ouksel, H.; Callebert, J.; Lisdero, C.; Aubier, M.; Boczkovicz, J. 2001. Decreased pulmonary and tracheal smooth muscle expression and activity of type 1 nitric oxide synthase (nNOS) after ovalbumin immunization and multiple aerosol challenge in guinea pigs. *Am J Respir Crit Care Med. 164,* 149-154.

[73] Schuiling, M.; Meurs, H.; Zuidhof, A.B.; Venea, N.; Zaagsma, J. 1998. Dual action of iNOS-derived nitric oxide in allergen-induced airway hyperreactivity in conscious, unrestrained guinea pigs. *Am J Respir Crit Care Med. 158,* 1442-1449.

[74] Singh, S.; Evans, T.W. 1997. Nitric oxide, the biological mediator of the decade: fact or fiction? *Eur Respir J. 10,* 699-707.

[75] Singh, D.; Richards, D.; Knowles, R.G.; Schwartz, S.; Woodcock, A.; Langley, S.; O'Connor, B.J. 2007. Selective inducible nitric oxide synthase inhibition has no effect on allergen challenge in asthma. *Am J Respir Crit Care Med. 176,* 988–993.

[76] Taylor, D.A.; McGrath, J.L.; Orr, L.M.; Barnes, P.J.; O'Connor, B.J. 1998. Effect of endogenous nitric oxide inhibition on airway responsiveness to histamine and adenosine-5'-monophosphate in asthma. *Thorax. 53,* 483-489.

[77] Taylor, D.A.; McGrath, J.L.; O'Connor, B.J.; Barnes, P.J. 1998. Allergen-induced early and late asthmatic responses are not affected by inhibition of endogenous nitric oxide. *Am J Respir Crit Care Med. 158,* 99–106.

[78] Vallance, P. 2001. Nitric oxide. *Biologist. 48,* 153-158.

[79] Venugopalan, C.S.; Krautmann, M.J.; Holmes, E.P.; Maher, T.J. 1998. Involvement of nitric oxide in the mediation of NANC inhibitory neurotransmission of guinea-pig trachea. *J Auton Pharmacol. 18,* 281-286.

[80] Víteček, J.; Lojek, A.; Valacchi, G.; Kubala, L. 2012. Arginine-Based Inhibitors of Nitric Oxide Synthase: Therapeutic Potential and Challenges. *Mediators of Inflammation. Article ID 318087,* 22 pp.

[81] Walter, R.; Schaffner, A.; Schoedon, G. 1994. Differential regulation of constitutive and inducible nitric oxide production by inflammatory stimuli in murine endothelial cells. *Biochem Biophys Res Commun. 202,* 450-455.

[82] Warner, R.L.; Paine, R.; Christensen, P.J.; Marletta, M.A.; Richards, M.K.; Wilcosen, S.E.; Ward, P.A. 1995. Lung sources and cytokine requirements for in vivo expression of inducible nitric oxide synthase. *Am J Resp Cell Mol Biol. 12,* 649-661.

Reviewed by:

Assoc. Prof. Miloš Jeseňák, M.D., Ph.D. et Ph.D., MBA – Department of Pediatrics, Jessenius Faculty of Medicine in Martin and University Hospital Martin, Comenius University in Bratislava, Martin, Slovak Republic

In: Advances in Respiratory Therapy Research
Editor: Miloš Jeseňák

ISBN: 978-1-63463-004-7
© 2015 Nova Science Publishers, Inc.

Chapter 3

Gastroesophageal Reflux Disease and Bronchial Asthma in Children – Current Therapeutic Approach

Zuzana Havlicekova, Miloš Jeseňák, Renata Szepeova
and Peter Banovcin*

Department of Pediatrics, Centre of Experimental and Clinical Respirology,
Comenius University Jessenius Faculty of Medicine, Martin, Slovakia

Abstract

Bronchial asthma and gastroesophageal reflux disease are common conditions, which often coexist together. The association should be considered in the presence typical esophageal symptoms, nocturnal cough and insufficient asthma control. The causality of this relationship has not been clearly explained. Still remains unclear, whether the reflux causes asthma, asthma triggers reflux disease, or both coexist simultaneously in one patient. Patients with gastroesophageal reflux disease, including asthmatics, are usually treated with the combination of dietary management, lifestyle modifications and pharmacological therapy. The main problem with the acid suppression treatment is the change of acidic reflux to nonacidic, but it doesn´t resolve the reflux, that can still produce respiratory symptoms. Clinical studies focused on the effect of treatment of GERD, mainly with proton pump inhibitors, in asthmatic patients gave inconsistent results. Double-blind prospective controlled trials demonstrated that treatment of asymptomatic GERD does not improve asthma control in children. In addition, long term PPIs use has been associated with increased risk of side effects (community-acquired

---

* Corresponding Author address: Zuzana Havlicekova, M.D., Ph.D., Department of Pediatris, Centre of Experimental and Clinical Respirology, Jessenius Faculty of Medicine in Martin, Comenius University in Bratislava, University Hospital, Kollarova 2, 036 59, Martin, Slovak Republic, e-mail: zhavlicekova@gmail.com

pneumonia and other respiratory infections, gastrointestinal infections, higher risk of bone fractures).

Keywords: Bronchial Asthma, Extraeosophageal Reflux, Gastroesophageal Reflux, Protone Pump Inhibitors

1. Introduction

Gastroesophageal reflux (GER) is a physiological phenomenon and term gastroesophageal reflux disease (GERD) is defined as condition which develops when the reflux of stomach contents causes troublesome symptoms and/or complications. It usually presets with the classic manifestations like heartburn, regurgitation and non-cardiac chest/epigastric pain, but also with extraesophageal manifestations. Bronchial asthma and GERD are common conditions, which often coexist together [19]. The association should be considered in a presence typical esophageal symptoms, nocturnal cough and insufficient asthma control. Numerous studies have described association between gastroesophageal reflux and bronchial asthma and other respiratory diseases and symptoms. But the causality of this relationship has not been clearly explained. Still, it remains unclear whether the reflux causes asthma, asthma triggers reflux disease, or both coexist simultaneously in one patient. Gastroesophageal reflux is more frequent in patients with nonalergic idiopathic bronchial asthma.

2. Epidemiology

The prevalence of gastroesophageal reflux in asthmatic children evaluated by 24-hour pH-monitoring ranging between 43-87 %, but nearly half of the children are asymptomatic [7, 11]. Esophagitis has been found in 8.5% of paediatric patients with asthma [4].

3. Pathogenesis

There have been several theories explaining association between GERD and bronchial asthma. The relationship between asthma and reflux is complex.

Large group of studies pointed, that *gastroesophageal reflux can trigger or aggravate asthma*. Gastroesophageal reflux contributes to airflow obstruction in asthmatics by two main mechanisms: directly through microaspiration of gastric contents causing airway inflammation and/or indirectly through vagally mediated reflex [10]. Malfunction in any of the physiological protective mechanisms allows direct impact of noxious gastroduodenal contents with the airways. There are structural (lower and upper esophageal sphincter, diaphragm, phrenoesophageal ligament) and also functional (mucosal integrity, esophageal clearance mechanisms – esophageal motility, salivary bicarbonate) protective mechanism. Delayed gastric emptying seems to be other important pathogenetic factor in gastroesophageal reflux in infants and children [2]. Aspiration of gastric content is important stimulus of bronchospasm. Microaspirations can also damage the bronchial tree mucosa, which results in inflammation of the mucosa and bronchial hyper-responsiveness [12]. A lot of studies confirmed, that except of gastric content, refluxate can contain also duodenal material (pepsin, pesinogen, pancreatic enzymes, bile acids and salts). So, extraesophageal symptoms are not associated only with acidic, but also with weakly acidic/noncidic (ph 5-7) reflux episodes. The refluxate can be exclusively liquid, but also mixed with gas. Current studies have been focused on the influence of the nonacidic reflux on airway epithelium. Embryologic studies showed that esophagus and bronchial tree share a common embryologic origin and neural innervation. The parasympathetic nervous system (n. vagus) innervates esophagus and tracheobronchial tree. Influence of hydrochloric acid in distal esophagus increases airway hyperresponsiveness. Acid in the inflamed esophagus affects on exposed receptor and causes an increased airway hyperresponsiveness via the vagal reflex [22].

Another group of studies suppose that *high prevalence of gastroesophageal reflux in patients with asthma may be the consequence of asthma itself.* Asthma can induce reflux by several mechanisms. Poorly controlled asthma is associated with lung hyperinflation. Thoracic distension may result in decrease of diaphragm with an impairment of her function, as an important component of the antireflux barrier [14]. Descent of the diaphragm, caused by lung hyperinflation in increased work of breathing, increases the pressure gradient between abdomen and thorax that may cause herniation of the lower esophageal sphincter (LES) into thorax and impairment of barrier function [24]. Also some asthma medicaments may promote acid reflux. Beta-agonists, theophylline and corticosteroids may decrease LES tone [5, 6]. Above conclusions suggest a vicious cycle of GERD and associated bronchial asthma. Schematic representation of bilateral relationship between bronchial asthma and GERD is in Figure 1.

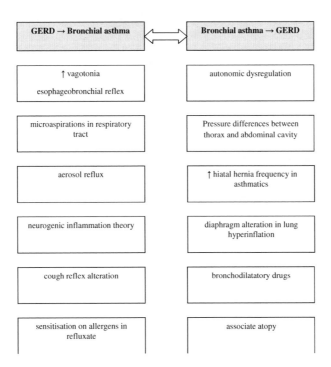

Figure 1. Bilateral relationship between bronchial asthma and GERD.

4. Diagnostic Procedures

The patient's history is very important part of the diagnosis of GERD-associated asthma. The diagnosis is important to consider in a presence of symptoms suggesting reflux: nocturnal cough, worsening of asthma symptoms after eating large meal, or being in the supine position. GERD should be considered in asthmatics who don´t respond to bronchodilator or steroid therapy. An additional clue may be the development of typical esophageal reflux symptoms [8]. Although 24-hour pH monitoring is considered the "gold standard" in the diagnosis of typical GERD, it is also increasingly used in establishing the diagnosis of GERD in patients with extraesophageal symptoms. The clinical utility of pH monitoring in this patient population, however, remains controversial. It´s the only esophageal test that can directly correlate acid reflux episodes with wheezing or other symptoms of bronchospasm. Because of high occurrence of nonacidic reflux episodes, sensitivity is improved using a combination of pH- and impedance-monitoring [1]. Gastroesophageal scintigraphy has a high specificity but low sensitivity, which limits its usefulness. Esophagogastroduodenoscopy has low sensitivity in patients with respiratory symptoms associated with GERD.

5. Treatment

Patients with GERD, including asthmatics, are usually treated with the combination of dietary management, lifestyle modifications and pharmacological therapy. It´s recommended avoidance of foods and drinks that decrease lower esophageal sphincter tone and increase acid production (greasy and spicy foods, citrus juices, chocolate, and caffeine). Smoking (nicotine), also passive, stimulates acid production and participates on transient lower esophageal sphincter relaxations. Carbonated drinks can provoke gastric distension, which stimulate transient lower esophageal sphincter relaxations. Eating smaller, more frequent portions through the day, not before the bedtime, is recommended. Some patients can benefit from raising the head of the bed. Weight loses in obese patients decreased risk of reflux episodes.

Premise, that gastroesophageal reflux can worsen asthma control trough microaspiration of acidic gastric contents is the base of the acid suppression treatment concept. Acid suppression is the mainstay of therapy for GERD and proton pump inhibitors, less histamine type-2 receptor antagonists are the most potent drugs. Prescriptions for proton pump inhibitors in patients with insufficient asthma control have increased markedly in the past decade. The main problem with the acid suppression treatment is the change of acidic reflux to nonacidic, but it doesn´t resolve the reflux, that can still produce respiratory symptoms. Clinical studies focused on the effect of treatment of GERD, mainly with proton pump inhibitors, in asthmatic patients revealed inconsistent results. Proton pump inhibitors (PPIs) are often prescribed for poorly controlled asthma regardless of reflux symptoms. There have been large increases in the use of PPIs among children last years. However, many recent clinical studies demonstrate that treatment of GERD with proton-pump inhibitors did not improve asthma control. Clinical studies were focused on pulmonary functions, rate of asthma exacerbations, asthma symptoms frequency and quality of life. Some earlier clinical trials in children symptomatic with gastroesophageal reflux and respiratory symptoms, including asthma, indicate benefit of PPIs treatment on respiratory outcomes [13]. Some authors even speak about different disease entity, calling GERD-induced bronchial asthma [21]. Double-blind prospective controlled trials demonstrated that treatment of asymptomatic GERD does not improve asthma control in children. Holbrook et al. (2012) assessed effectivity of lansoprasole in reduction of asthma control in children without overt GERD. In this trial of children with poorly controlled asthma without typical symptoms of GER, who were using inhaled corticosteroids, the addition of lansoprazole, compared with placebo, improved neither symptoms nor lung function but was associated with increased adverse events. Children treated with lansoprazole reported more respiratory infections [11]. Because of conflicting results of studies concerning the effects of lower esophageal acidification as a trigger of asthma systematic review by the Cochrane Collaboration was published in 2000 and then in 2003. The objective of this review was to evaluate the effectiveness of treatments for gastro-oesophageal reflux in terms of their benefit on asthma. Randomised controlled trials of gastroesophageal reflux treatment in adults and children with a diagnosis of both asthma and gastroesophageal reflux was realized. Twelve trials met the inclusion criteria. Patients were treated with proton pump inhibitors (6 studies), H2 antagonists (5 studie), surgery (1 study) and conservative management (1 study). Treatment duration ranged from 1 week to 6 months. Anti-reflux treatment did not consistently improve lung function, asthma symptoms, nocturnal asthma or the use of asthma medications [9]. In addition, PPIs use has been associated with increased risk of community-acquired pneumonia and other respiratory symptoms (sore throat, bronchitis), gastrointestinal infections in adults and children, which is thought to be related to a reduction in the host defence against bacterial colonization imparted by low gastric acid [16]. Patients with acid suppression therapy, especially with PPIs, have higher risk of activity related bone fractures [23].

Metoclopramide and domperidon are dopaminergic antagonists that have also been used as prokinetic agents for gastrointestinal dysmotility. But side effect limited their use in pediatric patients. Development of novel therapeutic agents has focused on the underlying mechanisms of GERD, such as transient lower esophageal sphincter relaxation, motility disorder, mucosal protection, and esophageal hypersensitivity. Newer PPI with faster and longer duration of action and potassium-competitive acid blocker, a newer acid suppressant, have also been investigated in clinical trials [21]. Fundoplication is an effective technique in the treatment of the severe atypical symptoms of GERD, including asthma [17].

Conclusion

Asymptomatic gastroesophageal reflux identified by 24-hour pH monitoring is very common in paediatric patients with asthma. But the relationship remains unclear. A lot of theories explaining this association were published. Majority of recent clinical studies demonstrate that treatment of GERD with proton-pump inhibitors did not improve asthma control. Although treatment benefit was described in selected group of patients. Further randomized controlled clinical studies, focusing also on safety concerns of long-term PPIs use in children, should be realized to better evaluate the role of antireflux therapy in asthmatics. Despite of higher GERD incidence among children with bronchial asthma, current studies don´t support routine esophageal pH testing in asymptomatic asthmatics. Current evidence also does not support routine long-term use of PPIs in asthmatics, which do not also have symptomatic gastroesophageal reflux. But some authors recommend the initial empiric trial of twice daily PPI's for 2–3 months at the beginning of treatment. In those responsive to therapy for both heartburn and/or asthma symptoms, PPI's should be tapered to the minimal dose necessary to control symptoms. In unresponsive patients testing for reflux (24- hour pH/impedance monitoring) may be needed.

Acknowledgments

This work was supported with project VEGA 1/0252/14 and with project "Centre of Experimental and Clinical Respirology", co-financed from EU sources.

References

[1]   Ahmed, T.; Vaezi, M.F. 2005. The role of pH monitoring in extraesophageal gastroesophageal reflux disease. *Gastrointest Endosc Clin N Am. 15*, 319-31.

[2]   Argon, M.; Duygun, U.; Daglioz, G.; Omür, O.; Demir, E.; Aydogdu, S.; 2006. Relationship between gastric emptying and gastroesophageal reflux in infants and children. *Clin Nucl Med. 31*, 262-5.

[3]   Boeckxstaens, G.E.; Smout, A. 2010. Systematic review: role of acid, weakly acidic and weakly alkaline reflux in gastro-oesophageal reflux disease. *Aliment Pharmacol Ther. 32*, 334-43.

[4]   Cinquetti, M.; Micelli, S.; Voltolina, C.; Zoppi, G.; 2002. The pattern of gastroesophageal reflux in asthmatic children. *J Asthma. 39*, 135-42.

[5]   Crowell, M.D.; Zayat, E.N.; Lacy, B.E.; Schettler-Duncan, A.; Liu, M.C. 2001. The effects of an inhaled beta(2)-adrenergic agonist on lower esophageal function: a dose-response study. *Chest. 120*, 1184-9.

[6]   Ekström, T.; Tibbling, L. 1988. Influence of theophylline on gastro-oesophageal reflux and asthma. Eur J Clin Pharmacol. *35*, 353-6.

[7]   Farcău, D.; Dreghiciu, D.; Chereches-Panța, P.; Popa, M.; Farcău, M.; Nanulescu. M. 2004. Effectiveness of antireflux therapy in asthmatic children with gastroesophageal reflux disease. *Pneumologia. 53*, 207-11.

[8]   Gaude, G.S., 2009. Pulmonary manifestations of gastroesophageal reflux disease. Ann Thorac Med. *4*, 115-23.

[9]   Gibson, P.G.; Henry, R.L.; Coughlan, J.L. 2003. Gastro-oesophageal reflux treatment for asthma in adults and children. *Cochrane Database Syst Rev. 2*: CD001496.

[10] Harding, S.M.; Richter, J.E.; 1997. The role of gastroesophageal reflux in chronic cough and asthma. *Chest. 111*, 1389-402.

[11] Holbrook, J.T.; Wise, R.A.; Gold, B.D.; Blake, K.; Brown, E.D.; Castro, M.; Dozor, A.J.; Lima, J.J.; Mastronarde, J.G.; Sockrider, M.M.; Teague, W.G. 2012. Lansoprazole for children with poorly controlled asthma: a randomized controlled trial. *JAMA. 307*, 373-81.

[12] Jiang, S.P.; Huang, L.W. 2005. Role of gastroesophageal reflux disease in asthmatic patients. *Eur Rev Med Pharmacol Sci. 9,* 151-160.

[13] Khoshoo, V.; Le, T.; Haydel, R.M.; Landry, L.; Nelson, C. 2003. Role of gastroesophageal reflux in older children with persistent asthma. *Chest. 123,* 1008-13.

[14] Mittal, R.K.; Balaban, D.H. 1997. The esophagogastric junction. *N Engl J Med. 27,* 924-32.

[15] Saritas Yuksel, E.; Vaezi, M.F., 2012. Extraesophageal manifestations of gastroesophageal reflux disease: cough, asthma, laryngitis, chest pain. Swiss Med Wkly. http://www.smw.ch/content/smw-2012-13544.

[16] Sheen, E.; Triadafilopoulos, G. 2011. Adverse Effects of Long-Term Proton Pump Inhibitor Therapy. *Digestive Diseases and Sciences. 56,* 931-950.

[17] Tashjian, D.B.; Tirabassi, M.V.; Moriarty, K.P.; Salva, P.S.; 2002. Laparoscopic Nissen Fundoplication for Reactive Airway Disease. *J Pediatr Surg, 37,*1021-1023.

[18] Thakkar, K.; Boatright, R.O.; Gilger, M.A.; El-Serag, H.B., 2010. Gastroesophageal reflux and asthma in children: a systematic review. *Pediatrics. 125,* 925-30.

[19] Vakil, N.; van Zanten, S.V.; Kahrilas, P.; Dent, J.; Jones, R.; Globale Konsensusgruppe. 2006. The Montreal definition and classification of gastroesophageal reflux disease: a global evidence-based consensus. *Am J Gastroenterol. 101,* 1900 – 1920.

[20] Wang, Y.K.; Hsu, W.H.; Wang, S.S.; Lu. C.Y.; Kuo, F.C.; Su, Y.C.; Yang, S.F.; Chen, C.Y.; Wu, D.C.; Kuo, C.H. 2013. Current pharmacological management of gastroesophageal reflux disease. *Gastroenterol Res Pract.,* http://www.ncbi.nlm.nih.gov /pmc/articles/PMC3710614/pdf/GRP2013-983653.pdf

[21] Wang, Z.; Kotwal, R.M.; 2012. Is GERD-induced asthma a different disease entity? *Ther Adv Respir Dis. 6,* 57.

[22] Wu, D.N.; Tanifuji, Y.; Kobayashi, H.; Yamauchi, K.; Kato, C.; Suzuki, K.; Inoue, H. 2000. Effects of esophageal acid perfusion on airway hyperresponsiveness in patients with bronchial asthma. *Chest. 118,* 1553-6.

[23] Yu, E.W.; Bauer, S.R.; Bain, P.A.; Bauer, D.C.; 2011. Proton pump inhibitors and risk of fractures: a meta-analysis of 11 international studies. *Am J Med. 124,* 519-26.

[24] Zerbib, F.; Guisset, O.; Lamouliatte, H.; Quinton, A.; Galmiche, J.P.; Tunon-De-Lara, J.M. 2002. Effects of bronchial obstruction on lower esophageal sphincter motility and gastroesophageal reflux in patients with asthma. *Am J Respir Crit Care Med. 166,* 1206-11.

Reviewed by:
Peter Banovcin, M.D., Ph.D. – Clinic of Gastroenterological Internal Medicine, Comenius University in Bratislava, Jessenius Faculty of Medicine in Martin, Slovakia

In: Advances in Respiratory Therapy Research
Editor: Miloš Jeseňák

ISBN: 978-1-63463-004-7
© 2015 Nova Science Publishers, Inc.

Chapter 4

Acute Cough Related to Upper Airway Diseases in Children, Understanding of Mechanisms and Therapeutical Implications

*Jana Plevkova**

Department of Pathophysiology,
Jessenius Faculty of Medicine in Martin, Comenius University in Bratislava,
Martin, Slovak Republic

Abstract

Cough – a phenomenon completely absent at birth develops quickly as one of the most important and powerful airway defensive reflexes in humans. Its maturation is characterized by high susceptibility to endogenous and exogenous factors, known as cough plasticity. Cough in children is also one of the most frequent reasons parents seek medical attention, in case that cough leads to sleep impairment, school absences or inability to play with other children. A high rate of cough prevalence among children is a consequence of relative immaturity of the immune system and high susceptibility to upper and lower respiratory tract infections. The cough concept is a parental problem.

A cough is exclusively a vagal phenomenon. There are two types of airway afferents mediating cough – no dose Aδ fibers responding basically to mechanical stimulation and acid, and C – fibers, responding to chemical signals. Both types of neural pathways are important in airway physiology. Maturation of cough-related pathways is strongly influenced by air pollution, lower respiratory tract infection and gender. Although the

---

* Corresponding Author address: Assoc. Prof. Jana Plevkova, M.D., Ph.D., Department of Pathophysiology, Jessenius Faculty of Medicine in Martin, Comenius University in Bratislava, Sklabinska 26, 036 01, Martin, Slovak Republic, e-mail: jplevkova@gmail.com

mechanisms of first and second factors on coughs are more or less understood, the gender differences, normally seen in adult population were not yet satisfactorily explained.

The most common causes of pediatric cough are upper respiratory tract infections, which are in a majority of cases induced by a virus. Successful symptom relief can be achieved by understanding the mechanisms by which the upper airway diseases influence coughing, thus reducing their impact on the airway physiology. Over-the-counter medication for common cold & cough relief must be administered with caution and in a way to diminish the factors influencing coughing in URTI such as postnasal drip, lack of nasal functions or increased afferent drive from the nasal mucosa. The effects, safety and tolerability of antitussives, antihistamines, decongestants, mucolytic and herbal products in general need to be reconsidered.

Keywords: Cough, Cough Reflex and Receptors, Over-the-Counter Medication, Symptomatic Therapy, Upper Respiratory Tract Infections

1. Introduction

A cough is the most important airway defensive reflex which protects the airways from accumulation of secretions, tissue debris, invasion of foreign bodies and participates on elimination of chemical irritants either produced in the airways (inflammatory mediators) or entering the airways from the surrounding environment (airborne irritants) [140]. Therefore, a cough is fulfilling its physiological role which is of substantial importance for the human airways.

A cough is, however one of the most common symptoms of respiratory diseases, the presence of which leads to a consultation of pediatricians. Parental and teacher concerns are usually superior to the complaint of a child, and these factors can considerably modify the information necessary to establish a diagnosis, with a tendency to aggravate the cough as a symptom and its impact on sleep, school performance and spare time of the affected child [87].

The most common causes of coughs in children with normal immune profiles without congenital lung and/or heart diseases are upper respiratory tract infections (URTI) [4]. Two out of three children younger than four years are visiting pediatricians at least once in a year with URTI, where the cough is the main complaint [39]. Some data indicates that even otherwise healthy children may complain with URTI several times in a year, usually during the winter or at a period of changes in season [87].

Upper respiratory tract infections are in approximately 90% of causes induced by respiratory viruses, the other 10% is caused either by bacteria or atypical microorganisms. Symptoms of such diseases in otherwise healthy children have a tendency for spontaneous resolution with time, although bothersome coughs and nocturnal coughs are the most prominent bothersome symptoms that require attention [28, 56].

As was previously supposed by a clinical branch of cough researchers, a cough in URTI was believed to be a consequence of the effect of inflammatory mediators and mucus excess on upper airway afferents, thus inducing their activation with a reflex response – coughing [57]. The recent understanding of the airway sensory system provides substantial evidence that it is not possible to induce coughing by stimulation of any afferents in the upper airways (nose, sinuses), because these "cough relevant" afferents are located in the larynx, trachea and main bronchi [103-5, 124]. If the cough belongs to the spectrum of clinical presentation of these diseases, there must be mechanisms responsible for up-regulation of coughing in children with URTI.

This review summarizes the recent understanding of the physiology of the cough reflex, and consequences of URTI for regulation of the cough reflex subjects with common cold. As a majority of children with URTI receive only symptomatic treatment to alleviate a cough, it would be beneficial to understand "up-regulation" mechanisms during URTI to achieve normalization and "down regulation" of the cough reflex parameters to pre-disease value. Understanding these mechanisms could be a reasonable and logical background for symptomatic treatment of coughs in a child with URTI and troublesome daily or nocturnal coughs.

2. Cough As a Reflex

Cough reflex is exclusively a vagal phenomenon, with the polysynaptic reflex arch consisting of several parts. They are airway afferent nerves, afferent neural pathways and brainstem circuits, which are responsible for processing the afferent information. If the information is relevant and reaches the threshold to induce reflex response, cough motor pattern is generated by the brainstem center, activated by efferent pathways and finally receives effectors of the cough reflex [17].

The first part of the reflex arch involves airway sensory nerves. Afferent nerves innervating the airways belong to the vagus nerve predominantly; however there is some recent data suggesting that airways are innervated also by fibers derived from dorsal root ganglia (DRG). Neurons responsible for mediation and modulation of a cough were identified using retrograde neuronal tracing methods and they are located in vagal nodose and jugular ganglia, while their terminals are broadly distributed within the airway mucosa in so- called tussigenic areas in the larynx, trachea and bronchi [141]. Airway afferent nerves are the most studied parts of the cough reflex arch and the recent understanding of their function will be explained in detail, so as they rise as a promising target for antitussive therapy.

Afferent pathways carrying the information towards the central nervous system run to the brainstem within the vagus nerve and superior laryngeal nerve, entering the ventrolateral parts of the medulla. It is believed that the glossopharyngeal nerve and auricular branch of the vagus nerve may represent potential sources of cough relevant afferent drives out of the respiratory system [61].

Based on the recent data, cough patterns are generated in complex polyfunctional neuronal network localized in the brainstem. A cough pattern generator is not an anatomically defined structure, but rather a neuronal network spread in rostrocaudal direction in the brainstem. These neuronal populations are not exclusively responsible for airway defensive reflexes, but they also regulate normal breathing patterns and its modification based on different signaling (chemosensory, nociceptive, airway signaling etc.) [12]. The system is holarchial, specifically orchestrated and gated, which processes afferent impulses from and out of the respiratory system. Information for the airway enters this network via the nucleus of the solitary tract (nTS), which is believed to be the most important site where airway afferents terminate and are synaptically connected to second order neurons. If information reaches the threshold and is relevant for coughing, the neuronal network will initiate the motor pattern via activation of premotor and motor neurons located in caudal and ventral respiratory groups. Neurogenesis of the cough is further related to the lateral tegmental field, pontine respiratory group and lateral reticular nucleus [13, 61, 120]. The motor act of coughing consists of the inspiratory phase, then the compressive phase when the glottis is closed, but expiratory muses are activated already rising the intrathoracic pressure, which will be the driving force for the expulsion of the air in the expiratory phase [120].

Efferent pathways and effectors are not specific only for coughs, but also for breathing, sneezing and other respiratory defensive reflexes. Motor drive is initiated in the premotor and motor neurons and conducted to peripheral motoneurons via reticulospinal tracts to the particular segments of the spinal cord at the cervical, thoracic and lumbar levels. Final efferent signaling is conducted via phrenic, intercostal and lumbal nerves. The efferent innervation of pharyngeal and laryngeal muscles provided by vagus nerves and other cranial nerves is a very important component. Airway smooth muscles and glands also belong to the effectors of the cough reflex, and these are innervated by sympathetic and parasympathetic nerves [60, 138]. Lessons learned from patients with neuromuscular diseases clearly demonstrate that reduced effort of expiratory muscles lead to less effective cough expulsions, thus increasing the risk of airway diseases such as aspiration pneumonia. The motor act of coughing is perfectly orchestrated with spatiotemporal sequential activation of diaphragm, chest, abdominal, lumbal and laryngeal muscles and their role was documented by EMG studies and endoscopic analysis of the vocal cords during coughing [43, 115].

3. Novel Approach to Classification of Airway Sensory Nerves Mediating Cough

Afferent nerve subtypes in the airways could be characterized and classified into several categories based on their myelinization, sensitivity to chemical or mechanical stimuli, adaptation to lung inflation, conduction velocity and more. The most known and frequently used classification of airway sensors divides them into slowly adapting receptors (SAR), rapidly adapting receptors (RAR) and C-fibers (bronchial and pulmonary C-fibers) [18, 49, 78].

New approaches to the classification of the airway sensors relevant for coughing were introduced recently, and consider embryologic origin of the airway sensors. Vagal neurons innervating airway mucosa are located in the nodose and jugular ganglia of the vagus nerve, and the majority of tracing studies, neurophysiological and neuropharmacological studies were completed on guinea pigs. It was documented, that the guinea pig vagus nerve is very similar to the human vagus nerve; therefore a guinea pig animal model is the best available model for cough translational studies. Functional specification of nodose and jugular neurons can clearly distinguish two main types of airway afferents responsible for mediation and modulation of coughs [18, 78, 141].

3.1. Airway Sensory Nerves Responding to Mechanical Stimulation

Airway mechanosensors adapt to the lung inflation either rapidly or slowly; thus we can recognize two main types of airway mechanosensors – rapidly adapting receptors (RAR), which reduce the burst of action potentials during prolonged lung inflation; and slowly adapting receptors (SAR), which adapt to this stimulation slowly [19, 53, 76]. Both types originate from the nodose and jugular ganglia of the vagus nerve and terminate in the airway and lungs. Conduction velocity typical for these fibers is 10-20m/s. The burst of action potentials appears after activation by relevant mechanical stimuli such as lung volume changes (inflation/deflation), contraction of airway smooth muscles and edema of the airway wall [18, 19, 53, 140]. RARs and SARs are generally not sensitive to chemical substances unless these substances are able to induce airway wall edema, increase mucus output or induce changes on airway muscle tone. This is indirect activation by chemical substances [125-127,139]. RARs and SARs can be distinguished by their response to the mechanical forces, while RARS are activated by lung inflation/deflation; SARS are activated during the inspiration, with the peak activity at the end of inspiration and early expiration [53, 60, 61, 119]. Reflex response to the activation of RARs is tachypnea and airway smooth muscle contraction, while SARs participate on Hering-Breuer inflation reflex, which is responsible for termination of inspiratory effort switching to the expiration after the optimal stretch of the airways is recognized [119, 137, 138].

Specific types of mechanosensors were identified in the guinea pig airways. It is an Aδ mechanosensor with lower conduction speed (5m/s) located mainly in the extrapulmonary airways (larynx, trachea and main bronchi) responding to mechanical punctual stimulation and acid by burst of action potential. These stimuli are relevant to induce coughing in anaesthetized guinea pigs. Interestingly, this type of nerve ending is different from RARs, SARs and C-fibers, and it originates from the vagal nodose ganglia. Based on the data from animal studies this type of the nerve ending could be attributed to what is called a "cough receptor" [19].

3.2. Afferent Nerve Endings Responding to Chemical Stimuli

Chemosensitive afferents are broadly distributed all over the airways and lungs. These fibers are not activated during regular breathing cycles, but are rather activated by different chemical stimuli such as inflammatory mediators, oxidizing substances or air-borne irritants. Airway chemosensory neurons are located in the vagal nodose and jugular ganglia, and also dorsal root ganglia [70, 78, 79]. Majority of these fibers are nonmyelinated C-fibers and their activation by chemical substances, either exogenous or endogenous for the release of tachykinins [6, 64, 65]. Tachykinins containing C-fibers are located mainly in extra pulmonary airways, while intrapulmonary airways are innervated by the C-fibers which do not release tachykinins after activation. These may respond to high threshold mechanical stimulation – stimulation with nociceptive relevance (lung hyperinflation, strong punctual stimulus) [83].

Thin unmyelinated C-fibers conduct impulses with slow speeds (1m/s) and they represent the majority of nerve fibers innervating airways and lungs. These neurons are located in the vagal nodose and jugular ganglia, and also the dorsal root ganglia [79].

Peripheral terminals of these afferents are located in the airways, lung interstitium and interalveolar septa. The role of C-fibers in a cough remains controversial and needs to be further clarified. Activation of C-fibers in anaesthetized guinea pigs by chemical stimuli does not induce a cough. Conscious subjects respond to the activation of jugular C-fibers by coughing; however activation of nodose C-fibers has an inhibitory effect on coughing in the guinea pig model. Circumstantial evidence suggests that their effects in humans are comparable to those identified in guinea pigs [20]. Activation of jugular C-fibers by stimuli which does not reach the threshold for induction of cough motor pattern can induce in humans the specific sensation of the urge-to-cough. This is complex cortical interpretation of airway nociceptive signaling, which proceeds the cough motor pattern [37].

3.3. What is the Cough Receptor?

Studies in experimental animals clearly document that different types of airway sensory nerves participate on mediation and modulation of a cough in experimental conditions. Mechanical and chemical stimuli applied to the tussigenic areas of the airways can provoke coughing, in case those stimuli reach the cough threshold. It is possible that cough-related pathways are many, and there is also circumstantial evidence about primary and secondary cough-related pathways [31, 79, 123].

Although it is not possible to translate all results obtained in animal models to human conditions, it is possible to assume that diseases such are respiratory tract infections or other inflammatory processes initiate coughing by different mechanisms which are complex and overlapping during the time of disease. Both mechanosensors and chemosensors in the airways may play important role in inception and modulation of the cough.

So what is the "cough receptor" after all? Rapidly adapting receptors in the airways were considered primary afferent fibers relevant for coughing induced by mechanical stimuli such as punctual stimulation, bronchoconstriction, and bronchial wall edema [116] and also by secondary consequences of the action of certain substances, like bradykinin [84]. However, there is a pool of evidence suggesting that RARs are not the "cough receptors" as many substances with ability to activate RARs (metacholin, leukotriene, neurokinins, and histamine) do not induce coughing. In some species (not guinea pigs and probably also not in humans) RARs are active during the breathing cycle and they are activated only by certain specific stimuli [116, 140].

The most reliable candidate for the cough receptor is the mechanosensor from nodose ganglia, slowly conducting Aδ fiber sensitive to mechanical punctual stimulation and acid, identified and further characterized by Canning and co-workers in 2004.

Evidence also supports the role of chemosensory fibers in the cough reflex in humans. Chemical substances known to be activators of airway chemosensors such as bradykinin, citric acid, capsaicin are also known as the most potent tussive agents in humans and animal models, however only in conscious state [21, 63]. These substances fail to induce coughing in anesthetized subjects; their inhalation leads to a reduction of respiratory rate and inhibits intensity of cough elicited by mechanical punctual stimulation [116, 140].

These conflicting evidences lead to an assumption that coughing induced by chemical agents depends on cortical activity, which is suppressed by general anaesthesia and this assumption correlates with the conception of the urge-to-cough. Therefore, coughing induced by chemical substances is not "strictly" of reflex origin, but it may also be a voluntary response to conscious perception of airway irritation (urge-to-cough) [37].

Based on the data about the most common stimuli inducing coughing (mechanical stimuli and chemical substances) and characterized properties of the airway sensory afferents, it is possible to conclude that humans are equipped by two types of cough reflex. One type is the cough to mechanical stimuli and acid substances mediated via Aδ nodose neurons [19, 22]. Phylogenetic studies suggest that this type of cough is an old airway defensive mechanism developed as a protection against aspiration of boluses of "acidic" substances – which is meant to be gastroesophageal reflux [14]. The second type of cough in humans is mediated by airway chemosensors – mainly C-fiber Chemosensors – nerve fibers of C nonmyelinated types are derived predominantly from the jugular ganglion. These fibers are sensitive to chemical factors such as capsaicin, bradykinin, adenosine, cinnamaldehyde, allylisothiocyanate, and these fibers are relatively insensitive to mechanical stimulation [23, 53, 83]. This type of cough – cough to chemical stimulation— is phylogenetically a younger type of the airway defense.

4. Cough Plasticity

The definition of coughing clearly shows that coughing is a reflex phenomenon. However reflex must not be understood as a complete stereotype. There is a growing pool of literature since 2002 about so-called cough plasticity, or neuroplasticity. This term describes changes in a structure of nerves mediating and modulating coughing. Eventually, there is a functional change at the level of airway sensory nerves, afferent pathways, ganglia, and the central nervous system. Coughing, if precisely regulated prevents the individual from aspiration and contribution to the airway cleaning. In terms of plasticity, a cough can be regulated up and down. Up-regulation of a cough is usually present in a majority of respiratory system diseases, and it may also develop as a consequence of extrapulmonary [67]. Cough reflex may be up-regulated in subjects suffering from airway inflammatory diseases, or extra pulmonary processes (GERD). In turn, cough reflex could be suppressed (down-regulated) in the elderly, new-borns, anaesthetized subjects, lung transplant recipients, paralyzed subjects, or patients with neuromuscular disorders [142].

Studies of the cough up-regulation may be helpful to understand the pathogenesis of chronic cough syndromes, and studies of the down-regulation may bring new insight to the cough modulation with potential clinical application.

How does plasticity work and what are the main mechanisms responsible for so-called neuroplastic changes?

It is not only one type of nerve fiber activated in case of different pathological processes in the airways. Inflammation, for instance, activated C and also Aδ fibers by direct and indirect mechanisms (release of inflammatory mediators, prostaglandins, increased mucus output, airway wall swelling etc.). Interaction of afferent nerve subtypes can lead to modulation of the cough. Activation of jugular C-fibers may interfere with Aδ fibers, thus potentiating the cough response. This would explain why coughing is significantly augmented in subjects with airway inflammation. Synergistic interactions between C and Aδ sensory drives leading to augmented cough responses are based on the mechanism of convergence [15, 20, 85]. It was documented that activation of nonmyelinated C-fibers induces the release of tachykinins not only at the peripheral terminals in the airway mucosa, but also at the central projections site. Increased release of neurokinin on the sites of projections to second and higher order neurons in the brainstem can thus increase central synaptic transmission.

A second type of neuroplastic change is related to the increased expression of cation channels which are responsible for activation and action potential discharge in cough relevant afferents. These ion channels are TRPV1 and TRPA1 abundantly expressed on airway terminals. Inflammation of various aetiologies leads to increased expression of ion channels, thus increasing irritability and responsiveness of airway sensors. Neuroplastic changes were observed in subjects with allergic airway inflammation [94, 136] and also there are some recent data about up-regulation of TRP channels in airway sensory nerves induced by respiratory viruses.

Mechanisms of signal transduction in vagal afferents are not entirely understood [66]. The majority of inflammatory mediators affects airway sensory nerves in either activation (production of action potential discharge) or modulation of their neurophysiological properties, for example in membrane excitability. For example, bradykinin induces single discharge of action potentials in airway Aδ fibers. Administration of PGE2 does not activate Aδ terminals, but increases the effect of administered bradykinin. Based on similar studies it was documented that not all inflammatory mediators can activate cough fibers. Bradykinin is an activator, but the majority of them – prostaglandins, leukotriene can "modulate" their membrane excitability, thus reducing the threshold for other tussigenic stimuli. The result of this interaction is augmented cough response [66, 83].

Central neuronal interactions seem to play a substantial role in cough plasticity [30, 80]. Coughing is often present in subjects suffering from extrapulmonary diseases such as reflux or rhinosinusitis. Interactions of airway afferents with afferents innervating oesophagus or nose may potentiate cough responses at the central level [62, 85, 106]. Coughing in reflux patients could be an excellent example for such interactions of vagal afferents. Infusion of the acid to esophagus does not induce coughing, but it potentiates the cough response induced by an airway challenge in healthy volunteers. Similar effects were observed in subjects with stimulation of nasal afferents in experimental settings. Stimulation of trigeminal terminals does not provoke coughing, but it facilitates coughing induced simultaneously from the lower airways [106]. Mechanisms proposed for these central interactions are based on the convergence of afferent inputs to the similar or close sites in the central nervous system.

Another hypothesis describes interaction between so-called primary cough pathways, which represents basic line of airway defense against acute injury from aspiration or mechanical stimulation. Probably, coughing present in subjects with different airway diseases (COPD, airway inflammation, fibrosis etc.) and chronic irritation of the airways may contain so-called secondary cough pathways, which may evoke or modify coughing by the interactions between primary and secondary cough pathways [85]. The understanding of a central neuroplastic mechanism is broadly limited by the lack of information about the neuronal cooperation at the brainstem level.

Recent evidence obtained in animal models suggests that interaction of afferent inputs from airway chemosensors interfere with the afferent drive from the "cough receptor" thus increasing the cough response [81, 86]. Similar results were obtained for convergence and synergistic interaction between chemosensors for esophagus and nose with the primary cough pathway in the brainstem [23, 103, 105]. All of these observations suggest that activation of airway chemoreceptors with subsequent rise of the excitability of the central cough pattern generator may lead to coughing is up-regulated and is a part of clinical presentation of many diseases, for example airway inflammation, diseases of the nose and esophagus [23]. Based on these observations, it is suggested that if a rise of the afferent drive to the brainstem circuits regulating cough may facilitate coughing, reduction of this afferent drive and/or its reduced central processing may have potential clinical application.

5. Airway Defensive Mechanisms at Birth and Maturation of the Cough Reflex

It is not known whether human fetus coughs, however it performs "respiratory-like movements" exchanging boluses of amniotic fluid between the airways and surroundings. "Cough-like" movement has never been detected in fetus; in fact this information is not available in relevant literature. Coughing is not present at birth; however it is very frequent in the first months and years of the childhood Coughing requires extremely high flow rates to clean the airways, which is hardly achieved in liquid-filled lungs in new-borns [11].

It would be naive to assume that new-borns miss airway protection. There are well-described neonatal aspiration syndromes, so the new-borns are equipped with pharyngeal and laryngeal protective mechanisms against potential hazards. For example, low chloride solutions such as water, gastric fluid, saliva have potential to provoke laryngeal chemoreflex as one of the reflex tools of the airway protection.

Studies performed by Perkell and co-workers in sleeping human infants showed that administration of 0.1 ml bolus of water instilled through the nasal catheter induced swallows in 55%, obstructed breaths in 40%, apnea in 40%, arousal in 18%, and coughing in only 1-2% of children. Responses to this stimulation differ between term and preterm infants. Later, during the neonatal period, coughing is usually associated with diseases such as tuberculosis, pertussis and chlamydia pneumonia infection or aspiration of a foreign body [24, 54, 118]. Preterm children with respiratory virus infection display rather laryngeal chemoreflex apnea instead of a cough [101].

Studies performed in animals in early postnatal period document that coughing appears several days (10-14 days) after the birth and this interval is different for rabbits, kittens and rats. In these experimental animals 2-4 days old, mechanical stimulation of the airways induces apnea/hypopnea. Older new-born animals respond to the mechanical stimulation of the airways with sporadic coughing, and these reflex responses are replaced after 14 days of age by regular cough reflex [68].

With maturation of a new-born, apnea and swallowing components of laryngeal chemoreflex decrease while coughing becomes increasingly prominent [129]. Coughing develops quickly as a substantial airway defensive reflex and its presence as the most prominent symptom of airway diseases is of importance during childhood. For example at the age of 2-4 months children lose the protection of maternally-acquired antibodies and become susceptible to upper respiratory tract infections. At the age of three years children have four to five episodes of upper respiratory tract infections per year [71]. It is also reported that 17-20% of infants at preschool age have recurring cough. Neural pathways responsible for regulation of coughing may undergo changes in structure and function in response to exposure to cigarette smoke, inflammation and allergens [74, 132]. There is indirect evidence that a child's neuronal system is more plastic - there is no direct evidence whether a cough pathway can undergo such plasticity during development.

The process of maturation of the cough reflex is very sensitive to neuroplastic changes, and it is believed that different influences during the maturation process may lead to definite status of the cough reflex physiology and regulation. During this period, coughing is influenced by several factors such as exposure to air pollutants, airway inflammatory diseases and endogenous factors related to the gender and puberty [135].

Air pollutants – like particulate matter, mixed pollutants and molds are strongly associated with increased coughing and wheezing, and association with coughing is stronger than association with wheezing [7, 34, 113]. On the other hand, exposure to irritant gasses is associated with chest tightness and more wheezing than coughing [7, 8, 118, 134]. Although the population is exposed to air-borne pollutants in general, children seem to be more exposed than adults, because the dose of air pollutants in the airways is likely increased compared to adults.

There are several reasons for this difference. Children have higher lung/airway surface area per kilogram (kg) of body weight. Under normal breathing rate, their tidal volume calculated to kg of body weight is 50% higher compared to adults and children spend more time outdoors performing activities that increase ventilatory rate, thus inhaling air-borne pollutants. An interesting study was performed in northern Slovakia with approximately 60,000 inhabitants on non-atopic, non-wheezing children with no URTI within two weeks. This study identified that pubertal development plays a significant role in changes of the cough threshold during childhood. Children with late puberty revealed the gender differences. The impact of air pollution was studied as well. Rural children displayed no significant differences in cough threshold among age groups, while urban children showed significant differences in cough threshold between 8-10 years compared to 11-14 years and 15-18 years. In general, urban children had lower cough threshold which means they would cough to the stimuli [135].

Except for air pollution, the role of lower airway infection on cough sensitivity during development was studied. Significant differences were found in 8-10 year old children (p< 0.03) but not in older children, suggesting that repeated infections of lower respiratory tract influence have stronger neuroplastic changes in younger children. Respiratory morbidity does not differ between urban and rural children. Coughing in healthy children is influenced by living area, lower respiratory tract infections with most significant changes observed in youngest children suggest higher plasticity of the cough reflex [135].

Cough reflex sensitivity to capsaicin in adult population is significantly influenced by gender; however, the mechanism responsible for reduced capsaicin threshold in female still remains elucidated. The general idea of increased sensitivity of the female airways to tussive agents is considered to be an evolutional feature. It is hypothesized that increased airway sensitivity in female subjects is related to the higher risk for aspiration of a refluxate as a consequence of the pregnancy. This protective mechanism was probably of high importance in the past when conception was not regulated and the average count of pregnancies in individual female was higher than now. However, this is only a speculation based on the physiological understanding of the airway sensors sensitive either to the inflammatory mediators, air-borne irritants (C fiber mediated cough) and bolus of acids (Aδ fiber mediated cough) [14].

The etiology of the gender difference in cough reflex sensitivity remains speculative. Previous analysis has shown that enhanced cough sensitivity in women is not explained on the basis of age, height, weight or pulmonary function. The observation that postmenopausal women have a lower cough threshold than premenopausal women argues against the possibility that enhanced cough sensitivity in women is attributed to hormonal factors [44, 98].

It appears likely, therefore, that women have an intrinsically more sensitive cough reflex. This hypothesis is supported by the observation that coughing because of ACE inhibitors occurs more commonly in women [45, 88]. Recent studies demonstrate that gender differences in airway wall structure may lead to further elucidation of this question [44].

6. Cough As a Symptom

Coughing is one of the most common reasons why parents seek medical advice. Even otherwise healthy children can cough 0-141 cough epochs daily, and this result obtained from objective assessment of a cough is not conclusive for a disease condition [50, 52]. Children are more susceptible to respiratory tract infections and to the airborne irritants induced by airway dysfunction; therefore coughing children is a frequent finding. The most common cause of coughing in children are infections of the upper respiratory tract, which are in immunocompetent children without associated comorbidities solved up to three weeks on average [47]. The problem could be a child with episodes of recurrent or chronic coughing, which is a diagnostic and therapeutic challenge.

Several types of cough could be recognized in children. Acute cough typically lasts fewer than two weeks, and is considered a symptom most frequently related to a respiratory tract infection. A cough lasting 4 - 8 weeks is increasingly recognized as prolonged acute cough, in relation to protracted bacterial bronchitis (PBB) [35]. Chronic cough lasts more than four weeks in children versus eight weeks in adults [27], and the quality - dry or productive, the latter suggesting a more serious condition – must be specified. It may be associated with other signs or symptoms, called "cough pointers". Thus cough may be specific or nonspecific, depending on presence or absence of these pointers.

Clearly there is a "grey" area between acute and chronic cough, sometimes called "subacute cough" [28, 128]. An example of such a situation would be a child with pertusis or post-viral cough whose cough may be slowly resolving over a 3–8-week period.

Although the chronic cough syndrome is a well-defined condition in adults, it is debatable in children. The reasons are many, including lack of epidemiological data, methodological bias and frequent, commonly repeated episodes of acute or subacute respiratory conditions. In this situation coughing is the main complaint with inability to clearly recognize, whether the condition is "chronic cough" or an accumulation and summation of "acute cough" episodes. Chronic cough is associated with high morbidity in children and their families. In contrast to adults, the child with chronic cough does not report feelings of anxiety or depression, but parents feel stressed, frustrated and helpless when confronted with their child and their own sleepless nights [77]. When forceful, this cough may determine symptoms like syncope [48], pneumo-mediastinum, pneumothorax, urinary incontinence or vomiting. It decreases the quality of life and affects daily activities, responsible for significant absenteeism at school [56].

Epidemiological studies of chronic cough in adults identified three most common diseases which are associated with chronic intractable cough. They are upper airway diseases (rhinitis and/or sinusitis), gastroesophageal reflux and asthma with its clinical phenotypes. These three causes are known as the diagnostic triad, and the majority of diagnostic protocols either confirm or exclude the most probable cause of coughing [93].

Situations in children are different. Although some diseases of the airways affect both adult and pediatric populations, there are considerable differences. Prominent causes of chronic cough in children include frequently recurring simple viral bronchitis, "cough variant asthma" and post-infectious cough. The common conditions when associated with prolonged periods of coughing but no wheezing can be difficult to clinically differentiate and were extensively reviewed elsewhere [24, 25, 29].

7. Acute Cough Related to Upper Respiratory Tract Infections

Acute cough in children is defined as an episode of cough which lasts less than two weeks, and in a majority of these children upper respiratory tract infection is a cause of the cough. In case of lack of tachypnea, fever and X-ray findings, it is possible to expect that no complication will appear in the primary pediatric care [121]. However, even coughing in children can be distressing and has a major impact on a child's sleep, school performance and ability to play. Community-based surveys show that parental-reported cough as an isolated symptom has a high prevalence. Reported cough with colds has a prevalence of 28% in boys and 30% in girls.

Upper respiratory tract infections (URTI) are the most common causes of coughing in children. They are in more than 90% of cases induced by viruses alone, with or without secondary bacterial infection [51, 52]. Statistical data suggest that even children with normal immune profiles have approximately 4-6 episodes of respiratory infections per year with average duration of 7-9 days. Coughing is one of the most common symptoms of URTI, with children coughing 28-63 days in a year. Some children may also suffer from post-infectious cough, which could be responsible for the rise of the concern [28].

Position paper of the EAACI – The Children Rhinitis Task Force's published results of the ISAAC study phase three revealed an average prevalence of rhinitis 8.5% (range 1.8-20.4%) in 6- to 7- year old children and 14.6% (range 1.4-33.3%) for 13-14 year old children. The most common disease is acute inflammation of the upper airways induced by a virus infection. This information by the ISAAC study documents the growing importance of rhinitis of any etiology in pediatric populations [114, 122].

Diseases of the upper airways are the most commonly identified causes of chronic cough in adults. Despite the differences in studied populations and diagnostic protocols, it has been consistently reported to be the main cause for chronic cough (20-40%) among patients attending the specialized cough clinics [92]. The term "upper airway cough syndrome" was suggested for association of the cough and upper respiratory tract diseases in adults. In fact, "upper airway cough syndrome" has never been defined in children despite frequent association between the upper airway diseases and cough in children.

Pathogenesis of upper airway cough syndrome was systematically studied and it has been recognized that simple mechanistic theory of "post-nasal drip syndrome" is not the only mechanism that provokes coughing in subjects with rhinitis. Complex pathogenesis involves the combination of mechanisms such as microaspiration, post-nasal drip of the mucus, spreading of the inflammation via systemic circulation, nasobronchial reflex, sinobronchial reflex, and lack of nasal functions in subjects with rhinitis together with mechanisms of central and peripheral cough plasticity [106, 107].

7.1. Cough Sensitivity in Children with URTI

Cough reflex sensitivity is defined as the lowest concentration of tussive agent inducing a cough. The values are further classified into C2 – the lowest concentration of capsaicin inducing two or more coughs, and C5 – the lowest concentration of capsaicin inducing five or more coughs. The test is performed using gradually increasing concentrations of tussive agent – TRPV1 agonist capsaicin. This parameter is usually changed in airway diseases and all states characterized by up-regulation of cough. Heightened cough reflex sensitivity means that lower concentration of capsaicin is needed to achieve C2 and C5 compared to normal values [29].

A study performed in children with common cold and allergic rhinitis during the pollen season and out of it showed that inflammation located in the upper airways led to significant reduction of the cough threshold [107]. The data obtained in the capsaicin cough challenge are suggestive for modulation of cough sensitivity which was reported also for adults with different types of upper airway diseases [40, 95, 100].

Capsaicin cough sensitivity was also tested in children with normal immune profiles and normal counts of blood eosinophils, without congenital lung/heart diseases, no current medication and free from URTI for at least three weeks. Children were tested three times, once before the URTI (pre disease measurement), again the second day of URTI (disease) and finally after the complete recovery from URTI was achieved (recovery). Children were included in the study only in case coughing was their parental main complain. The data showed that cough sensitivity to capsaicin is significantly reduced during the URTI, with normalization of the threshold to pre-disease value after recovery [102]. Interestingly, there were children in whom the cough was still present after 2-3 weeks, instead of in already normalized cough threshold. Analysis of these groups (parental smoking, air pollution, more frequent respiratory tract infections) did not elucidate this finding. The differences between coughers (cough still present after stabilization of C2) and no coughers (absolute resolution of cough) suggest the role of other, probably central mechanisms participating on cough in children with already normalized thresholds [102].

It was previously suggested by clinical respirologists that coughing can be elicited directly by the activation of the nasal afferents. This assumption was not correct. The upper airways are innervated by the trigeminal nerve, and stimulation of these nerve endings in the nasal mucosa by mechanical and chemical stimuli (capsaicin, AITC, cinnamon aldehyde, histamine) fail to provoke coughing in experimental and clinical settings [16, 103-105]. Primary responses to this stimulation are sneezing, itching/irritation, nasal congestion and rhinorrhoea. Animal models, studies in human healthy volunteers and subjects with upper airway diseases indicate that it is not possible to induce coughing from the upper airways. Augmented cough response however indicates that there must be a mechanisms/mechanisms responsible for up-regulation of coughing [107, 108].

It is known that inflammation in the upper airways potentiate either coughing induced by stimulation of putative TRPV1-expressing capsaicin- sensitive fibers or coughing initiated by capsaicin-insensitive mechanosensitive Aδ nodose fibers [106]. Recent understanding of the airway sensors and their neurophysiology together with the evidence about peripheral and central cough plasticity may explain why children with URTI cough, even though the primary pathological process is located in the upper airways, while cough- related nerve fibers are located in the larynx, trachea and main bronchi.

Reactivity of nasal mucosa to any considered pathological process is activation of defensive and protective mechanisms with the tendency to do the following:

1. eliminate potentially harmful noxae – sneezing
2. dilute the noxious stimulus if applicable and eliminate it by mucocilliary transport (rhinorrhoea)
3. prevent further inhalation of noxious stimulus – reduction of nasal patency [117].

To achieve dilution and increase mucus output, nasal vessels and glands are activated by immune, neural and humoral signaling. Therefore the most common upper airway symptoms are sneezing, rhinorrhoea and nasal congestion with reduced nasal patency. All of these mechanisms may influence cough reflex arch either at the peripheral level (sensors) or central level (brainstem circuits, cortex) [106].

7.2. Mechanisms Influencing Cough Sensitivity in Children with URTI

7.2.1. Complete Obstruction of the Nasal Passages - Lack of Nasal Functions

The nose is the first part of the respiratory system which is in contact with ambient air. It serves many important functions including warming, moistening and filtering inhaled air. Normal individuals prefer inhalation through the nasal passages even though the resistance of the nasal passages is higher than resistance of the oral cavity. At the rest and mild physical exercise children breathe through the nose, and they switch to oral breathing during speech, laughter, singing or exercise. Optimal nasal patency is critical for successful breast or bottle feeding in smallest infants [97].

Nasal obstruction is subjective phenomenon however it can be objectively measured. In case of complete nasal obstruction children switch to oral breathing which is not optimal for air conditioning. An example could be a child with hyperplastic adenoids. Oral breathing leads to inhalation of cold dry air, which is not optimally filtered in the upper airways. Deposition of inhaled chemicals, air-borne irritants and particulate matter, together with changes of osmolality of superficial fluid may lead to the functional and/or morphological impairment of the lower airway mucosa with increased cough reflex sensitivity. Additional warming and moistening of inhaled air in the lower airways lead to the lack of superficial mucosal fluids with hypertonicity, which could also modulate activity of cough related pathways [69]. Inhalation of poorly filtered and unconditioned air may lead to initiation of inflammation either based on immune system signaling or via initiation of neurogenic inflammation by inhaled irritants [6, 10].

7.2.2. Post-Nasal Drip

Since the term post-nasal drip (PND) is rather associated with chronic upper airway diseases (rhinosinusitis) it may appear also in children with URTI [55, 57, 72]. Increased production of mucus in the nose and sinuses in URTI subjects leads to the nasal discharge. Only 30% of secretion is transported forward to the nostril and drips out of them. 70% of the mucus produced in the nose and sinuses moves to the nasopharynx and pharynx as a consequence of anatomical conditions and orientation of mucocilliary transport [33, 94]. Previously, it was thought that dripping of the mucus down to the laryngeal aperture can reach the larynx, trachea, or eventually more distal airways. Studies using radiolabelled material applied to the sinuses demonstrated that no mucus reaches the larynx or more distal airways. Radio labeled marker was detected in the upper gastrointestinal tract 24 hours after its sinonasal administration [5]. There are effective laryngeal reflexes, which probably provide sufficient defense and prevent the mucus against entering the lower airways [106].

Even though, post-nasal drip can activate mechanosensors in the pharynx and hypopharynx by its presence on the mucosa's surface. Signal molecules, inflammatory mediators, cells and their products which are present in the mucus can be a massive source for activation or sensitization of the chemosensors in the pharynx and hypopharynx [36]. Literature about post-nasal drip share conflicting evidence, as majority of patients with clinically diagnosed PND do not cough. It is also difficult to establish diagnosis of PND based on finding mucus on the dorsal pharyngeal wall dripping down to the hypopharynx [72, 99].

7.2.3. Incomplete Nasal Obstruction with Microaspiration

The lack of objective evidence about transportation of the macroscopic amount of mucus from nose to tussigenic areas together with the benefits of nasal decongestants on cough in common cold subjects led to postulation of a hypothesis of microaspiration [36]. Similar hypothesis of aspiration of refluxate in "gaseous" form was implied for reflex related coughing [90]. The hypothesis explains that increased airflow resistance of nasal passages increases the turbulent pattern of the airflow through the nasal passages. These conditions may lead to formation of polydisperse aerosol out of the nasal secretions.

Indirect evidence was obtained to prove this phenomenon. In animals with experimentally induced rhinitis animals were either tracheotomised immediately after rhinitis was induced, or were allowed to remain with intact airways for 20 minutes, while ventilation was enhanced by CO_2 admixture to the inhaled air. The data suggested that breathing through intact airways with increased respiratory drive necessary to pass the air through "swollen nasal passages" may potentially contribute to the microaspiration of aerosol with mixture of inflammatory mediators to the distal portion of the airways [106].

Similar results were reproduced in human healthy volunteers with histamine induced nasal discharge and obstruction; both parameters were objectively measured and quantified. The subjects were instructed to breathe through the nose with force to overcome increased resistance, and the other group was instructed to breathe through the mouth wearing a nose clip. Intensified nasal breathing may augment cough response probably by the mechanism of microaspiration of inflammatory aerosol [104].

These results can be supported by the observation of the effect of medication reducing nasal mucosal swelling and secretion on cough in humans – subjects with reduced secretion and nasal resistance cough less [36].

7.2.4. Nasobronchial/Sinobronchial Reflex

Reflex interactions between the nose and lower airways are frequently subjected to the discussion. There are conflicting evidences whether sinobronchial and nasobronchial reflexes exist. While some authors describe the rise of lower airway resistance in the subjects with activation of nasal trigeminal afferents, some other authors failed to prove their existence [73, 75, 131]. The data are indicative for existence of nasobronchial/sinobronchial interactions, but rather in the subjects with already present airway hyperesponsivenss.

Activation of neural trigeminal – vagal responses in URTI depends on activation of trigeminal afferents by mechanical and chemical stimuli, such is the presence of the mucus in the nasal passages and also the presence of inflammatory mediators, tachykinis etc. Nasobronchial reflex in the sense it is defined can therefore result in narrowing the airway. It was previously believed that bronchoconstriction can activate cough related fibers by the mechanical forces produced by the change of the airway lumen. It is recognized, that cough and bronchoconstriction are different reflex processes, but they may potentiate each other by the mechanism of central convergence and synergistic interactions of cough and bronchoconstriction related pathways [85].

Upper airway infection with extension to the sinuses may lead to reduced production of nitric oxide, which is synthetized in sinuses and reaches the lower airways with every inspiration. Physiological levels of nitric oxide modulate bronchomotor responses and prevent bronchoconstriction [2].

7.2.5. The Role of Central Neuronal Pathways - Convergence

Apart from the nasal discharge with potential microaspiration and decreased nasal patency which were the dominant factors for cough in the previous paragraphs, there is also direct evidence that cough is sensitized more importantly by the neural mechanisms. Local pre-treatment with 1% mesocain inhibited previously augmented cough responses in animal models and intranasal administration of irritants which activate trigeminal nerves enhances urge-to-cough [16]. Therefore, the role of the nasal afferents in this process of sensitization is strongly suggested [30]. Inflammatory mediators released during the URTI are known as potent activators (histamine, bradykinin) and sensitizers (prostaglandins, leukotrienes) of nasal trigeminal afferents [110, 111]. In the light of cough plasticity concept, we started to hypothesize that cough reflex could be considerably modulated by afferent drives from the nose.

Intranasal administration of different chemical substances known as activators of trigeminal afferents in animal and human studies documented that if cough is induced simultaneously from the lower airways, it is significantly augmented. Parameters of cough sensitivity are typically shifted towards lower concentrations. Total and cumulative count of coughs is increased together with considerably enhanced urge-to-cough [16, 103-105].

'Urge-to-cough' is a subjective interpretation of airway irritation, which precedes cough motor pattern. It represents cortical conscious contribution to the airway defense. It is difficult to say, whether it is voluntary cough, because subjects may cough to a request, if you ask them to without any perceived airway irritation. Taken together these facts, 'urge-to-cough' is specific sensation of airway irritation, which leads to coughing [44,45]. It was documented that adult subjects with URTI have significantly heightened urge to cough [41, 42].

7.2.6. The Role of Virus - Virus Induced Neuroplasticity

Hand in hand with the penetration to the mucosa and after the contact with pattern recognition receptors on epithelial cells and mucosal dendritic cells, the immune system will initiate the response, recruiting immune cells inflammatory mediators and signal molecules. Many of them have the ability to either activate or sensitize cough mediating afferents. These mediators will activate also C-fibers leading to release of tachykinins with their further proinflammatory effects and also effects on the cough mediating afferent.

Penetration of the microorganisms and initiation of the inflammatory process can lead to the activation of cough related afferents by both direct and indirect effects.

Based on the results from animals research and human cough challenges it was assumed that cough is induced by airway afferent nerves expressing TRPV1 and TRPA1 channels [9, 46]. It was previously hypothesized by A.H. Morice [89] that respiratory viruses share ability to induce coughing to spread from one host to another. During a common cold, patients experience bouts of coughing as the result of minor environment insults such as change in air temperature or exposure to noxious stimuli like cigarette smoke. Objective evidence of this "virus-induced" cough hypersensitivity relies on challenge experiments. A shift in the cough dose response curve with a lower threshold in URTI has been demonstrated in adults and also in children [95, 102]. Recovery of the cough reflex to a more normal level is seen as the infection abates. Prof. Morice suggested that cough reflex hypersensitivity induced by viruses is a fundamental part of the pathogenesis of URTI enabling the viruses to disseminate themselves through the population using droplet transmission, however the evidence remained [95].

Recently published data showed that respiratory viruses have the ability to up-regulate cough reflex. The authors showed for the first time that rhinovirus can infect neuronal cells. Furthermore, infection causes up-regulation of TRP channels by channel-specific mechanisms. The increase in TRPA1 and TRPV1 levels can be mediated by soluble factors induced by infection whereas TRPM8 requires replicating virus [1]. Knowing the role of the TRPA1 channels in the modulation of cough reflex (V1 and A1 for up-regulation) and TRPM8 (menthol receptor for down-regulation), the hypothesis can be made that viruses regulate coughing by their replication cycle inside the host organism. This information is very interesting as the TRP channels appear to be very promising targets to manage coughing [16, 46]. The data from expression systems are highly suggestive for the role of the virus itself in the up-regulation of the cough reflex.

It was documented that viral infection leads to increase expression of TRPV1 channel on airway sensory nerves. TRPV1 channel is known to be activated by capsaicin, the pungent extract of red pepper [9] and its increased expression on airway afferent nerves is associated with increased sensitivity of the airways to tussive stimuli.

There are also speculations that increased expression of the TRPV1 by the virus is an integral part of the virus life cycle, as it starts after the replication of the virus is terminated. This may lead to robust coughing, which causes the virus to spread from one host to another across the population. When the synthesis of the soluble particles of the virus is terminated, the nerves increase the TRPM8 which is known as a channel responsible for massive down-regulation of cough (Table 1) [1].

Table 1. Proposed mechanisms of cough and cough reflex targets

Proposed Mechanism & Intervention	Cough Reflex Targets
Complete nasal obstruction → lack of nasal functions in oral breathing	Inhalation of cold dry and unfiltered air * Damage of the superficial mucosal layers with increased penetration of tussigenic factors to the nerves * Neurogenic and/or immune factors initiated inflammation
Overproduction of mucus & post nasal drip	Activation of mechanosensitive Aδ fibres in the pharynx and laryngeal aperture * Activation/sensitization of chemosensitive C fibres by mediators and signal molecules in the mucus
Incomplete nasal obstruction → nasal breathing with increased nasal resistance	Formation of polydisperse aerosol of secretions and inflammatory mediators, cells and their products - microaspiration to the lower airways * Activation/sensitization of chemosensitive C fibres
Nasobronchial/sinobronchial reflex	Modulation of activity of airway afferents by increased tone of the smooth muscle cells
Irritation of nasal trigeminal afferents by ongoing inflammation	Convergence of trigeminal and vagal afferent drive with up-regulation of cough pattern generator activity
Virus induced neuroplastic changes	Peripheral plasticity of putative cough fibres in the airway – increased expression of TRPV1 and TRPA1 ion channels

8. Therapeutical Implications

Acute coughing in children suffering from URTI can be an intractable problem; however, it has self-limiting characteristics with typical resolution with time [32]. Upper airway symptoms and coughing can be troublesome, especially at night, disturbing the child's and parent's sleep, and limiting the school performance and ability to play during the day. Since the majority of URTI is induced by virus, antibiotics are not a solution for uncomplicated URTI, although symptomatic treatment for upper airway symptoms and coughing are frequently recommended by pediatricians or by parents themselves [58, 59].

Over-the-counter medication seems to have no documented benefit in children under the age of five. Therapeutic options for the management of acute cough in children are limited because of the lack of data to support efficiency of currently available antitussives, as well as safety concerns associated with these agents. All cough suppressants currently marketed to adult patients present an unacceptable risk/benefit profile for pediatric use, because of potential for excessive sedation (narcotics, dextromethorphan, first-generation antihistamines) or hyperstimulation (pseudoephedrine, phenylephrine) (Table 2) [38, 39].

Table 2. Modes of action of over-the-counter medication

Medication	Modes of Action
Antitussives	Centrally acting – inhibition of neuronal populations responsible for cough pattern generation (codeine, dextromethorphan) * Peripherally acting (dropropizine, levodropropizine, butamirate)
Mucolytics	Heterogeneous group of compounds increasing the volume of mucus with reducing its viscosity by hydration of the mucus layer or hydrolysis of chemical bonds in the mucus macromolecules with anti-inflammatory, and antioxidative activity (ambroxol, N-acetyl cysteine, erdosteine)
Antihistamine-decongestants	Combination of histamine H1 receptor inverse agonists with anti-inflammatory action and α adrenoreceptor agonist which cause vasoconstriction of nasal mucosal vessels
Antihistamines H1	Histamine H1 inverse agonists are promiscuit substances having antihistamine and anticholinergic effects. Their ability to penetrate hematoencephalic barrier is responsible for light sedative effect which can be of help in intense coughing
Other drug combination	Fixed drug combination using different ingredients

The American College of Chest Physicians does not recommend pharmacological treatment of acute cough in children. Instead, they support care with analgesics, hot beverages, lozenges, herbal products and honey [58].

Unfortunately, for a persistent or severe cough in URTI these non-pharmacological strategies are ineffective; thus safe and effective antitussive medication should be considered.

Understanding mechanisms responsible for augmentation of coughs in children with URTI can be the key to the management of the clinical presentation. Patent nasal passages, reduced mucus and activation of nasal sensory afferents may alleviate coughing. Data from basic research confirms that the magnitude of nasal symptoms positively correlates with the magnitude of coughing; thus suppression of nasal inflammation and its consequences (nasal obstruction, rhinorrhea, activation of nerves) could be the main target for therapeutic strategies.

Metaanalysis of Cochrane database sources and systemic reviews of randomized controlled trials using over-the-counter medication suggest that over-the-counter common cold and cough medicines do not appear to be more effective than placebos in relieving symptoms of acute cough. Even if statistically significant, effect sizes were small and of doubtful clinical relevance. The number of trials on each category was small and the results must be interpreted with a caution [3, 130].

Over-the-counter medication for acute cough can be categorized according to their modes of actions into several categories – antitussives, mucolytics, antihistamine-decongestant combination, other drug combination, and antihistamines H1 [122]. Since the guidelines are generalized, and do not respect individual circumstances of individual pediatric patients and their families, it would be beneficial to use individualized and personalized approaches to every single child with URTI, to relieve their symptoms, and to suppress acute cough if applicable. Generalized administration of over-the-counter medication in each category should be carefully reconsidered, with the understanding that coughing, sneezing and nasal swelling with discharge are natural airway defensive processes, and they undoubtedly have significance, even though they influence the quality of life in pediatric URTI subjects.

Acknowledgments

This work was supported with project "Center of Experimental and Clinical Respirology", co-financed from EU sources.

References

[1]   Abdullah, H.; Heaney, L.G.; Cosby, S.L.; et al. (2014). Rhinovirus upregulates transient receptor potential channels in a human neuronal cell line: implications for respiratory virus-induced cough reflex sensitivity. *Thorax*, 69(1):46-54.

[2]   Antosova, M.; Plevkova, J.; Strapkova, A.; Buday, T (2012). Nitric oxide—Important messenger in human body. *Open J Mol & Integr Physiol*, 2, 98-106.

[3]   Arrol, B. (2005). Non- antibiotic treatment for upper – respiratory tract infections (common cold). *Respiratory Medicine*, 99: 1477-1484.

[4]   Ayers, J.G.; Noah, N.D.; Flemming, D.M. (1993). Incidence of episodes of acute asthma and acute bronchitis in general practice. *Br J Gen Pract*, 43 (374) 361-364.

[5]   Bardin, P.G.; Van Heerden, B.B.; Joubert, J.R. (1990). Absence of pulmonary aspiration of sinus contents in patients with asthma and sinusitis. *J Allergy Clin Immunol,* 86(1):82-8.

[6] Barnes, P. (2001). Neurogenic inflammation in the airways. *Respir Physiol,*125(1-2):145-54.

[7] Bayer-Oglesby, L.; Grize, L.; Gassner, M.; et al. (2005). Ambient air pollution levels and improved respiratory health in Swiss children. *Environ Health Perspect,* 113(11):1632-7.

[8] Belanger, K.; Gent, J.F.; Triche, E.W.; et al. (2006). Association of indoor nitrogen dioxide exposure with respiratory symptoms in children with asthma. *Am J Respir Crit Care Med,* 173(3):297-303.

[9] Bessac, B.F.; Jordt, S.E. (2008). Breathtaking TRP Channels: TRPA1 and TRPV1 in Airway Chemosensation and Reflex Control. *Physiol,* 23: 360-370.

[10] Biringerova, Z.; Buday, T.; Calkovsky, V.; et al. (2011). The Nose as a Target of Air Pollution, Physiological Aspects and Clinical Relevance of Nasal TRPA1 Receptors. *Acta Med Martiniana,* 11:3: 13-19.

[11] Boileau, S.; Deschildre, A. (2010). Acute respiratory distress in the newborn and the child. Foreign bodies of the upper respiratory tract. *Rev Prat,* 20;60(5):715-20.

[12] Bolser, D.C.; Hey, J.A.; Chapman, R.W. (1999). Influence of central antitussive drugs on the cough motor pattern. *J Appl Physiol,* 86: 1017-1024.

[13] Bolser, D.C.; Poliacek, I.; Jakus, J.; et al. (2006). Neurogenesis of cough, other airway defensive behaviors and breathing: A holarchical system? *Respir Physiol Neurobiol,* 28;152(3):255-65.

[14] Brooks, S.M. (2011). Perspective on the human cough reflex. *Cough* 7: 10.

[15] Brozmanova, M.; Plevkova, J.; Tatar, M.; et al. (2008). Cough reflex sensitivity is increased in the guinea pig model of allergic rhinitis. J Physiol Pharmacol. 59 Suppl 6:153-61.

[16] Buday, T.; Brozmanova, M.; Biringerova, Z.; et al. (2012).Modulation of cough response by sensory inputs from the nose - role of trigeminal TRPA1 versus TRPM8 channels. *Cough,* 3; 8(1):11.

[17] Canning, B.J. (2006). Anatomy and neurophysiology of the cough reflex: ACCP Evidence-Based Clinical Practice Guidelines. *Chest,* 129: 33-47.

[18] Canning, B.J. (2010). Afferent nerves regulating the cough reflex: Mechanisms and mediators of cough in disease. *Otolaryngol Clin North Am*; 43 (1): 15-vii.

[19] Canning, B.J.; Mazzone, S.B.; Meeker, S.B.; et al. (2004). Identification of tracheal and laryngeal afferent neurons mediating cough in anaesthetized guinea-pigs. *J Physiol,* 557: 543-558.

[20] Canning, B.J.; Mazzone, S.B.; Mori, N.; et al. (2004). Identification of the tracheal and laryngeal afferent neurons mediating cough in anaesthetized Guinea apigs. *J Physiol,* 557 (2), 543-558.

[21] Canning, B.J.; Mori, N, Mazzone, S.B. (2006). Vagal afferent nerves regulating the cough reflex. *Respir Physiol Neurobiol,* 152: 223-242.

[22] Canning, B.J.; Mori, N.; Farmer, D. (2004). Permissive but not essential role of capsaicin-sensitive afferent nerves in citric acid-induced cough in anesthetized guinea pigs. *Am J Repsir Crit Care Med*; 169: A799.

[23] Canninng, B.J.; Chou, Y.L. (2009). Cough sensors. I. Physiological and pharmocological properties of the afferent nerves regulating cough. *Handb Exp Pharmacol,* 187: 23-47.

[24] Chang, A.B. (2005). Cough: are children really different to adults? *Cough*; 1: 7.

[25] Chang, A.B. (2006). The physiology of cough. *Paediatr Respir Rev,* 7 (1): 2-8.

[26] Chang, A.B.; Eastburn, M.M.; Gafney, J.; et al (2005). Cough quality in children: a comparison of subjective vs. bronchoscopic findings. *Respiratory Research,* 6: 3.

[27] Chang, A.B.; Glomb, W.B. (2006). Guidelines for evaluating chronic cough in pediatrics. *Chest,* 129: 260S-283S.

[28] Chang, A.B.; Landau, L.I.; Van Asperin, P.P.; et al. (2006). Cough in children: definitions and clinical evaluation. Position statement of the Thoracic Society of Australia and New Zealand. *MJA* 2006; 184: 398-403.

[29] Chang, A.B.; Phelan, P.D. Roberts, R.G. (1996). Capsaicin cough receptor sensitivity test in children. *Eur Respir J,* 9 (11): 2220-2223.

[30] Chen, C.Y.; Joad, J.P. Bonham, A.C. et al. (2009). Central mechanisms I: plasticity of central pathways. *Hand Exp Pharmacol,* (187): 187-201.

[31] Chou, Y.L, Scarupa, M.D. Mori, N. (2008). Differential effect of airway afferent nerve subtypes on cough and respiration in anesthetized guinea pigs. *Am J Physiol Regul Integr Comp Physiol,* 295 (5): R1572-1584.

[32] Chung, K.F.; Widdicombe, J.G. (2009). Pharmacology and Therapeutics of Cough. *Handbook of experimental Pharmacology.* Berlin Heidelberg, Springer-Verlag.

[33] Cole, P. (1998). Physiology of the nose and paranasal sinuses. *Clin Rev Allergy Immunol 1998,16: 33-51.*

[34] Couriel, J.M. (1994). Passive smoking and the health of children. *Thorax,* 49: 731-734.

[35] Craven, V.; Everard, M.L. (2013). Protracted bacterial bronchitis: reinventing an old disease. *Arch Dis Child,* 98(1):72-76.

[36] Curley, F.J.; Irwin, R.S.; Pratter, M.R. et al. (1988). Cough an the common cold. *Am Rev Respir Dis 1988, 138: 305 – 311.*

[37] Davenport, P.W. (2008). Urge-to-cough: what can it teach us about cough? *Lung.,*186 Suppl 1:S107-11.

[38] De Sutter, A.I.; van Driel, M.L.; Kumar, A.A.; et al. (2012). Oral antihistamine-decongestant-analgesic combinations for the common cold. *Cochrane Database Syst Rev,*15;2:CD004976.

[39] DeBlasio, F.B.; Dicpinigaitis, P.V.; DeDanieli, G.; et al. (2012). Efficacy of levodropropizin in pediatric cough. *Pulm Pharmacol & Ther,* (25): 337-342.

[40] Dicpinigaitis PV, Rhoton WA, Bhat R, NegassA A.Investigation of the urge-to-cough sensation in healthy volunteers. 2011 *Respirology.* 17, 337–341.

[41] Dicpinigaitis, P.V. (2007). Experimentally induced cough. *Pulm Pharmacol Ther,* 20 (4): 319-324.

[42] Dicpinigaitis, P.V.; Bhat, R.; Rhoton, W.A.; et al. (2011). Effect of viral upper respiratory tract infection on the urge-to-cough sensation. Respir Med. 105(4):615-618.

[43] Fontana, G.A. (2003). Motor mechanisms and the mechanics of cough. In: Chung, K.F.; Widdicombe, J.G.; Boushey, H.A., eds. *Cough: Causes, Mechanisms and Therapy.* Oxford, UK: Blackwell Publishing, 2003; 193-205, ISBN 1-4051-1634-X.

[44] Fujimura, M.; Kasahara, K.; Kamio, Y.; et al. (1996). Female gender as a determinant of cough threshold to inhaled capsaicin. *Eur Respir J,* 9:1624–1626.

[45] Gibson, G.R. (1989). Enalapril-induced cough. *Arch Intern Med,* 149:2701–2703.

[46] Grace, M.S.; Dubuis, E.; Birrell, M.A.; et al. (2013) Pre-clinical studies in cough research: Role of Transient Receptor Potential (TRP) channels. *Pulm Pharmacol Ther,* 26(5): 498–507.

[47] Gupta, A.; McKean, M.; Chang, A.B. (2007). Management of chronic non-specific cough in childhood: an evidence-based review. *Arch Dis Child Educ Pract Ed*, 92(2):33-39.

[48] Hallander, H.O.; Gnarpe, J.; Gnarpe, H.; et al. (1999). Bordetella pertussis, Bordetella parapertussis, Mycoplasma pneumoniae, Chlamydia pneumoniae and persistent cough in children. *Scand J Infect Dis*, 31: 281-286.

[49] Hanacek, J.; Davies, A.; Widdicombe. J.G. (1984). Influence of lung stretch receptors on the cough reflex in rabbits. *Respiration*, 45: 161-168.

[50] Hay, A.D.; Heron, J.; Ness, A.; ALSPAC study team. (2005). The prevalence of symptoms and consultations in pre-school children in the Avon Longitudinal Study of Parents and Children (ALSPAC): a prospective cohort study. *Fam Pract*, 22(4):367-374.

[51] Hay, A.D.; Schroeder, K.; Fahey, T. (2004). Acute cough in children. 10-minute consultation. *BMJ* 2004; 328: 1062.

[52] Hay, A.D.; Wilson, A.D. (2002). The natural history of acute cough in children aged 0 to 4 years in primary care: a systematic review. *Br J Gen Pract*, 52: 401-409.

[53] Ho, C.Y.; Gu, Q.; Lin, Y.S.; et al. (2001). Sensitivity of vagal afferent endings to chemical irritants in the rat lung. *Resp Physiol*, 127: 113-124.

[54] Holinger, L.D. (1986). Chronic Cough in Infants and Children. *Laryngoscope*, 96: 316-322.

[55] Huang, W.; You, Y. (2012). Treatment of chronic rhinosinusitis in children with main complaint of chronic cough. *Lin Chung Er Bi Yan Hou Tou Jing Wai Ke Za Zhi*, 26(21):993-994.

[56] Irwin, R.S.; Glomb, W.B.; Chang, A.B. (2006). Habit cough, tic cough, and psychogenic cough in adult and peddiatric populations: ACCP evidence-based clinical practice guidelines. *Chest*, 129 (suppl): 174S-179S.

[57] Irwin, R.S.; Pratter, M.R.; Holand, P.S. et al. (1984). Postnasal drip causes cough and is associated with reversible upper airway obstruction. *Chest*, 85: 346-352.

[58] Isbister, G.K.; Prior, F.; Kilham, H.A. (2012). Restricting cough and cold medicines in children. *J Paediatr Child Health*, 48(2):91-8.

[59] Jackson, A.P.; Simenson, S. (2013). Management of common cold symptoms with over-the-counter medications: clearing the confusion. *Postgrad Med*, 125(1):73-81.

[60] Jakus, J. (1999). *Neurónové mechanizmy dýchania a respiračných reflexov*. Bratislava: Univerzita Komenského; 5-60, ISBN 80-223-1379-3.

[61] Jakus, J.; Tomori, Z.; Stransky, A. (2004). *Neuronal determinants of breathing, coughing and related motor behaviours*. Martin, Slovakia: Wist, 95-186, ISBN 80-8049-381-2.

[62] Javorkova, N.; Varechova, S.; Pecova, R.; et al. (2008) Acidification of the esophagus acutely increases the cough sensitivity in patients with gastro-oesophageal reflux and chronic cough. *Neurogastroenterol Motil*, 20(2):119-24.

[63] Karlsson, J.A. (1996). The role of capsaicin-sensitive C-fibers afferent nerves in the cough reflex. *Pulm Pharmacol*, 9: 315-321.

[64] Kollarik, M.; Dinh, Q.T.; Fischer, A.; et al. (2003). Capsaicin-sensitive and –insensitive vagal bronchopulmonary C-fibers in the mouse. *J Physiol*, 551: 869-879.

[65] Kollarik, M.; Ru, F;, Undem. (2007). Acid-sensitive vagal sensory pathways and cough. *Pulm Pharmacol Ther*, 20 (4): 402-411.

[66] Kollarik, M.; Undem, B.J. (2006). Sensory transduction in cough-associated nerves. *Respir Physiol Neurobiol,* 152 (3): 243-254.

[67] Kollarik, M.; Undem, B.J. Plasticity of vagal afferent fibers mediating cough. In: Chung, K.F.; Widdicombe, J.G.; Boushey, H.A., eds. *Cough: Causes, Mechanisms and Therapy.* Oxford, UK: Blackwell Publishing, 2003; 181-192, ISBN 1-4051-1634-X.

[68] Korpas, J,; Tomori, Z. (1979). *Cough and Other Respiratory Reflexes.* Basel: S Karger, 1979; 356 s., ISBN 978-80-89182-22-0.

[69] Koskela, H.O.; Purokivi, M.K. (2013). Capability of hypertonic saline cough provocation test to predict the response to inhaled corticosteroids in chronic cough: a prospective, open-label study *Cough,* 9:15 doi: 10.1186/1745-9974-9-15.

[70] Kummer, W.; Fiecher, A.; Kurkowski, R. (1992). The sensory and sympathetic innervation of guinea-pig lung and trachea as studied by retrograde neuronal tracing and double-labelling immunohistochemistry. *Neuroscience,* 49: 715-737.

[71] Leder, K.; Sinclair, M.I.; Mitakakis, T.Z.; et al. (2003). A community-based study of respiratory episodes in Melbourne, Australia. *Aust N Z J Public Health,* 27(4):399-404.

[72] Leo, G.; Incorvaia, C.; Masieri, S,; et al. (2010). Imaging criteria for diagnosis of chronic rhinosinusitis in children. *Eur Ann Allergy Clin Immunol.* 42(6):199-204.

[73] Levi, L.R.; Tyler, G.R.; Olson, L.G.; et al.: (1990). Lack of airway response to nasal iritation in normal and asthmatic subjects. *Aus Nz J Med,* 20:578-582.

[74] Li, J.S.; Peat, J.K.; Xuan, W.; et al. (1999). Meta-analysis on the association between environmental tobacco smoke (ETS) exposure and the prevalence of lower respiratory tract infection in early childhood. *Pediatr Pulmonol,* 27: 5-13.

[75] Littel, N. T.; Carlisle, C.C.; Millman, R.P.; et al.: (1990). Changes in airway resistance following nasal provocation. *Am Rev Respir Dis, 141:580-583.*

[76] Lee, L.Y.; Pisari, T.E. (2001). Afferent properties and reflex functions of bronchopulmonary C- fibers. *Respir Physiol, 125, 47-65.*

[77] Marchant, J.M.; Newcombe, P.A.; Juniper, E.F.; et al. (2008). What is the burden of chronic cough for families? Chest, 134(2):303-9.

[78] Mazzone, S.B. (2004). Sensory regulation of the cough reflex. *Pulm Pharmacol Ther,* 17: 361-368.

[79] Mazzone, S.B. (2005). An overview of the sensory receptors regulating cough. *Cough,* 1: 2.

[80] Mazzone, S.B.; Canning, B.J. (2002). Central nervous system control of the airways: pharmacological implications. *Curr Opin Pharmacol*; 2: 220-228.

[81] Mazzone, S.B.; Canning, B.J. (2002). Plasticity of the cough reflex. *Eur Respir Rev,* 85: 236-242.

[82] Mazzone, S.B.; Canning, B.J. (2002). Synergistic interactions between airway afferent nerve subtypes regulating the cough reflex in guinea pigs. *Am J Physiol Reg Int Comp Physiol,* 283: R86-R98.

[83] Mazzone, S.B.; Canning, B.J.; Widdicombe, J.G. (2003). Sensory pathways for the cough reflex. In: Chung, K.F.; Widdicombe, J.G.; Boushey, H.A.; eds. *Cough: Causes, Mechanisms and Therapy.* Oxford, UK: Blackwell Publishing, 2003; 161-171, ISBN 1-4051-1634-X.

[84] Mazzone, S.B.; Mori, N.; Canning, B.J. (2002). Bradykinin-induced cough in conscious guinea-pigs. *Am J Respir Crit Care Med*; 165: A773.

[85] Mazzone, S.B.; Reynolds, S.M.; Mori, N.; at al. (2009).Selective expression of a sodium pump isozyme by cough receptors and evidence for its essential role in regulating cough. *J Neurosci,* 29 (43): 13662-13671.

[86] McAlexander, M.A.; Carr, M.J. (2009). Peripheral mechanisms I: plasticity of peripheral pathways. *Hand Exp Pharmacol,* (187): 129-154.

[87] McCormick, A.; Flemming, D.; Charlton, J. (1991-1992). *Morbidity statistics from general practice fourth national morbidity survey.* London, UK, MHSO, Office for National Statistics, 1991-92.

[88] McKay, K.O. (2000). Gender differences in airway wall structure in infant lungs (abstract). *Am J Respir Crit Care Med*; 161:A111.

[89] Morice, A.H. (2013). Chronic cough hypersensitivity syndrome. *Cough.* 13;9(1):14.

[90] Morice AH. Epidemilogy of cough (2002). *Pulm Pharmacol Ther,* 15:253-259.

[91] Morice, A.H.; Fontana, A.G.; Sovijarvi, A.R.A.; et al. (2004). The diagnosis and management of chronic cough. *Eur Respir J,* 24: 481-492.

[92] Morice, A.H.; Higgins, K.S.; Yeo, W.W. (1991). Adaptation of cough reflex with different types of stimulation. *Eur Respir J,* 5:841-847.

[93] Morice, A.H.; Fontana G.A.; Belvisi, M.; et al. (2007). ERS guidelines on the assessment of cough. *Eur Respir J,* 29: 1256-1276.

[94] Myers, A.C.; Kajekar, R.; Undem, B.J. (2002). Allergic inflammation induced neuropeptide production in rapidly adapting afferent nerves in guinea pig airways. *Am J Physiol Lung Cell Mol Physiol*, 282: 775-781.

[95] O' Connell, F.; Thomas, V.E.; Studham, J.M.; et al. (1996). Capsaicin cough sensitivity increases during upper respiratory infection. *Resp Med*, 9:279–286.

[96] O'Hara, J.; Jones, N.S. (2006). 'Post-nasal drip syndrome': most patients with purulent nasal secretions do not complain of chronic cough. *Rhinology*; 44 (4): 270-273.

[97] Olarinde, O.; Banerjee, A.R.; O'Callaghan, C. (2006). Effect of sleeping position on nasal patency in newborns. *Arch Dis Child Fetal Neonatal Ed,* 91(5): F365–F366.

[98] Os, I.; Bratland, B.; Dahlof, B.; et al. (1994). Female preponderance for lisinopril-induced cough in hypertension. *Am J Hypertens*, 7:1012–1015.

[99] Palmer, R.; Anon, J.B.; Gallagher, P. (2011). Pediatric cough: what the otolaryngologist needs to know. *Curr Opin Otolaryngol Head Neck Surg,* 19(3):204-209.

[100] Pecova, R.; Vrlik, M.; Tatar, M. (2005). Cough sensitivity in allergic rhinitis. *J Physiol Pharmacol.*, 56 Suppl 4:171-178.

[101] Pickens, D.L.; Schefft, G.; Thach, B.T. (1988). Prolonged apnea associated with upper airway protective reflexes in apnea of prematurity. *Am Rev Respir Dis,* 137(1):113-118.

[102] Plevkova J, Varechova S, Brozmanova M, Tatar M: Changes of the cough sensitivity in children with cough persisting after common cold from predisease testing to values after the recovery. *Acta Med Martiniana*, 2008 (7): 13-19.

[103] Plevkova, J.; Brozmanova, M.; Pecova, R.; et al. (2004). Effects of intranasal capsaicin challenge on cough reflex in healthy human volunteers. *J Physiol Pharmacol*, 55 (Suppl 3): 101-106.

[104] Plevkova, J.; Brozmanova, M.; Pecova, R.; et al. (2005). Effects of intranasal histamine on the cough reflex in subjects with allergic rhinitis. *J Physiol Pharmacol*, 56 Suppl 4:185-95.

[105] Plevkova, J.; Kollarik, M.; Brozmanova, M.; et al. (2004). Modulation of experimentally-induced cough by stimulation of nasal mucosa in cats and guinea pigs. *Respir Physiol Neurobiol*, 142 (2-3): 225-235.

[106] Plevkova, J.; Song, W.J. Chronic cough in subjects with upper airway diseases - analysis of mechanisms and clinical applications. (2013). *Asia Pac Allergy*, (2):127-35.

[107] Plevkova, J.; Varechova, S.; Brozamnova, M.; et al (2008). Changes f the cough sensitivity in children with cough persisting after common cold from pre-disease testing to values after the recovery of common cold symptoms. *Acta Med Martiniana*, 7 (3): 13-19.

[108] Plevkova, J.; Varechova, S.; Brozmanova, M.; et al. (2006). Testing of cough reflex sensitivity in children suffering from allergic rhinitis and common cold. J Physiol Pharmacol, 57 Suppl 4:289-296.

[109] Plevkova, J.; Kollarik, M.; Poliacek, I.; et al. (2013). The role of trigeminal nasal TRPM8-expressing afferent neurons in theantitussive effects of menthol. *J Appl Physiol*, 115, 268-274.

[110] Pratter, M.R. (2006). Chronic upper airway cough syndrome secondary to rhinosinus diseases (previously referred to as postasal drip syndrome). *Chest*; 129: 63S-71S.

[111] Pratter, M.R. (2006). Cough and the common cold: ACCP evidence-based clinical practice guidelines. *Chest*, 129 (suppl): 72S-74S.

[112] Pratter, M.R. (2006). Unexplained (idiopathic) cough: ACCP evidence-based clinical practice guidelines. *Chest*, 129 (suppl): 220S-221.

[113] Qian, Z.; Chapman, R.S.; Hu, W.; et al. (2004). Using air pollution based community clusters to explore air pollution health effects in children. Environ Int, 30(5):611-20.

[114] Roberts, G.; Xatzipsalti, M.; Borrego, L.M.; et al. (2013). Paediatric rhinitis: position paper of the *European Academy of Allergy and Clinical Immunology*, 68, 9:1102–1116.

[115] Sant´Ambrogio, G.; Kuna, S.T.; Vanoye, C.R.; et al. (1997). Activation of intrinsic laryngeal muscles during cough. *Am J Respir Crit Care Med*, 155: 637-641.

[116] Sant´Ambrogio, G.; Sant´Ambrogio, F.B.; Davies, A. (1984). Airway receptors in cough. *Bull Eur Physiolpathol Respir*, 20: 43-47.

[117] Sarin, S.; Undem, B.; Sanico, A.; et al. (2006).The role of the nervous system in rhinitis. J *Allergy Clin Immunol*, 118(5):999-1016.

[118] Schaad, U.B.; Rossi, E (1982). Infantile chlamydial pneumonia--a review based on 115 cases. *Eur J Pediatr*, 138(2):105-9.

[119] Schelegle, E.S.; Green, J.F. (2001). An overwiew of the anatomy and physiology of slowly adapting pulmonary stretch receptors. *Resp Physiol*, 125: 17-31.

[120] Shannon, R.; Baekey, D.M.; Morris K,F.; et al. (1998). Ventrolateral medullary respiratory network and a model of cough motor pattern generation. *J Appl Physiol*, 84: 2020-2035.

[121] Shields, M.D.; Bush, A.; Everard, M.L; et al. (2008). Cough Guideline Group. *Thorax* 2008; 63: 65.

[122] Shroeder, K.; Fahey, T. (2002). Should we advise parents to administer over the counter cough medicines for acute cough? Systemic review of randomized controlled trials. *Arch Dis Child*, 88: 170-175.

[123] Tatar M, Karcolova D, Pecova R, Kollarik M, Plevkova J, Brozmanova M: Experimental modulation of the cough reflex. Eu. Respir Rev 2002, 85: 264-269.

[124] Tatar, M.; Plevkova, J.; Brozmanova, M.; et al. (2009). Mechanisms of the cough associated with rhinosinusitis. *Pulm Pharmacol Ther*, 22 (2): 121-126.

[125] Tatar, M.; Webber, S.E.; Widdicombe, J.G. (1988). Lung C – fibre receptor activation and defensive reflexes in anaesthetized cats. *J Physiol* (London), 402:411-420.

[126] Tatar, M.; Webber,S.E.; Widdicombe, J.G. (1988). Lung C-fibre receptor activation and defensive reflexes in dogs. *J Physiol*, 402: 411-420.

[127] Tatar,M.; Karcolova, D.; Pecova ,R.; et al (2002). Experimental modulation of the cough reflex. *Eur Respir Rev*, 85: 264-269.

[128] Taussig, L.M.; Smith S.M.; Blumenfeld, R. Chronic bronchitis in childhood: what is it? *Pediatrics* 1981; 67: 1-5.

[129] Thach, B.T. (2007). Maturation of cough and other reflexes that protect the fetal and neonatal airway. *Pulm Pharmacol Ther*, 20(4):365-370.

[130] Thomson, F.; Mastrers, I.B.; Chang, A.B. (2002). Persistent cough in children – overuse of medications. *J Paediatr Child Health* 2002; 38: 578-581.

[131] Togias, A. (1999). Mechanisms of nose-lung interaction. *Allergy*, 54 Suppl 57:94-105.

[132] Undem, B.J.; Carr, M.J.; Kollarik, M. (2002) Physiology and plasticity of putative cough fibers in the guinea pig. *Pulm Pharmacol Ther*, 15: 193-198.

[133] Undem, B.J.; Carr, M.J.; Kollarik, M. (2002). Physiology and plasticity of putative cough fibers in the guinea pig. *Pulm Pharmacol Ther* 2002; 15: 193-198.

[134] van Strien, R.T.; Gent, J.F.; Belanger, K.; et al. (2004). Exposure to NO2 and nitrous acid and respiratory symptoms in the first year of life. *Epidemiology*, 15(4):471-8.

[135] Varechova, S.; Plevkova, J.; Hanacek, J.; et al. (2008). Role of gender and pubertal stage on cough sensitivity in childhood and adolescence. *J Physiol Pharmacol*, 59 Suppl 6:719-26.

[136] Weigand, L.A.; Undem, B.J.(2012). Allergen-induced neuromodulation in the espiratory tract. *Chem Immunol Allergy.*, 98:142-62.

[137] Widdcombe, J.G. (2001). Airway receptors. *Respir Physiol*, 125: 3-15.

[138] Widdicombe, J.G. (1954). Respiratory reflexes excited by inflation of the lungs. *J Physiol*; 123: 105-115.

[139] Widdicombe, J.G. (2003). Functional morphology and physiology of rapidly adapting receptors (RARs). *Anat Rec*; 270A: 2-10.

[140] Widdicombe, J.G. A brief overview of the mechanisms of cough. In: Chung, K.F.; Widdicombe, J.G.; Boushey, H.A. eds. *Cough: Causes, Mechanisms and Therapy*. Oxford, UK: Blackwell Publishing, 2003a; 17-23, ISBN 1-4051-1634-X.

[141] Widdocimbe, J.G. (1996). Sensory neurophysiology of the cough reflex. *J Allergy Clin Immunol*, 98 (5): 84-90.

[142] Woodcock, A.; Young, E.C.; Smith, J.A. (2010). New insights in cough. *Br. Med Bull*, 96:61-7.

Reviewed by:

Assoc. Prof. Ivan Poliacek, MSc., Ph.D. – Department of Medical Biophysics, Comenius University in Bratislava, Jessenius Faculty of Medicine in Martin, Slovakia

In: Advances in Respiratory Therapy Research
Editor: Miloš Jeseňák
ISBN: 978-1-63463-004-7
© 2015 Nova Science Publishers, Inc.

Chapter 5

Primary Ciliary Dyskinesia – Current Therapeutic Approach

Peter Durdik* and Peter Banovcin
Department of Pediatrics,
Center of Experimental and Clinical Respirology,
Comenius University Jessenius Faculty of Medicine, Martin, Slovakia

Abstract

Primary ciliary dyskinesia is a rare heterogeneous genetic disorder with an incidence estimated to be between 1:2000 and 1:40000. Over 250 proteins are involved in the formation of cilia and to date, the twenty-six genes have been identified in association with primary ciliary dyskinesia. However, despite the various genotypes that can cause primary ciliary dyskinesia, the clinical phenotypes are very similar. Affected ciliary function is characterized by ciliary immotility or dysmotility, impairing mucociliary clearance which is responsible for typical clinical symptoms (chronic recurrent upper and lower respiratory tract infections, male sterility and situs inversus in 40% - 50% of patients). Early diagnosis is essential to ensure specialist management and to reduce respiratory and ontological complications. The diagnosis of primary ciliary dyskinesia should be established on the presence of the characteristic clinical phenotype, appropriate screening tests, specific ultrastructural ciliary defects, evidence of abnormal ciliary function and genetic analysis. There is currently no specific pharmacological, non-pharmacological or surgical treatment that restores normal ciliary motility and improves mucus clearance. All treatment recommendations are based on very low level evidence. The guidelines for the management of primary ciliary dyskinesia in children, published by the ERS PCD Task Force in 2009, present the treatment based on periodic monitoring of the general condition, respiratory and auditory function, promotion of drainage of secretions through respiratory physiotherapy and physical exercise and aggressive

* Corresponding Author address: Peter Durdik, M.D., Ph.D., Department of Pediatris, Center of Experimental and Clinical Respirology, Jessenius Faculty of Medicine in Martin, Comenius University in Bratislava, University Hospital, Kollarova 2, 036 59, Martin, Slovak Republic, e-mail: Peter.Durdik@jfmed.uniba.sk

antibiotic treatment of respiratory infections. The curative treatment of primary ciliary dyskinesia is still unavailable, although gene therapy has major potential for treating ciliopathies. Other recently presented positive therapeutic modalities include alpha-1-antitrypsin, antiprotease and secretory immunoglobulin A.

Keywords: Ciliary Motility, Gene Therapy, Mucociliar Clearance, Pharmacotherapy, Physiotherapy, Primary Ciliary Dyskinesia

1. Introduction

Cilia are evolutionary conserved organelles localized on the surface of most human cell types. The specific and highly organized ultrastructure of microtubules gives this organelle an irreplaceable role in a plethora of cellular functions and normal developmental processes, from the flagella that propel the sperm and the nodal cilia that determine the left-right axis to the motile cilia that transport the egg through the fallopian tube or defend the upper and lower respiratory system. There is a typical "9+2" arrangement with nine doublets of peripheral microtubules, the central pair of single microtubules being specifically connected by nexin links and radial spokes and the ATPase activity of inner and outer dynein arms creates the sophisticated motile organelle [4, 25, 77, 86]. In healthy individuals, respiratory motile cilia with typical "9+2" arrangement are bathed in a layer of periciliary fluid and characteristically coordinated ciliary motility pattern propelling the overlying mucus towards the oropharynx where the mucus is swallowed or expectorated. Motile respiratory cilia and the character of respiratory mucus are the main components of mucociliary clearance playing a key role in the innate immunity of the respiratory system. The structure of the sperm flagella is similar to the ultrastructure of respiratory cilia while nodal cilia have a "9+0" arrangement, lacking the central pair of microtubules but still able to create a typical ciliary motility pattern [41, 63]. Apart from motile cilia, in other cell types throughout the body, primary or immotile cilia are utilized for the sensing of external stimuli (light, fluid flow, etc.) or are found on the tubular epithelial cells of the kidney (defective in polycystic kidney disease) [19, 43]. Alternation in the specific protein arrangement of cilia underlies a growing class of pleiotropic disorders termed ciliopathies [14]. A number of proteins creating and formatting cilia are responsible for the wide-ranging and expanding spectrum of ciliopathies [7, 24]. The mutations that affect structures or processes conserved between motile and primary cilia would result in a disease phenotype reflecting the function of both types of cilia, whereas mutations affecting pathways specific to one type of cilia would result in a more limited spectrum of disease. Primary ciliary dyskinesia is a subgroup of the family of ciliopathies affecting sperm flagella and motile cilia lining the respiratory epithelium, fallopian tubes and brain ventricles [89].

2. Definition

Primary ciliary dyskinesia is predominantly inherited as an autosomal recessive disorder characterized by chronic infection of the upper and lower respiratory tract and, in about 50% of cases, situs inversus and other forms of heterotaxy. In addition, male infertility is common.

The airway symptoms are mainly a result of impaired mucociliary clearance resulting in mucus accumulation often containing bacteria and allergens and leading to mucus stagnation, inflammation and chronic infection [2, 46].

Table 1. Summary of the most common molecular genetic testing used in primary ciliary dyskinesia [18, 38, 94]

Genetic Background of Primary Ciliary Dyskinesia

Gene/Locus Name	Ultrastructure Defect	Locus	Proportion of all PCD [%]
DNAI1 / CILD1	Outer dynein arms	9p13.3	2 - 9% [23, 94]
DNAAF3 / CILD2	Outer and Inner dynein arms	19q13.42	Unknown [57]
DNAH5 / CILD3	Outer dynein arms	5p15	15-21% [22, 60]
Unknown / CILD4	Normal	15q13.1-q15.1	Unknown
HYDIN / CILD5	Normal	16q22.2	Unknown [61]
NME8(TXNDC3) / CILD6	Outer dynein arms	7p14.1	Unknown [21]
DNAH11 / CILD7	Normal	7p15.3	6% [39]
Unknown / CILD8	Unknown	15q24-q25	Unknown
DNAI2 / CILD9	Outer dynein arms	17q25.1	2% [45]
DNAAF2(C14orf104,KTU,PF13) /ILD10	Outer and Inner dynein arms	14q21.3	<2% [62]
RSPH4A / CILD11	Central pair	6q22.1	Unknown [15]
RSPH9 / CILD12	Central pair	6q22.1	Unknown [15]
DNAAF1 (LRRC50) / CILD13	Outer and Inner dynein arms	16q23.3-q24.1	4-5% [20, 44]
CCDC39 / CILD14	Inner dynein arms and Axonemal organization	3q26.33	2-10% [56]
CCDC40 / CILD15	Inner dynein arms and Axonemal organization	17q25.3	1-8% [3, 6]
DNAL1 / CILD16	Outer dynein arms	14q24.3	Unknown
CCDC103 / CILD17	Outer and Inner dynein arms	17q21.31	Unknown [64]
HEATR2 / CILD18	Outer and Inner dynein arms	7p22.3	Unknown [31]
LRRC6 / CILD19	Outer and Inner dynein arms	8q24.22	3% [42]
CCDC114	Outer dynein arms	19q13.33	Unknown
CCDC164 (DRC1)	Nexin link and Axonemal organization	2p23.3	Unknown
RPGR	Mixed	Xp21.1	Unknown
OFD1	Unknown	Xq22	Unknown
ARMC4	Outer dynein arms	10p12.1	Unknown
DYX1C1 (DNAAF4)	Outer and Inner dynein arms	15q21.3	Unknown
ZMYND10	Outer and Inner dynein arms	3p21.31	Unknown
CCDC65	Inner dynein arms and nexin link	12q13.12	Unknown
RSPH1	Central pair and Radial spoke	21q22.3	Unknown
SPAG1	Outer and Inner dynein arms	8q22.2	Unknown

The impaired mucociliary clearance is the consequence of altered ciliary beat frequency (static cilia, reduced beat frequency or hyperfrequency) or asynchronous beating pattern or both that is usually, but not always, associated with structural abnormality of cilia [2, 10]. The incidence varies widely from 1:2000 to 1:40000 cases explained by the broad spectrum of clinical manifestation and severity and the lack of standard diagnostic procedures. In addition, many cases of primary ciliary dyskinesia are still undiagnosed [46]. Recent technological advances in biomedicine and technological improvement have increased the ability to recognize and establish the primary ciliary dyskinesia as the reason for chronic respiratory disease in youth followed by appropriate treatment. This creates an assumption for improved long-term prognosis [2, 28, 40].

3. Genetics of Primary Ciliary Dyskinesia

Primary ciliary dyskinesia is inherited in an autosomal recessive manner. The parents of the affected child are asymptomatic heterozygotes and therefore carry the mutant allele. Each child of such parents has a 25% chance of being affected, a 50% chance of being an asymptomatic carrier and a 25% chance of being fully healthy. Over 250 proteins are involved in the formation of cilia and so the disease-causing genes are commonly very large and mostly unrecognized. To date, the twenty six genes have been identified in association with primary ciliary dyskinesia, mainly leading to dynein arm or radial spoke defects. The most frequent are DNAH5 and DNAI1 [18, 23, 31, 37, 52].

4. Clinical Manifestation of Primary Ciliary Dyskinesia

The diagnosis of primary ciliary dyskinesia should be established in specialist centers based on the presence of a typical clinical phenotype, appropriate screening and diagnostic test and genetic analysis [2, 84]. The association of chronic sinopulmonary disease with situs inversus has been known for the last 100 years, having been first reported by SIEWART in 1904 as a case of bronchiectasis associated with situs inversus [81], and in 1933 Kartagener described cases of situs inversus and bronchiectasis that were all associated with sinusitis [36]. Typical Kartagener phenotype is chronic or recurrent sinusitis, infertility and situs inversus. Especially children with chronic sinopulmonary disease and situs inversus are highly suspected for the diagnosis of primary ciliary dyskinesia, otherwise known as Kartagener's syndrome. In general, children with primary ciliary dyskinesia often have chronic upper or lower respiratory tract symptoms, typically a chronic wet-sounding cough and occasionally symptoms of airway obstruction – wheezing or shortness of breath [14, 18, 46]. Chronic rhinitis, recurrent sinusitis or otitis, symptoms associated with ciliary dysfunction, are frequent in many various diseases in children and can delay diagnosis of primary ciliary dyskinesia. In addition to the presented results of clinical studies the ERS Task Force recommends [2] that primary ciliary dyskinesia should be considered when the following features are observed:

a) a positive family history of primary ciliary dyskinesia,

b) unexplained chronic sinusitis, otitis or rhinitis in children,

c) chronic productive cough and unexplained non-cystic bronchiectasis,

d) unexplained severe neonatal respiratory distress,

e) complex congenital heart disease, especially with disorders of laterality (e.g. atrial isomerism, transposition of great vessels, double-outlet right ventricle, anomalous venous return, interrupted inferior vena cava, bilateral superior vena cava) [95],

f) asplenia (right isomerism) or polysplenia (left isomerism) [74],

g) polycystic kidney or liver disease [1],

h) cerebral ventriculomegaly at any age in the absence of obvious cause [5],

i) biliary atresia [5],

j) severe esophageal disease (esophageal atresia and severe reflux),

k) retinal degeneration – retinitis pigmentosa [58],

l) oral-facial-digital syndrome type 1 [8],

m) infertility – immotile sperm in males or females with recurrent ectopic pregnancy.

Typical clinical symptoms of primary ciliary dyskinesia develop and change depending on the age of the child. The antenatal period is characterized by situs inversus, heterotaxy or mild fetal cerebral ventriculomegaly on ultrasound screening [14]. In the neonatal period more than 75% of full-term newborns exhibit neonatal respiratory distress requiring an oxygen supply for days to weeks. In addition, continuous rhinorrhea from the first day of life, mirror-image organ arrangement or hydrocephalus of unknown origin may reflect dysfunction of motile or immotile cilia [2, 59, 82]. Childhood is the period with a broad spectrum of typical or atypical clinical presentation. In infants and preschool children the chronic upper respiratory tract infections are frequent, especially due to socialization in playschools, but suspected ciliary dysfunction should induce daily rhinitis without remission, recurrent otitis media with effusion and often obstructive bronchitis, recurrent pneumonia, and chronic productive or a wet-sounding cough. In older children severe chronic sinusitis, atypical asthma that is non-responsive to treatment, idiopathic bronchiectasis or hearing abnormalities can be presented in patients with primary ciliary dyskinesia. Adolescence and adult life in patients with ciliary dysfunction is characterized by a worsening of the symptoms from childhood (chronic mucopurulent sputum, more evident bronchiectasis) and the appearance of infertility in males or ectopic pregnancy in females [2, 9, 17, 18].

Bronchiectasis is described in about 50-70% of children with primary ciliary dyskinesia and the middle lobe and lingula followed by the lower lobes are the most frequent distribution. The severity of bronchiectasis is age dependent and deteriorates with worsening lung function and colonization of airways [37, 76, 83]. The most frequent pathogens isolated from sputum in primary ciliary dyskinesia are Heamophilus influenza, Streptococcus pneumoniae, Staphylococcus aureus, P. aeruginosa or nontuberculous mycobacteria [59, 83]. Lung functions deteriorate with increasing age and are characterized by obstructive pulmonary impairment as reflected in spirometric and plethysmographic measurements. Restrictive pulmonary defects may occur after extensive lung resection typically due to severe bronchiectasis associated with frequent local inflammation and mucopurulent production [48, 51, 70, 88].

5. Screening Tests

Screening tests may select the patients with suspected ciliary dysfunction and requiring detailed diagnostic investigations of ciliate epithelial cells in order to assess function (frequency and pattern) and ultrastructure. The spectrum of screening tests includes the saccharin test, radioaerosol mucociliary clearance tests and nasal nitric oxide measurement, where a limitation of these tests is particularly patient compliance. Furthermore, there is insufficient clinical experience of the use of screening tests in children younger than 5 years and the screening tests do not evaluate ciliary dyskinesis selectively (they evaluate ciliary dyskinesis together with abnormalities of mucus) [2, 46]. The ERS PCD Task Force published in 2009 does not recommend using the *saccharin test* in children, because it is difficult to perform and unreliable in children aged less than 12 years [2]. A microtablet of saccharin is placed on the inferior turbinate and the time taken for it to taste sweet is recorded. Normally a time of less than 60 minutes can avoid the disturbance of mucociliary clearance. A positive test is evaluated as an extension of mucociliary clearance with maintaining the ability to detect sweet taste on the tongue, while prolonged MCC is caused by ciliary dyskinesia or abnormalities of mucus (especially the physical or chemical properties of mucus) [13, 46]. *Radioaerosol mucociliary clearance tests* use a radioactive tracer to assess pulmonary or nasal mucociliary clearance. Test sensitivity is high, but specificity low, and therefore both methods are supplementary tests in the diagnostic algorithm of primary ciliary dyskinesia since neither of the tests is diagnostic [2, 50]. In the last 20 years a number of clinical studies have shown that the *nasal nitric oxide concentrations* were lower in patients with primary ciliary dyskinesia. Test specificity of 89% and sensitivity of 100% with a positive predictive value of 89% for correctly diagnosing primary ciliary dyskinesia when using a nasal nitric oxide cut-off level of less than 105ppb predict measurement of nasal nitric oxide as a reliable screening method for primary ciliary dyskinesia [16, 90]. It has been included in the British and European consensus guidelines of primary ciliary dyskinesia. Nasal nitric oxide measurement is not yet approved for clinical use in the USA [2, 84]. The measurement is extremely helpful in guiding the diagnostic pathway, but the major disadvantages are the cost of equipment and consumables and the necessity of patient cooperation (patients' age limit is more than 5 years). The reduced nasal nitric oxide concentrations are explained by four hypotheses:

1. Increased breakdown of nitric oxide to metabolites due to trapped and broken down nitric oxide in viscous sputum or its consumption by denitrifying bacteria.
2. Reduced biosynthesis of nitric oxide caused by decreased expression of nitric oxide synthase isoenzymes, or loss of nitric oxide synthase activity via mechanochemical uncoupling or limitations to availability of the nitric oxide synthase substrate L-arginine.
3. Nitric oxide is trapped in the obstructed paranasal sinuses and decreases nitric oxide release from the paranasal sinuses into the nasal passage.
4. Reduced production and storage capacity of nitric oxide in the paranasal sinuses (hypoplasia or agenesis) [68, 69, 75, 90].

6. Diagnostic Tests

If there is a clinical suspicion of primary ciliary dyskinesia supported by a positive screening test, the diagnosis should be confirmed by analysis of the ciliated epithelium of the respiratory tract [2]. The techniques used to obtain the samples are nasal or bronchial brushing using a cytology brush, but patients should not be brushed within four weeks of an upper respiratory tract infection to avoid secondary dyskinesia or poor ciliate samples. Bronchial biopsy by flexible bronchoscope is also reported as a method of collecting samples. A diagnostic work-up requires the assessment of ciliary beat frequency and ciliary beat pattern with transmission electron microscopy to confirm ultrastructural abnormalities. Air-liquid interface in cell culture is indicated only for difficult diagnostic cases [2, 30, 72].

6.1. Ciliary Beat Pattern and Frequency Analysis

Normal ciliary beat frequency in humans is between 11-18Hz at 37°C (98.6°F) and normal ciliary beat pattern is in the two characteristic cycles: an effective movement phase, in which the cilium extends throughout its length, penetrates into the mucus layer (gel layer) and moves it orally. The second phase is a recovery phase, when the cilium bends in periciliary fluid (sol layer) and returns to the starting position prepared for the next beat [33]. The samples from the nose or bronchial epithelium, collected by the brushing method or biopsy at 37°C (98.6°F), are observed using a 100x objective by light microscopy, a digital high-speed video camera recording of more than 500 frames per second and appropriate software application [2, 29, 34, 85]. Ciliary beat frequency is analysed by using specific mathematical algorithms and ciliary beat pattern by a slow-motion-replay of recorded samples. It is generally accepted that the diagnosis of primary ciliary dyskinesia by ciliary beat frequency and ciliary beat pattern is a necessary diagnostic method and normal results can exclude this diagnosis [29, 33]. In addition, a limitation of this analysis is the necessity of doctor-specialist and still subjective evaluation; therefore, new clinical researches are focusing on the automated analysis of ciliary beat frequency and pattern. Patients with primary ciliary dyskinesia have markedly reduced ciliary beat frequency to approximately 3Hz or static (mainly in outer dynein arms defects or combined outer and inner dynein arms defects). Isolated inner dynein arms defects or radial spoke defects are characterized by a stiff beat pattern with reduced amplitude; ciliary transposition defects leading to circular beat at a frequency of about 10Hz and DNAH11mutation is presented by an altered beat pattern with a hyperkinetic beat frequency [2, 80].

6.2. Electron Microscopy

Electron microscopy was important in the diagnosis of primary ciliary dyskinesia in the recent past, but impaired ciliary beat with normal ciliary ultrastructure has reduced the importance of this diagnostic method as the gold standard in diagnostic procedure [2]. Ultrastructural defects are common but not present in all cases; about 70-80% of patients with primary ciliary dyskinesia have ultrastructural abnormalities involving absent inner or outer dynein arms, radial spoke defects, loss of microtubular arrangement, or missing central pair or transposition defects [65, 73]. The most frequent abnormalities are defects of the outer dynein arms that are well determined in electron microscope and predominantly associated with static or extremely decreased ciliary frequency. It is acknowledged that electron microscopy in the diagnosis of ciliary ultrastructural abnormalities has limitations. One is that specialist knowledge is required in order to interpret the various ultrastructural defects responsible for primary ciliary dyskinesia. In addition, defects of the inner dynein arms are difficult to determine since they are less electron-dense and less frequent along the ciliary axoneme. Furthermore, in normal individuals, primary defects are seen in about 5% of cilia and secondary defects caused by infection, inflammation, smoking and other various pollutants have been described in up to 10% of cilia. These ultrastructural abnormalities cause isolated alterations in ciliary beating or ciliary motility pattern but overall, the mucociliary transport is undisturbed [65, 73, 79, 87]. About 10% of patients with primary ciliary dyskinesia remain undiagnosed due to normal ciliary ultrastructure, particularly in centers where diagnosis depends on electron microscope, with no capacity for high-speed video analysis. This atypical form of primary ciliary dyskinesia with typical phenotype but ciliary hyperfrequency associated with normal ciliary ultrastructure can be caused by mutation in the dynein axonemal heavy chain (DNAH11) [80].

6.3. Air-Liquid Interface Cell Culture

This method is mostly used to reduce false positive diagnoses in patients with secondary ciliary dysfunction, to confirm less common phenotypes or when the sample from brushing or biopsy has possible secondary ciliary defects. Differentiation of basal epithelial cells to ciliated cells is achieved using culture at air-liquid interface. It allows a second diagnostic work-up with reduced environmental factors and the necessity for repeat brushing [2, 30, 35, 72].

6.4. Genetic Analysis

Genetic testing can offer a more profound evaluation of primary ciliary dyskinesia, but it should be reserved until after the clinical diagnosis has been proven and directed for the specific ciliary ultrastructural defects, and should not be part of the initial diagnostic testing. The numerous candidate genes for primary ciliary dyskinesia are identified; clinical genetic analysis is provided only for selected genes depending on the frequency in the specific population. DNAH5, DNAI1 or DNAH11 testing are the most commonly realized [2, 18, 38, 94].

7. Therapy

There is currently no specific pharmacological, non-pharmacological or surgical treatment that restores normal ciliary motility and improves mucus clearance but the main goals of management of primary ciliary dyskinesia should be to make the diagnosis early and start treatment as soon as possible in order to prevent development of secondary complications, especially deterioration in lung function. There are no randomized trials of primary ciliary dyskinesia treatment and, consequently, all treatment recommendations are based on very low-level evidence. The use of guidelines developed for cystic fibrosis patients, such as airway clearance techniques, regular inhaled antibiotics, rhDNase or hypertonic saline, is common in the management of patients with primary ciliary dyskinesia in many European pediatric centers; however, the pathophysiology of these two diseases is different [9, 10, 71]. In 2009 the guidelines for the management of primary ciliary dyskinesia in children were published by the ERS PCD Task Force [2].

Generally, the treatment of patients with primary ciliary dyskinesia can be based on three simultaneous actions:

1) Periodic monitoring of the general condition (every 2-3 months in children and 6-12 months in adults), respiratory function and auditory function including:
   a. regular visits to the pediatrician, pulmonologist, otolaryngologist and primary care physician,
   b. regular assessments of pulmonary functions to detect their early deteriorations,
   c. regular sputum cultures to monitor infectious flora,
   d. chest CT scan for the signs of disease progression,
   e. otoscopic and audiometric review,
   f. regular clinical assessment of chronic rhinosinusitis.
2) Promotion of drainage of secretions through respiratory physiotherapy and physical exercise.
3) Aggressive antibiotic treatment of respiratory infections [14, 54].

7.1. Respiratory Therapy

The respiratory system is dominantly affected in primary ciliary dyskinesia where its abnormalities are basic clinical symptoms presenting in children. Therefore, the management and also research focus is mainly on the treatment of the respiratory system. Respiratory treatment involves aggressive treatment of upper and lower airway infections, improvement of mucociliary clearance and management of chronic lung complications (deterioration of lung functions, development of bronchiectasis) [2, 46]. The lung function deteriorations do not exactly correlate with the time of diagnosis or treatment. Recent clinical studies showed that decreased FEV1 and development of bronchiectasis were presented in one-third of cases despite therapy and the early diagnosis. However, other publications showed lung function improvement with adequate management of primary ciliary dyskinesia [51].

Prevention and aggressive treatment of airway infection is essential to protect against chronic complications. The typical pathological colonization of airways in primary ciliary dyskinesia, as presented also in patients with cystic fibrosis or other chronic lung disease, varies depending on the patient's age. In children, the most common are Haemophilus influenzae and Staphylococcus aureus; in adults, they are Streptoccocus pneumoniae, P. aeruginosa and nontuberculous mycobacteria. Acute infection of the respiratory tract should be promptly treated with high-dose oral antibiotics, guided by microbiological examination of mucus. The ERS Task Force recommends performing regular culture of sputum, cough swabs or occasionally, in children who do not expectorate, a bronchoalveolar lavage in an approximately 3-4-month period. High-dose oral antibiotics should be prescribed at the first sign of worsening respiratory symptoms or deterioration of lung function and if it is possible for positive cultures and sensitivity, given continuously and for adequate therapeutic time. In particular, isolates of Pseudomonas aeruginosa should be treated with cystic fibrosis protocol. There are no dates on the significant improvement of intravenous antibiotics except in the case of persistent respiratory symptoms without response to oral antibiotics. Similarly continuous prophylactic oral antibiotics given in cycles are usually not recommended except in specific cases with very frequent recurrent infections [2, 12, 84]. Macrolides have long been recognized as exerting immunomodulary and anti-inflammatory actions. They are able to suppress the cytokines of inflammation and to confer an additional clinical benefit through their immunomodulatory properties. Recent clinical studies present a beneficial effect of macrolides in primary ciliary dyskinesia and might represent a therapeutic option [10, 59, 93].

Apart from treatment of the acute worsening of primary ciliary dyskinesia the management should focus on primary prevention to decrease the risk of infection and development of chronic lung diseases. Prevention should include the avoidance of active and passive smoking, minimization of exposure to outdoor and indoor pollutions, decreased contact with respiratory pathogens and immunization [67, 71]. Patients with primary ciliary dyskinesia should receive all protocol immunizations, especially against the influenza virus, *Streptococcus pneumoniae* and *Haemophilus influenzae* type b [14].

Airway clearance techniques are the main therapeutic objective in patients with primary ciliary dyskinesia, where the therapeutic opinion is focused on increased mucociliary clearance, modifying mucous viscosity or ciliary movement. Physiotherapy together with physical activity is considered an important component in the management of patients to improve mucociliary clearance. Strategies of physiotherapy vary with age, cooperation, changing clinical stage and local expertise and resources. It consists of postural drainage, breathing maneuvers, handling, chest percussion, cough and use of oscillating devices, but there is no evidence for the efficiency of any one particular technique [10, 46]. In addition, regular performance of physiotherapy twice daily at home, and with the regular support of a physiotherapist, is effective for airway clearance, although about one-fourth of patients do not perform it routinely. A combination of physical exercise before physiotherapy is encouraged as it induces better bronchodilation. All techniques should be more intensive during acute infection and often combined with inhalation and mucolytics. There is general agreement that routine hypertonic 3-7% nasal saline irrigations and anticholinergics improve symptoms but N-acetylcysteine is not effective and should not be indicated. Aerosols such as recombinant human deoxyribonuclease (rhDNase), hypertonic saline, or mannitol, L-arginine or uridine triphosphate (UTP) have questionable effectiveness in modifying mucous viscosity in primary ciliary dyskinesia [2, 11, 83]. In addition, application of rhDNase is an exceedingly expensive treatment and is used more in centers with a higher number of primary ciliary dyskinesia cases. Use of inhaled β2-agonists and corticosteroids should be withdrawn if they have been started by a misdiagnosis of asthma, because they do not appear to be beneficial in all patients with primary ciliary dyskinesia; hence, in some subgroups where FEV1 reversibility is observed they might be useful [14, 71, 84].

The complications of chronic lung diseases - particularly bronchiectasis - should be treated conservatively, including respiratory tract clearance with combinations of physiotherapy and physical exercise, an aggressive and prolonged antibiotic treatment of upper and lower respiratory tract infections and regular supervision by specialists [10]. Surgical treatment is reserved only for specific rare cases where morbidity can be clearly attributed to a localized area of severe bronchiectasis [14, 26, 47, 71].

7.2. Ear, Nose, and Throat Management

Recurrent infections of ear, nose and throat are frequent and together with respiratory symptoms and bronchiectasis make the diagnosis of primary ciliary dyskinesia in children. Altered ciliary movement is responsible for mucociliary clearance dysfunction associated with decreased evacuation of pathogens, mucus stagnation and the worsening of physiologic cleaning of the upper respiratory tract, leading to acute or chronic middle ear infection (otitis media) and chronic rhinosinusitis [12]. Episodes of acute middle ear infection presenting in more than 85% children must be promptly treated with antibiotics. Transition to chronic secretory otitis media is also common in children and the accumulation of mucus in the Eustachian tube can cause conductive hearing loss (10-30% of children with primary ciliary dyskinesia aged 1-3 years [2, 49, 91]. The aim of the treatment of secretory otitis media in young children is to improve hearing and to mitigate the effects of hearing loss on speech and language development. Conservative treatment with regular audiological assessment, hearing aids and hearing therapy is preferred against surgery. In many patients, placement of transtympanic drains (ventilation tubes) is often followed by a persistent mucoid otorrhea and developed tympanic perforations. Therefore, the surgical ventilation tubes should be reserved for children who are predisposed to secretory otitis media or with multiple risk factors, where the ventilation tubes can achieve normal hearing thresholds in these children [14, 27, 91].

Nasal secretion is present lifelong in most children with primary ciliary dyskinesia, often watery or mucoid and purulent during acute infection, and typically transported by gravity or airflow due to decreased mucociliary clearance. The severity of rhinosinusitis symptoms does not correlate with ultrastructural defects [2]. The most successful treatment of nasal secretion is regular clearance of nasal mucus including saline nasal douches and sometimes anticholinergics; mucolytics are not recommended. Long-term nasal corticosteroids may improve rhinosinusitis but there is no adequate effect on rhinorrhea. Acute sinusitis has to be managed promptly by prolonged antibiotic therapy specifically against typical bacteria in patients with primary ciliary dyskinesia. In addition, the underdevelopment of frontal and sphenoidal sinuses and nasal polyps are also more common [92]. Indications for surgical management, typically endoscopic sinus surgery and debridement of sinonasal polyps, include nasal obstruction, polyposis, headache, lateral nasal wall deformities, pulmonary exacerbations or declining pulmonary function tests that correlate with sinusitis refractory to medical therapy. Adenoidectomy may still have utility, particularly in younger children, although the effectiveness has not been widely reported [55, 66].

7.3. Infertility Treatment

A semen analysis should be offered for all men with primary ciliary dyskinesia. New in vitro fertilization techniques, especially intracytoplasmic sperm injection, are useful, but the appropriate genetic counseling should be included in standard care. In women close pregnancy monitoring is required due to the increased possibility of ectopic pregnancy [2, 14, 46].

7.4. Other Therapeutic Options

The curative treatment of primary ciliary dyskinesia is still unavailable, although gene therapy has major potential for treating ciliopathies, because all mutations are loss-of-function alleles. Also, recent advances in gene delivery and endogenous gene and transcript repair enhance the prospects of this new therapeutic option in the near future [52, 53].

Other recently presented hypotheses about the positive therapeutic and protector modalities include alpha-1- antitrypsin, antiprotease and secretory immunoglobulin A. The wild type (PiMM) of the alpha-1-antitrypsin genotype is associated with the upper limit of alpha-1-antitrypsin concentration and might inhibit neutrophil elastase in the lung interstitium and the alveolar space reflecting a beneficial change of the protease-antiprotease balance [78].

Acknowledgments

This work was supported by the project "Measurement of kinetics of cilia in respiratory tract", co-financed by EU sources.

References

[1] Badano, J.L., Mitsuma, N., Beales, P.L., Katsanis, N., (2006). The ciliopathies: an emerging class of human genetic disorders. *Annu. Rev. Genomics. Hum. Genet.* 7, 125–48.

[2] Barbato, A., Frischer, T., Kuehni, C.E., Snijders, D., Azevedo, I., Baktai, G., Bartoloni, L., Eber, E., Escribano, A., Haarman, E., Hesselmar, B., Hogg, C., Jorissen, M., Lucas, J., Nielsen, K.G., O'Callaghan, C., Omran, H., Pohunek, P., Strippoli, M.P., Bush, A., (2009). Primary ciliary dyskinesia: a consensus statement on diagnostic and treatment approaches in children. *Eur. Respir. J.* 34, 1264–76.

[3] Becker-Heck, A., Zohn, I.E., Okabe, N., Pollock, A., Lenhart, K.B., Sullivan-Brown, J., McSheene, J., Loges, N.T., Olbrich, H., Haeffner, K., Fliegauf, M., Horvath, J., Reinhardt, R., Nielsen, K.G., Marthin, J.K., Baktai, G., Anderson, K.V., Geisler, R., Niswander, L., Omran, H., Burdine, R.D., (2011). The coiled-coil domain containing protein CCDC40 is essential for motile cilia function and left-right axis formation. *Nat. Genet.* 43, 79–84.

[4]   Berbari, N.F., O'Connor, A.K., Haycraft, C.J., Yoder, B.K., (2009). The primary cilium as a complex signaling center. *Curr. Biol.* 19, R526–R535.

[5]   Bisgrove, B.W., Yost, H.J., (2006). The roles of cilia in developmental disorders and disease. *Development.* 133, 4131–43.

[6]   Blanchon, S., Legendre, M., Copin, B., Duquesnoy, P., Montantin, G., Kott, E., Dastot, F., Jeanson, L., Cachanado, M., Rousseau, A., Papon, J.F., Beydon, N., Brouard, J., Crestani, B., Deschildre, A., Désir, J., Dollfus, H., Leheup, B., Tamalet, A., Thumerelle, C., Vojtek, A.M., Escalier, D., Coste, A., de Blic, J., Clément, A., Escudier, E., Amselem, S., (2012). Delineation of CCDC39/CCDC40 mutation spectrum and associated phenotypes in primary ciliary dyskinesia. *J. Med. Genet.* 49, 410–6.

[7]   Blouin, J., Meeks, M., Radhakrishna, U., Sainsbury, A., Gehring, C., Saïl, G.D., Bartoloni, L., Dombi, V., O'Rawe, A., Walne, A., Chung, E., Afzelius, B.A., Armengot, M., Jorissen, M., Schidlow, D.V., van Maldergem, L., Walt, H., Gardiner, R.M., Probst, D., Guerne, P.A., Delozier-Blanchet, C.D., Antonarakis, S.E., (2000). Primary ciliary dyskinesia: a genome-wide linkage analysis reveals extensive locus heterogeneity. *Eur. J. Hum. Genet.* 8, 109-18.

[8]   Budny, B., Chen, W., Omran, H., Fliegauf, M., Tzschach, A., Wisniewska, M., Jensen, L.R., Raynaud, M., Shoichet, S.A., Badura, M., Lenzner, S., Latos-Bielenska, A., Ropers, H.H., (2006). A novel X-linked recessive mental retardation syndrome comprising macrocephaly and ciliary dysfunction is allelic to oral-facial-digital type I syndrome. *Hum. Genet.* 120, 171–78.

[9]   Bush, A., Hogg, C., (2012). Primary ciliary dyskinesia: recent advances in epidemiology, diagnosis, management and relationship with the expanding spectrum of ciliopathy. *Expert. Rev. Respir. Med.* 6, 663–82.

[10]   Bush, A., Chodhari, R., Collins, N., Copeland, F., Hall, P., Harcourt, J., Hariri, M., Hogg, C., Lucas, J., Mitchison, H.M., O'Callaghan, C., Phillips, G., (2007). Primary ciliary dyskinesia: current state of the art. *Arch. Dis. Child.* 92, 1136–40.

[11]   Campbell, R., (2012). Managing upper respiratory tract complication of primary ciliary dyskinesia in children. *Curr. Opin. Allergy Clin. Immunol.* 12, 32–38.

[12]   Campbell, R.G., Birman, C.S., Morgan, L., (2009). Management of otitis media with effusion in children with primary ciliary dyskinesia: a literature review. *Int. J. Pediatr. Otorhinolaryngol.* 73, 1630–1638.

[13]   Canciani, M., Barlocco, E.G., Mastella, G., de Santi, M.M., Gardi, C., Lungarella, G., (1988). The saccharin method for testing mucociliary function in patients suspected of having primary ciliary dyskinesia. *Pediatr. Pulmonol.* 5, 210–4.

[14]   Carceller, M.A., Roig, M.M., Payá, X.M., Gimenoc, J.C., (2010). Primary ciliary dyskinesia. Ciliopathies. *Acta Otorrinolaringol Esp.* 61, 149−159.

[15]   Castleman, V.H., Romio, L., Chodhari, R., Hirst, R.A., de Castro, S.C., Parker, K.A., Ybot-Gonzalez, P., Emes, R.D., Wilson, S.W., Wallis, C., Johnson, C.A., Herrera, R.J., Rutman, A., Dixon, M., Shoemark, A., Bush, A., Hogg, C., Gardiner, R.M., Reish, O., Greene, N.D., O'Callaghan, C., Purton, S., Chung, E.M., Mitchison, H.M., (2009). Mutations in radial spoke head protein genes RSPH9 and RSPH4A cause primary ciliary dyskinesia with central-microtubular-pair abnormalities. *Am. J. Hum. Genet.* 84, 197–209.

[16]   Corbelli, R., Bringolf-Isler, B., Amacher, A., Sasse, B., Spycher, M., Hammer, J.,
       (2004). Nasal nitric oxide measurements to screen children for primary ciliary
       dyskinesia. *Chest.* 126, 1054–9.

[17]   Coren, M., Meeks, M., Buchdahl, R., Buchdahl, R.M., Bush, A., (2002). Primary ciliary
       dyskinesia (PCD) in children: age at diagnosis and symptom history. *Acta Paediatr.* 91,
       667-9.

[18]   Djakow, A., O'Callaghan, C., (2014). Primary ciliary dyskinesia. *Breathe.* 10, 123-33.

[19]   Driscoll, J.A., Bhalla, S., Liapis, H., Ibricevic, A., Brody, S.L., (2008). Autosomal
       dominant polycystic kidney disease is associated with an increased prevalence of
       radiographic bronchiectasis. *Chest.* 133, 1181–8.

[20]   Duquesnoy, P., Escudier, E., Vincensini, L., Freshour, J., Bridoux, A.M., Coste, A.,
       Deschildre, A., de Blic, J., Legendre, M., Montantin, G., Tenreiro, H., Vojtek, A.M.,
       Loussert, C., Clément, A., Escalier, D., Bastin, P., Mitchell, D.R., Amselem, S., (2009).
       Loss-of-function mutations in the human ortholog of Chlamydomonas reinhardtii
       ODA7 disrupt dynein arm assembly and cause primary ciliary dyskinesia. *Am. J. Hum.
       Genet.* 85, 890–6.

[21]   Duriez, B., Duquesnoy, P., Escudier, E., Bridoux, A.M., Escalier, D., Rayet, I., Marcos,
       E., Vojtek, A.M., Bercher, J.F., Amselem, S., (2007). A common variant in
       combination with a nonsense mutation in a member of the thioredoxin family causes
       primary ciliary dyskinesia. *Proc. Natl. Acad. Sci. U S A.* 104, 3336–41.

[22]   Failly, M., Bartoloni, L., Letourneau, A., Munoz, A., Falconnet, E., Rossier, C., De
       Santi, M.M., Santamaria, F., Sacco, O., Delozier-Blanchet, C.D., Lazor, R., Blouin,
       J.L., (2009). Mutations in DNAH5 account for only 15% of a non-preselected cohort of
       patients with primary ciliary dyskinesia. *J. Med. Genet.* 46, 281–6.

[23]   Failly, M., Saitta, A., Munoz, A., Falconnet, E., Rossier, C., Santamaria, F., De Santi,
       M.M., Lazor, R., Delozier-Blanchet, C.D., Bartoloni, L., Blouin, J.L., (2008). DNAI1
       mutations explain only 2% of primary ciliary dykinesia. *Respiration.* 76, 198–204.

[24]   Geremek, M., Uit, M., (2004). Primary ciliary dyskinesia: genes, candidate genes and
       chromosomal regions. *J. Appl. Genet.* 45, 347-61.

[25]   Goetz, S.C., Anderson, K.V., (2010). The primary cilium: a signalling centre during
       vertebrate development. *Nat. Rev. Genet.* 11, 331–44.

[26]   Graeter, T., Schäfers, H.J., Wahlers, T., Borst, H.G., (1994). Lung transplantation in
       Kartagener's syndrome. *J. Heart Lung Transplant.* 13, 724–6.

[27]   Hadfield, P., Rowe-Jones, J., Bush, A., Mackay, I.S., (1997). Treatment of otitis media
       with effusion in children with primary ciliary dyskinesia. *Clin. Otolaryngol.* 22, 302-6.

[28]   Hargaš, L., Koniar, D., Hrianka, M., Jošková, M., Ďurdík, P., Bánovčin, P., (2013).
       Contactless Parameters Measurement of Motion Object by Virtual Instrumentation,
       Applied Electronics 2013, International Conference, Pilsen, 10-12 September 2013,
       IEEE Catalog Number CFP1369A-PRT, ISBN 978-80-261-0166-6, ISSN 1803-7232

[29]   Hargaš, L., Koniar, D., Štofan, S., Hrianka, M., (2010). Ciliary Frequency and
       Trajectory Determination Using Image Analysis. *Acta Pneumonologica et Allerglogica
       Pediatrica*, 13, 3-4.

[30]   Hirst, R.A., Rutman, A., Williams, G., O'Callaghan, C., (2010). Ciliated air-liquid
       cultures as an aid to diagnostic testing of primary ciliary dyskinesia. *Chest.* 138: 1441–
       7.

[31] Horani, A., Druley, T.E., Zariwala, M.A., Patel, A.C., Levinson, B.T., Van Arendonk, L.G., Thornton, K.C., Giacalone, J.C., Albee, A.J., Wilson, K.S., Turner, E.H., Nickerson, D.A., Shendure, J., Bayly, P.V., Leigh, M.W., Knowles, M.R., Brody, S.L., Dutcher, S.K., Ferkol, T.W., (2012). Whole-Exome Capture and Sequencing Identifies HEATR2 Mutation as a Cause of Primary Ciliary Dyskinesia. *Am. J. Hum. Genet.* 91, 685–93.

[32] Hornef, N., Olbrich, H., Horvath, J., Zariwala, M.A., Fliegauf, M., Loges, N.T., Wildhaber, J., Noone, P.G., Kennedy, M., Antonarakis, S.E., Blouin, J.L., Bartoloni, L., Nusslein, T., Ahrens, P., Griese, M., Kuhl, H., Sudbrak, R., Knowles, M.R., Reinhardt, R., Omran, H., (2006). DNAH5 mutations are a common cause of primary ciliary dyskinesia with outer dynein arm defects. *Am. J. Respir. Crit. Care Med.* 174, 120–6.

[33] Chilvers, M.A., Rutman, A., O'Callaghan, C., (2003). Ciliary beat pattern is associated with specific ultrastructural defects in primary ciliary dyskinesia. *J. Allergy Clin. Immunol.* 112, 518-24.

[34] Chilvers, M.A., Rutman, A., O'Callaghan, C., (2003). Functional analysis of cilia and ciliated epithelial ultrastructure in healthy children and young adults. *Thorax.* 58, 333–8.

[35] Jorissen, M., Willems, T., Van der Schueren, B., Verbeken, E., De Boeck, K., (2000). Ultrastructural expression of primary ciliary dyskinesia after ciliogenesis in culture. *Acta Otorhinolaryngol. Belg.* 54, 343–56.

[36] Kartagener, M., (1933). "Zur Pathogenese der Bronchiektasien: Bronchiektasien bei Situs viscerum inversus". *Beiträge zur Klinik der Tuberkulose.* 83, 489–501

[37] Kennedy, M.P., Noone, P.G., Leigh, M.W., Zariwala, M.A., Minnix, S.L., Knowles, M.R., Molina, P.L., (2007). High-resolution CT of patients with primary ciliary dyskinesia. *AJR Am. J. Roentgenol.* 188, 1232–8.

[38] Knowles, M.R., Daniels, L.A., Davis, S.D., Zariwala, M.A., Leigh, M.W., (2013). Primary ciliary dyskinesia. Recent advances in diagnostics, genetics, and characterization of clinical disease. *Am. J. Respir. Crit. Care Med.* 188, 913-22.

[39] Knowles, M.R., Leigh, M.W., Carson, J.L., Davis, S.D., Dell, S.D., Ferkol, T.W., Olivier, K.N., Sagel, S.D., Rosenfeld, M., Burns, K.A., Minnix, S.L., Armstrong, M.C., Lori, A., Hazucha, M.J., Loges, N.T., Olbrich, H., Becker-Heck, A., Schmidts, M., Werner, C., Omran, H., Zariwala, M.A., (2012). Mutations of DNAH11 in patients with primary ciliary dyskinesia with normal ciliary ultrastructure. *Thorax.* 67, 433–41.

[40] Koniar, D., Hargaš, L., Štofan, S., Hrianka, M., (2010). High Speed Video System for Tissue Measurement Based on PWM Regulated Dimming and Virtual Instrumentation. *Electronics And Electrical Engineering*, 10 (106), ISSN 1392-1215 (print), ISSN 2029-5731 (online)

[41] Kotov, N.V., Bates, D.G., Gizatullina, A.N., Gilaziev, B., Khairullin, R.N., Chen, M.Z.Q., Drozdov, I., Umezawa, Y., Hundhausen, C., Aleksandrov, A., Yan, X., Spurgeon, S.K., Smales, C.M., Valeyev, N.V., (2011). Computational modelling elucidates the mechanism of ciliary regulation in health and disease. *BMC Syst. Biol.* 5, 143.

[42] Kott, E., Duquesnoy, P., Copin, B., Legendre, M., Moal, F.D., Montantin, G., Jeanson, L., Tamalet, A., Papon, J., Siffroi, J., Rives, N., Mitchell, V., de Blic, J., Coste, A., Clement, A., Escalier, D., Touré, A., Escudier, E., Amselem, S., (2012). Loss-of-function mutations in LRRC6, a gene essential for proper axonemal assembly of inner

and outer dynein arms, cause primary ciliary dyskinesia. *Am. J. Hum. Genet.* 91, 958–64.

[43] Leigh, M.W., Pittman, J.E., Carson, J.L., Ferkol, T.W., Dell, S.D., Davis, S.D., Knowles, M.R., Zariwala, M.A., (2009). Clinical and genetic aspects of primary ciliary dyskinesia/Kartagener syndrome. *Genet. Med.* 11, 473-87.

[44] Loges, N.T., Olbrich, H., Becker-Heck, A., Häffner, K., Heer, A., Reinhard, C., Schmidts, M., Kispert, A., Zariwala, M.A., Leigh, M.W., Knowles, M.R., Zentgraf, H., Seithe, H., Nürnberg, G., Nürnberg, P., Reinhardt, R., Omran, H., (2009). Deletion and point mutations of LRRC50 cause primary ciliary dyskinesia due to dynein arms defects. *Am. J. Hum. Genet.* 85, 883–9.

[45] Loges, N.T., Olbrich, H., Fenske, L., Mussaffi, H., Horvath, J., Fliegauf, M., Kuhl, H., Baktai, G., Peterffy, E., Chodhari, R., Chung, E.M., Rutman, A., O'Callaghan, C., Blau, H., Tiszlavicz, L., Voelkel, K., Witt, M., Zietkiewicz, E., Neesen, J., Reinhardt, R., Mitchison, H.M., Omran, H., (2008). DNAI2 mutations cause primary ciliary dyskinesia with defects in the outer dynein arm. *Am. J. Hum. Genet.* 83, 547–58.

[46] Lucas, J.S.A., Walker, W.T., Kuehni, C.E., Layor, R., (2011). Primary ciliary dyskinesia. *Eur. Respir. Monogr.* 54, 201–217.

[47] Macchiarini, P., Chapelier, A., Vouhé, P., Cerrina, J., Ladurie, F.L., Parquin, F., Brenot, F., Simonneau, G., Dartevelle, P., (1994). Double lung transplantation in situs inversus with Kartagener's syndrome. Paris-Sud University Lung Transplant Group. *J. Thorac Cardiovasc. Surg.* 108, 86–91.

[48] Madsen, A., Green, K., Buchvald, F., Hanel, B., Nielsen, K.G. (2013). Aerobic Fitness in Children and Young Adults with Primary Ciliary Dyskinesia. *PLoS One.* 8, e71409.

[49] Majitha, A., Fong, J., Hariri, M., Harcourt, J., (2005). Hearing outcomes in children with primary ciliary dyskinesia-a longitudinal study. *Int. J. Pediatr. Otorhinolaryngol.* 69, 1061-4.

[50] Marthin, J.K., Mortensen, J., Pressler, T., Nielsen, K.G., (2007). Pulmonary radioaerosol mucociliary clearance in diagnosis of primary ciliary dyskinesia. *Chest.* 132, 966–76.

[51] Marthin, J.K., Petersen, N., Skovgaard, L.T., Nielsen, K.G., (2010). Lung function in patients with primary ciliary dyskinesia: a cross-sectional and 3-decade longitudinal study. *Am. J. Respir. Crit. Care Med.* 181, 1262–8.

[52] McIntyre, J.C., Davis, E.E., Joiner, A., Williams, C.L., Tsai, I.C., Jenkins, P.M., McEwen, D.P., Zhang, L., Escobado, J., Thomas, S., Szymanska, K., Johnson, C.A., Beales, P.L., Green, E.D., Mullikin, J.C.; NISC Comparative Sequencing Program, Sabo, A., Muzny, D.M., Gibbs, R.A., Attié-Bitach, T., Yoder, B.K., Reed, R.R., Katsanis, N., Martens, J.R., (2012). Gene therapy rescues cilia defects and restores olfactory function in a mammalian ciliopathy model. *Nat. Med.* 18, 1423-8.

[53] McIntyre, J.C., Williams, C.L., Martens, J.R., (2013). Smelling the roses and seeing the light: gene therapy for ciliopathies. *Trends Biotechnol.* 31, 355-63.

[54] McManus, I., Mitchison, H., Chung, E.M., Stubbings, G.F., Martin, N., (2003). Primary ciliary dyskinesia (Siewert's/Kartagener's syndrome): respiratory symptoms and psycho-social impact. *BMC Pulm. Med.* 3:4.

[55] Mener, D.J., Lin, S.Y., Ishman, S.L., Boss, E.F., (2013). Treatment and outcomes of chronic rhinosinusitis in children with primary ciliary dyskinesia: where is the evidence? A qualitative systematic review. *Int. Forum Allergy Rhinol.* 3, 986–991.

[56] Merveille, A.C., Davis, E.E., Becker-Heck, A., Legendre, M., Amirav, I., Bataille, G., Belmont, J., Beydon, N., Billen, F., Clément, A., Clercx, C., Coste, A., Crosbie, R., de Blic, J., Deleuze, S., Duquesnoy, P., Escalier, D., Escudier, E., Fliegauf, M., Horvath, J., Hill, K., Jorissen, M., Just, J., Kispert, A., Lathrop, M., Loges, N.T., Marthin, J.K., Momozawa, Y., Montantin, G., Nielsen, K.G., Olbrich, H., Papon, J.F., Rayet, I., Roger, G., Schmidts, M., Tenreiro, H., Towbin, J.A., Zelenika, D., Zentgraf, H., Georges, M., Lequarré, A.S., Katsanis, N,, Omran, H., Amselem, S., (2011). CCDC39 is required for assembly of inner dynein arms and the dynein regulatory complex and for normal ciliary motility in humans and dogs. *Nat. Genet.* 43, 72–8.

[57] Mitchison, H.M., Schmidts, M., Loges, N.T., Freshour, J., Dritsoula, A., Hirst, R.A., O'Callaghan, C., Blau, H., Al Dabbagh, M., Olbrich, H., Beales, P.L., Yagi, T., Mussaffi, H., Chung, E.M., Omran, H., Mitchell, D.R., (2012). Mutations in axonemal dynein assembly factor DNAAF3 cause primary ciliary dyskinesia. *Nat. Genet.* 44, 381–9.

[58] Moore, A., Escudier, E., Roger, G., Tamalet, A., Pelosse, B., Marlin, S., Clément, A., Geremek, M., Delaisi, B., Bridoux, A.M., Coste, A., Witt, M., Duriez, B., Amselem, S., (2006). RPGR is mutated in patients with a complex X linked phenotype combining primary ciliary dyskinesia and retinitis pigmentosa. *J. Med. Genet.* 43, 326–33.

[59] Noone, P.G., Leigh, M.W., Sannuti, A., Minnix, S.L., Carson, J.L., Hazucha, M., Zariwala, M.A., Knowles, M.R., (2004). Primary ciliary dyskinesia: diagnostic and phenotypic features. *Am. J. Respir. Crit. Care Med.* 169: 459–67.

[60] Olbrich, H., Haffner, K., Kispert, A., Volkel, A., Volz, A., Sasmaz, G., Reinhardt, R., Hennig, S., Lehrach, H., Konietzko, N., Zariwala, M., Noone, P.G., Knowles, M., Mitchison, H.M., Meeks, M., Chung, E.M., Hildebrandt, F., Sudbrak, R., Omran, H., (2002). Mutations in DNAH5 cause primary ciliary dyskinesia and randomization of left-right asymmetry. *Nat. Genet.* 30, 143–4.

[61] Olbrich, H., Schmidts, M., Werner, C., Onoufriadis, A., Loges, N.T., Raidt, J., Banki, N.F., Shoemark, A., Burgoyne, T., Al Turki, S., Hurles, M.E., (2012). Recessive HYDIN Mutations Cause Primary Ciliary Dyskinesia without Randomization of Left-Right Body Asymmetry. *Am. J. Hum. Genet.* 91, 672–84.

[62] Omran, H., Kobayashi, D., Olbrich, H., Tsukahara, T., Loges, N.T., Hagiwara, H., Zhang, Q., Leblond, G., O'Toole, E., Hara, C., Mizuno, H., Kawano, H., Fliegauf, M., Yagi, T., Koshida, S., Miyawaki, A., Zentgraf, H., Seithe, H., Reinhardt, R., Watanabe, Y., Kamiya, R., Mitchell, D.R., Takeda, H., (2008). Ktu/PF13 is required for cytoplasmic pre-assembly of axonemal dyneins. *Nature.* 456, 611–6.

[63] Ostrowski, L.E., Dutcher, S.K., Lo, C.W., (2011). Cilia and Models for Studying Structure and Function. *Proc. Am. Thorac. Soc.* 8, 423–9.

[64] Panizzi, J.R., Becker-Heck, A., Castleman, V.H., Al-Mutairi, D.A., Liu, Y., Loges, N.T., Pathak, N., Austin-Tse, C., Sheridan, E., Schmidts, M., Olbrich, H., Werner, C., Häffner, K., Hellman, N., Chodhari, R., Gupta, A., Kramer-Zucker, A., Olale, F., Burdine, R.D., Schier, A.F., O'Callaghan, C., Chung, E.M., Reinhardt, R., Mitchison, H.M., King, S.M., Omran, H., Drummond, I.A., (2012). CCDC103 mutations cause primary ciliary dyskinesia by disrupting assembly of ciliary dynein arms. *Nat. Genet.* 44, 714–9.

[65] Papon, J.F., Coste, A., Roudot-Thoraval, F., Boucherat, M., Roger, G., Tamalet, A., Vojtek, A.M., Amselem, S., Escudier, E., (2010). A 20-year experience of electron microscopy in the diagnosis of primary ciliary dyskinesia. *Eur. Respir. J.* 35, 1057–63.

[66] Parsons, D.S., Greene, B.A., (1993). A treatment for primary ciliary dyskinesia: efficacy of functional endoscopic sinus surgery. *Laryngoscope.* 103, 1269–1272.

[67] Philips, G., Thomas, S., Heather, S., Bush, A., (1998). Airway response of children with primary dyskinesia to exercise and beta-2 agonists challenge. *Eur. Respir. J.* 11, 1389-91.

[68] Piacentini, G.L., Bodini, A., Peroni, D., Rigotti, E., Pigozzi, R., Pradal, U., Boner, A.L., (2008). Nasal nitric oxide for early diagnosis of primary ciliary dyskinesia: practical issues in children. *Respir. Med.* 102, 541–7.

[69] Pifferi, M., Bush, A., Caramella, D., Di Cicco, M., Zangani, M., Chinellato, I., Macchia, P., Boner, A.L., (2011). Agenesis of paranasal sinuses and nasal nitric oxide in primary ciliary dyskinesia. *Eur. Respir. J.* 37, 566–71.

[70] Pifferi, M., Bush, A., Pioggia, G., Caramella, D., Tartarisco, G., Di Cicco, M., Zangani, M., Chinellato, I., Maggi, F., Tezza, G., Macchia, P., Boner, A., (2012). Evaluation of pulmonary disease using static lung volumes in primary ciliary dyskinesia. *Thorax.* 67, 993–9.

[71] Pifferi, M., Di Cicco, M., Piras, M., Cangiotti, A.M., Saggese, G., (2013). Up to date on primary ciliary dyskinesia in children. *Early Hum. Dev.* 89, S45-8.

[72] Pifferi, M., Montemurro, F., Cangiotti, A.M., Ragazzo, V., Di Cicco, M., Vinci, B., Vozzi, G., Macchia, P., Boner, A.L., (2009). Simplified cell culture method for the diagnosis of atypical primary ciliary dyskinesia. *Thorax.* 64, 1077–81.

[73] Plesec, T.P., Ruiz, A., McMahon, J.T., Prayson, R.A., (2008). Ultrastructural abnormalities of respiratory cilia: a 25-year experience. *Arch. Pathol. Lab. Med.* 132, 1786–91.

[74] Raman, R., Al-Ali, S.Y., Poole, C.A., Dawson, B.V., Carman, J.B., Calder, L., (2003). Isomerism of the right atrial appendages: clinical, anatomical, and microscopic study of a long surviving case with asplenia and ciliary abnormalities. *Clin. Anat.* 16, 269–76.

[75] Santamaria, F., De Stefano, S., Montella, S., Barbarano, F., Iacotucci, P., Ciccarelli, R., Sofia, M., Maniscalco, M., (2008). Nasal nitric oxide assessment in primary ciliary dyskinesia using aspiration, exhalation, and humming. *Med. Sci. Monit.* 14, CR80–CR85.

[76] Santamaria, F., Montella, S., Tiddens, H.A., Guidi, G., Casotti, V., Maglione, M., de Jong, P.A., (2008). Structural and functional lung disease in primary ciliary dyskinesia. *Chest.* 134, 351–7.

[77] Satir, P., (1980). Structural basis of ciliary movement. *Environ Health Perspect.* 35, 77–82.

[78] Serapinas, D., Staikūnienė, J., Barkauskienė, D., Jackutė, J., Sakalauskas, R., (2013). An unusual regression of the symptoms of Kartagener syndrome. *Arch. Bronconeumol.* 49, 28-30.

[79] Shoemark, A., Dixon, M., Corrin, B., Dewar, A., (2012). Twenty-year review of quantitative transmission electron microscopy for the diagnosis of primary ciliary dyskinesia. *J. Clin. Pathol.* 65, 267-71.

[80] Schwabe, G.C., Hoffmann, K., Loges, N.T., Birker, D., Rossier, C., de Santi, M.M., Olbrich, H., Fliegauf, M., Failly, M., Liebers, U., Collura, M., Gaedicke, G., Mundlos,

S., Wahn, U., Blouin, J.L., Niggemann, B., Omran, H., Antonarakis, S.E., Bartoloni, L., (2008). Primary ciliary dyskinesia associated with normal axoneme ultrastructure is caused by DNAH11 mutations. *Hum. Mutat.* 29, 289–98.

[81] Siewart, A.K., (1904). Ueber einen Fall von Bronchiectasie bei einem Patientem mit Situs Inversus Viscerum [A case of bronchiectasis in a patient with situs inversus viscerum]. *Berliner Klin. Wochenschr.* 41, 139–41.

[82] Stannard, W.A., Chilvers, M.A., Rutman, A.R., Williams, C.D., O'Callaghan, C., (2010). Diagnostic testing of patients suspected of primary ciliary dyskinesia. *Am. J. Respir. Crit. Care Med.* 181: 307–14.

[83] Stillwell, P.C., Wartchow, E.P., Sagel, S.D., (2011). Primary Ciliary Dyskinesia in Children: A Review for Pediatricians, Allergists, and Pediatric Pulmonologists. *Pediatr. Allergy Immunol. Pulmonol.* 24, 191–6.

[84] Strippoli, M.P., Frischer, T., Barbato, A., Snijders, D., Maurer, E., Lucas, J.S., Eber, E., Karadag, B., Pohunek, P., Zivkovic, Z., Escribano, A., O'Callaghan, C., Bush, A., Kuehni, C.E.; ERS Task Force on Primary Ciliary Dyskinesia in Children, (2012). Management of primary ciliary dyskinesia in European children: recommendations and clinical practice. *Eur. Respir. J.* 39, 1482-91.

[85] Štofan, S., Koniar, D., Hargaš, L., Hrianka, M., Radvan, R., (2011). Design of lighting unit for inverse microscopewith high-speed video capture. *Applied Electronics*, Pilsen, ISBN 978-80-7043-865-7, ISSN 1803-7232

[86] Takeda, S., Narita, K., (2012). Structure and function of vertebrate cilia, towards a new taxonomy. *Differentiation.* 83, S4–S11.

[87] Theegarten, D., Ebsen, M., (2011). Ultrastructural pathology of primary ciliary dyskinesia: report about 125 cases in Germany. *Diagn. Pathol.* 6, 115.

[88] Valerio, G., Giallauria, F., Montella, S., Vaino, N., Vigorito, C., Mirra, V., Santamaria, F., (2012). Cardiopulmonary assessment in primary ciliary dyskinesia. *Eur. J. Clin. Invest.* 42, 617–22.

[89] van Reeuwijk, J., Arts, H.H., Roepman, R., (2011). Scrutinizing ciliopathies by unraveling ciliary interaction networks. *Hum. Mol. Genet.* 20, R149–R157.

[90] Walker, W.T., Jackson, C.L., Lackie, P.M., Hogg, C., Lucas, J.S., (2012). Nitric oxide in primary ciliary dyskinesia. *Eur. Respir. J.* 40, 1024–32.

[91] Wolter, N.E., Dell, S.D., James, A.L., Campisi, P., (2012). Middle ear ventilation in children with primary ciliary dyskinesia. *Int. J. Pediatr. Otorhinolaryngol.* 76, 1565-8.

[92] Yoo, Y., Koh, Y., (2004). Current treatment for primary ciliary dyskinesia conditions. *Expert Opin. Pharamcother.* 5, 369–377.

[93] Yoshioka, D., Sakamoto, N., Ishimatsu, Y., Kakugawa, T., Ishii, H., Mukae, H., Kadota, J., Kohno, S., (2010). Primary ciliary dyskinesia that responded to long-term, low-dose clarithromycin. *Intern. Med.* 49, 1437–40.

[94] Zariwala, M.A., Leigh, M.W., Ceppa, F., Kennedy, M.P., Noone, P.G., Carson, J.L., Hazucha, M.J., Lori, A., Horvath, J., Olbrich, H., Loges, N.T., Bridoux, A.M., Pennarun, G., Duriez, B., Escudier, E., Mitchison, H.M., Chodhari, R., Chung, E.M., Morgan, L.C., de Iongh, R.U., Rutland, J., Pradal, U., Omran, H., Amselem, S., Knowles, M.R., (2006). Mutations of DNAI1 in primary ciliary dyskinesia: evidence of founder effect in a common mutation. *Am. J. Respir. Crit. Care Med.* 174, 858–66.

[95] Zhu, L., Belmont, J.W., Ware, S.M., (2006). Genetics of human heterotaxias. *Eur. J. Hum. Genet.* 14, 17–25.

Reviewed by:

Jaroslav Fabry, M.D., Ph.D. – Department of Pediatric Pneumology and Phthisiology, Srobar's Institute for Children Tuberculosis and Respiratory Diseases, Dolny Smokovec, High Tatras, Slovakia

In: Advances in Respiratory Therapy Research
Editor: Miloš Jeseňák

ISBN: 978-1-63463-004-7
© 2015 Nova Science Publishers, Inc.

Chapter 6

Obstructive Sleep Apnea Syndrome in Children – The Recent View on the Treatment

---

Anna Sujanska[1,2], Peter Durdik[1], Miloš Jeseňák[1], Peter Banovcin[1],
Jole Rabasco[2], Ottavio Vitelli[2], Nicoletta Pietropaoli[2]
and Maria Pia Villa[2]*

[1]Department of Pediatrics, Centre of Experimental and Clinical Respirology,
Comenius University Jessenius Faculty of Medicine, Martin, Slovak Republic
[2]Neuroscience, Mental Health and Sense Organs Department, Pediatric Sleep Disease
Centre, S. Andrea Hospital, "Sapienza" University of Rome, Italy

Abstract

During the past decade obstructive sleep apnea syndrome has become widely recognized as a frequent and relatively common disorder with potentially serious clinical implications in childhood and has emerged as a public health problem. Recently it has been reported that delayed diagnosis of this syndrome can lead to neurobehavioral consequences and even serious cardiorespiratory morbidity, metabolic complications, as well as an increase in insulin resistance, high blood pressure and the development of OSAS in adulthood. This condition must be diagnosed and manage aggressively with the appearance of these new repercussions.

Interventions of pediatric OSAS are varied, complex and multidisciplinary. The goal of the treatment is to restore optimal breathing during the night and to relieve associated symptoms. Evidence suggests that surgical intervention involving the removal of the tonsils and adenoids will lead to significant improvements in the most uncomplicated

---

* Corresponding Author address: Anna Sujanska, M.D., Department of Pediatrics, Centre of Experimental and Clinical Respirology, Jessenius Faculty of Medicine in Martin, Comenius University in Bratislava, University Hospital, Kollarova 2, 036 59, Martin, Slovak Republic, e-mail: anna.sujanska@gmail.com

cases, as recently reported from a meta-analysis. However, post-operative persistence of this syndrome in the pediatric population is more frequent than expected, which supports the idea of the complexity of this syndrome. Adenotomy alone may not be sufficient in children with OSAS, because it does not address oropharyngeal obstruction secondary to tonsillar hyperplasia. Continuous positive airway pressure can effectively treat this syndrome in selected groups of children, improving both nocturnal and daytime symptoms, but poor adherence is a limiting factor. For this reason, CPAP is not recommended as a first-line therapy for OSAS when adenotonsillectomy is an option. The incorporation of nonsurgical approaches for milder forms and for residual OSAS after surgical intervention is now being investigated. Although adenotonsillar hypertrophy is the most common treatment for OSAS in children; obesity is emerging as an equally important etiological factor. Therefore, an intensive weight reduction program and adequate sleep hygiene are also important lifestyle changes that may be very effective in mitigating the symptoms of this syndrome. Pharmacological therapy (topical nasal steroids, leukotriene antagonists) is usually use for mild forms of OSAS and in children with associated allergic diseases. Rapid maxillary expansion is a relatively new special orthodontic treatment in selected groups of children with OSAS and malocclusion. Myofunctional therapy may be also a promising alternative therapeutic modality used in children with this condition.

Keywords: Obstructive sleep apnea syndrome, Adenotonsillectomy, Orthodontic treatment, Myofunctional therapy

Obstructive Sleep Apnea Syndrome in Children

Sleep is a primary essential physiological phenomenon particularly during childhood. It is associated with restitution of somatic, neural structures and various metabolic processes in children. Therefore, any obstacle present during sleep that leads to sleep disturbance has a negative impact on a child´s development [23].

Obstructive Sleep Apnea Syndrome (OSAS) is a sleep disordered breathing (SDB) characterized by a combination of repeated episodes of prolonged partial upper airway obstruction (obstructive hypopnoea) and/or intermittent complete obstruction (obstructive apnoea) that disturbs the normal sleep pattern, normal ventilation during sleep and results in disruption of normal gas exchange (intermittent hypoxia and hypercapnia) [21]. During the past decade, OSAS has become widely recognized as a frequent and relatively common disorder with potentially serious clinical implications in childhood and has emerged as a major public health problem [36].

The majority of children can suffer from a physical obstruction of the nasal airway caused by enlarged adenoids and of the oropharyngeal airway by enlarged tonsils, resulting in increased airway resistance. The peak incidence of OSAS in this group occurs in those aged 3 to 6 years, when the adenoids and tonsils undergo hypertrophy. However, the situation is more complex than simple obstruction by hypertrophy of lymphoid tissues, because not all children with large lymphoid tissues have OSAS. This reflects a variation between individual pharyngeal muscle tone and other anatomical differences (narrow palate). Due to increasing prevalence of obesity in the pediatric population, has led to the emergence of a second group in whom OSAS can occur. Pharyngeal adipose tissue and decreased respiratory capacity can contribute to the pathogenesis of this syndrome. The third group consists of children with craniofacial abnormalities, genetic syndromes such as Down syndrome and children with neuromuscular diseases [30].

Snoring, difficulty breathing and apnoeic pauses during sleep, restless sleep, frequent awakening during sleep and neurobehavioral disturbances are the typical symptoms usually present in children with OSAS. Other common nocturnal findings are frequently changing sleep positions, sleeping in a position with the head extended in an effort to open his or her airway and increased diaphoresis as a sign of increased effort of breathing at night and changed activity of autonomous system. Classic symptoms during the daytime are usually present as behavioural disturbances - from subtle impairments of learning, attention and behaviour to prominent neurobehavioral deficits that may mimic attention-deficit/hyperactivity disorder (ADHD) or learning disabilities. More severe causes of OSAS may be associated with a failure to thrive, growth retardation and with many deadly diseases such as systemic hypertension, metabolic syndrome, cor pulmonale, pulmonary hypertension and developmental delay. The presentation in children is much more varied and often difficult to diagnose based on individual symptoms compared with adults. Recently it has been reported that delayed diagnosis of OSAS can lead to neurobehavioral consequences and even serious cardiorespiratory morbidity, metabolic complications, as well as an increase in insulin resistance, high blood pressure and the development of OSAS in adulthood [14, 25, 28, 36]. Clinical manifestations, diagnostic criteria, pathophysiology, treatment approaches and the polysomnography findings of pediatric OSAS differ significantly from adults.

2. Epidemiology

Prevalence of OSAS has been traditionally estimated to be 1% to 5% in the pediatric population. This syndrome is observed in children of all ages and there is no significant gender difference. Most children with obstructive sleep apnea syndrome are aged 3-6 years, which coincides with adenotonsillar lymphatic tissue growth [21, 30].

3. Pathogenesis

According to the current understanding, OSAS is a dynamic process in which increased upper airway collapsibility is present and results from a combination of structural and neuromotor abnormalities, rather than from structural abnormalities alone [30]. Although the pathophysiology of pediatric OSAS is still not well understood, there are some elements such as anatomical structure, neuromotor tone and inflammation, which seems to be important in the development of this syndrome. The etiology of OSAS is multifactorial. Pathophysiologic determinants include structural factors (in non-obese healthy children the hypertrophied adenoids and tonsils), which may lead to anatomical obstruction in the pharyngeal airway, role of upper neuromotor tone, genetic predisposition or combination of these factors. Children with OSAS usually have structurally narrow airways, which predisposes them to having increased resistance and collapsibility when they sleep that leads to a reduced or absent airflow resulting in apneas/hypopneas [25, 35, 36]. In obese children, an increase of adipose tissue in the neck, throat and chest wall creates an increase in the work of breathing and an increase in the upper airway resistance [28]. Systematic and local inflammation can also contribute to the increased resistance at the adenotonsillar level in children. However, the situation is more complex than simple obstruction by hypertrophy of lymphoid tissues, because not all children with large lymphoid tissue have OSAS. Studies of family cohorts suggest that the genetic factors also play an important role in the pathophysiology of OSAS (affect anatomic features and ventilator drive). This reflects a variation between individual pharyngeal muscle tone and other anatomical differences. It appears that pediatric OSAS is a dynamic process that involves interactions between sleep state, upper airway mechanics and respiratory drive [30].

4. Diagnostic Procedures

Obstructive sleep apnea syndrome in children has completely different clinical features and requires a different management strategy from adults [30]. The process of diagnosing pediatric OSAS continues to evolve as more morbidity is recognized and more precise diagnostic methodologies become available [24]. Diagnosis of this condition is usually based on physical examination, history and clinical evaluation confirmed by the polysomnography (PSG) [21]. Standard overnight PSG is considering as a gold-standard test for establishing the presence and severity of OSAS in children (Figure 1) [3].

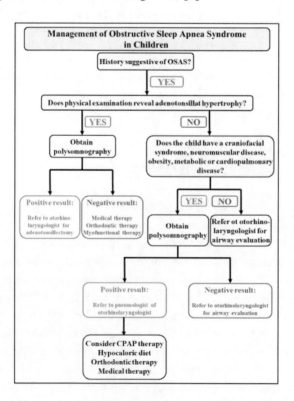

Figure 1. Management of Obstructive Sleep Apnea Syndrome in Children, (Adapted from Chan J. et al., 2004).

Evaluation of a child with suspected obstructive sleep apnea syndrome is as follows: All children and adolescents should be screened for symptoms of OSAS, as a part of routine health maintenance visits. If signs or symptoms of OSAS are present, clinicians should perform a more focused evaluation (Figure 2).

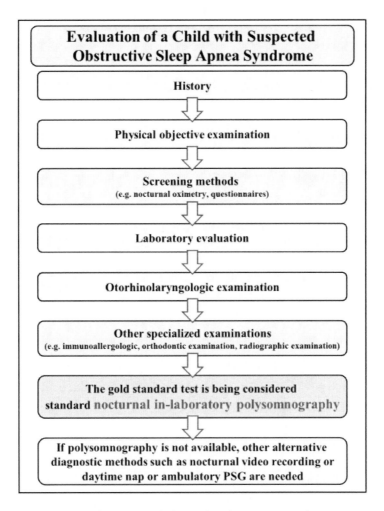

Figure 2. Evaluation of a child with suspected obstructive sleep apnea syndrome.

5. Treatment

Interventions for pediatric OSAS are varied, complex and often multidisciplinary. The goal of the treatment is to restore optimal breathing during the night and to relieve associated symptoms - improve daytime functioning and minimize negative impact. An early therapy based on the result of PSG plays an important role in a management of children with OSAS. Early identification of obstructive sleep apnea syndrome in the pediatric population is desirable, because it is a high-prevalence condition and identification and treatment can result in alleviation of current symptoms, prevention of sequelae, improved quality of life and decreased health care utilization [21]. The therapy needs to be evaluated carefully as the

OSAS in children is likely to be multifactorial [30]. A proposal treatment algorithm of pediatric OSAS is provided in Table 1.

Table 1. A proposal treatment algorithm of pediatric OSAS (Adapted from Villa M.P. et al., 2012). SDB - Sleep Disordered Breathing, CPAP - Continuous Positive Airway Pressure, AHI - Apnea Hypopnea Index

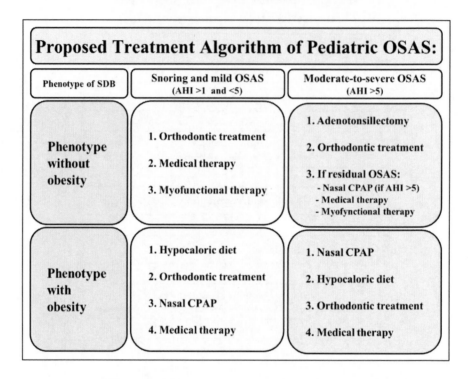

Proposed Treatment Algorithm of Pediatric OSAS:

Phenotype of SDB	Snoring and mild OSAS (AHI >1 and <5)	Moderate-to-severe OSAS (AHI >5)
Phenotype without obesity	1. Orthodontic treatment 2. Medical therapy 3. Myofunctional therapy	1. Adenotonsillectomy 2. Orthodontic treatment 3. If residual OSAS: - Nasal CPAP (if AHI >5) - Medical therapy - Myofynctional therapy
Phenotype with obesity	1. Hypocaloric diet 2. Orthodontic treatment 3. Nasal CPAP 4. Medical therapy	1. Nasal CPAP 2. Hypocaloric diet 3. Orthodontic treatment 4. Medical therapy

5.1. Surgical Therapy

5.1.1. Classic Otorhinolaryngologic (Surgical) Therapy

Adenotonsillar hypertrophy is the most common cause of OSAS in children. Therefore, surgical intervention involving the removal of the tonsils and/or adenoids is an effective definitive treatment, which provides more airway space [21]. Outcome-based data reports the effectives of adenotonsillectomy (AT) as the first-line surgical procedure for uncomplicated OSAS in children with hypertrophy of lymphoid tissues. AT leads to an improvement in polysomnographic parameters, in behaviour and attention and an improvement in cognitive abilities in the vast majority of patients. Although, AT in most children with OSAS is associated with a low complication rate, there are some at-risk groups of pediatric patients with this syndrome, who have an increased risk of postoperative complications. Risk factors include severe OSAS (apnoe/hypopnoe index – AHI > 10 events/hour), age <3 years, obesity, recurrent infections of upper airways, presence of cardiac complications, neuromuscular diseases and craniofacial abnormalities [13]. An important advantage of the objective documentation of the severity of OSAS by using nocturnal polysomnography should be the ability to predict the need for more intensive care after AT on the basis of a higher risk of postoperative complications (postoperative respiratory complications and haemorrhage) [33]. High-risk patients should be monitored as inpatients postoperatively [21]. Although the definition of postoperative respiratory compromise varies, most studies require that an intervention such as intubation, supplemental oxygen, nasopharyngeal tube or CPAP be performed in the high-risk groups [42]. Despite improvement in polysomnographic parameters after AT in the majority of patients, a significant proportion of patients are left with residual OSAS. In a relatively low-risk population, the estimate of this proportion ranges from a low of 13% to 29% when using an AHI ≥5/hour as the criterion to a high of 73% when including obese children and adolescents and a conservative AHI ≥1/hour. Absence of snoring postoperatively is reassuring but may not be 100% specific; it may therefore be advisable to obtain a postoperative PSG in the high-risk pediatric population even in the absence of reported persistent snoring [21]. The present of residual OSAS after treatment in children with OSAS is still an open and often discussed question. At present, there is no clear answer to the question, which kind of therapeutic modality to choose for children with residual OSAS.

Partial tonsillectomy (PT), in which a portion of the tonsil tissue is left to cover the musculature of the tonsillar fossa, is one of the possible techniques to decrease the morbidity associated with traditional tonsillectomy methods. There are only a few studies comparing PT with a total tonsillectomy in children with OSAS [8]. Some studies found that patients who undergo a partial tonsillectomy have a quicker recovery and less pain during the first few days compared with the children undergoing a total tonsillectomy. However, PT may be associated with the possibility of tonsillar regrowth, greater intraoperative blood loss and with a higher risk of recurrent infections [5, 43]. Pediatric patients undergoing PT should be monitored carefully long-term to ensure that symptoms of OSAS related to tonsillar regrowth do not occur [21].

Adenotomy alone may not be sufficient in children with this syndrome, because it does not address oropharyngeal obstruction secondary to tonsillar hyperplasia [21].

In summary, adenotonsillectomy emerges as the leading treatment approach for OSAS in children. However, post-operative persistence of this syndrome in the pediatric population is more frequent than expected, which supports the idea of the complexity of this syndrome [19].

5.1.2. Various Alternative Surgical Therapies

Various alternative surgical treatments (craniofacial surgery such as uvulopalatopharyngoplasty, uvulectomy, epiglottoplasty, distraction osteogenesis, mandibular advancement, tongue reduction, septoplasty, and turbinectomy) are used on an individualised basis that cannot replace the first-line therapies for OSAS in children.

Currently, tracheostomy is rarely indicated in the pediatric population with OSAS, because of the development of non-invasive approaches to maintain upper airway patency during sleep. It remains an effective surgical option for life-threatening obstructive apnea that is not amenable to other therapies. In the past, when surgery did not relieve the degree of sleep-associated respiratory disturbance, a tracheotomy was often performed [19].

5.2. Non-Surgical Therapy

5.2.1. Positive Airway Pressure

Positive airway pressure (PAP) is the mainstay of therapy for most adults, as well as in selected groups of pediatric patients with OSAS. The term CPAP - continuous (permanent) positive airway pressure means the application of ventilatory support in the form of continuous positive pressure generated by the device. It can be applied by a non-invasive nasal (nCPAP), nasal-oral or a facemask. Treatment with CPAP is a safe, effective and well-tolerated therapeutic modality in children as well [7]. Continuous distending airway pressure is applied during sleep using a nasal, nasal – oral or facemask and a small compressor. CPAP acts as a pneumatic splint to maintain airway patency. By simultaneously increasing the functional residual capacity, this pressure also helps prevent oxygen desaturation even if airway obstruction breaks through. CPAP or bi-level positive airway pressure (BiPAP) are used for children who are not good surgical candidates, have sleep disordered breathing associated with major craniofacial deformities, have residual OSAS after upper airway surgery or who have failed previous surgical treatment. Studies demonstrated significant improvement in sleeplessness, snoring, polysomnography parameters and oxyhemoglobin saturation while using PAP during the 6-month follow-up period [20, 21].

An alternative procedure for CPAP is the use of BiPAP. With this method, the inspiratory pressure is identical to the effective CPAP pressure and the expiratory pressure is lower. A randomised control trial of CPAP versus BiPAP in children with OSAS who were unsuitable for AT found no difference between these methods. There were also no significant differences in adherence between the CPAP and BPAP groups in children. CPAP pressures change over time in children, presumably because of growth and development. Therefore, it is recommended that CPAP pressures be frequently reassessed in children [20].

In summary, CPAP is recommended as a treatment if AT is not performed or if OSAS persists postoperatively in the pediatric population. Several studies have confirmed that nasal CPAP is effective in the treatment of both symptoms and polysomnographic evidence of OSAS, even in young children and selected groups of pediatric patients with OSAS [20]. However, adherence can be a main barrier to effective CPAP use and for this reason; CPAP is not recommended as a first-line therapy for OSAS when adenotonsillectomy is an option [17, 20]. This therapy is often not tolerated well by young children, children with Down and Prader-Willi syndrome and by their parents. It is important to train the family and child, use behavioural modification techniques and daytime training as well as finding the appropriate nasal interface [7, 17, 36].

5.2.2. Medical Therapy

Increased activation of inflammatory processes and oxidative stress have been proposed to explain the morbid consequences of sleep disordered breathing, which may be further modulated by lifestyle, genetic and environmental factors. Therefore, the incorporation of nonsurgical approaches for children with OSAS that target those inflammatory processes is now being investigated. Pharmacological therapy is usually used for mild forms of OSAS (AHI < 5events/hour), in children with associated allergic diseases and for residual obstructive sleep apnea syndrome [16]. There is still debate about the possibility of using topic nasal steroids and leukotriene antagonists in the treatment of OSAS in the pediatric population. An older study did not demonstrate a therapeutic effect of systemic corticosteroid use in this condition [2]. Only a few works have been published that retrospectively evaluated the use of local nasal corticosteroids, leukotriene antagonists or combination of both in children with OSAS. This treatment can improve the symptoms (reduce mucosal edema and volume of adenoids and tonsils) of mild forms of OSAS and in children with allergies, but the clinical effect is small. Based on these studies, intranasal steroids may be considered for treatment of mild OSAS (AHI <5/hour), but should not be used as the primary treatment of moderate or severe OSAS. The long-term effects of intranasal steroids are not known, follow-up evaluation is needed to monitor for adverse effects and to ensure that the OSAS does not recur. There is an absence of studies that specifically evaluated children who had atopy or chronic rhinitis, although one study mentioned that similar improvements were seen in children who had a history of allergic symptoms compared with those without [1, 15]. There is a need for further study to determine whether children who have atopy are more likely to respond to this therapy. Data are insufficient at this time to recommend treatment in children of OSAS with leukotriene antagonists [21]. Good nose hygiene and the lavage of the nasal cavity with a hypertonic solution are recommended as support for local therapy especially in mild forms of OSAS. Local and systemic activations of leukotrienes and corticosteroid receptors play a significant role in the pathophysiology of this syndrome in children, there are not enough data to conclude whether the inflammatory mechanisms are a component of the cause of OSAS or rather a consequence of the recurrent upper airway collapse and mechanical trauma [16].

5.2.3. Myofunctional Therapy

Upper airway muscle function plays an important role in the maintenance of upper airway patency and contributes to the genetics of obstructive sleep apnea syndrome in children [16]. Oropharyngeal exercises are a set of repetitive isotonic and isometric exercises for the tongue, soft palate and lateral pharyngeal walls, leading to an increased throughput to the upper respiratory tract and thus to obtain good breathing habits, speech, swallowing and chewing. These exercises are derived from speech–language pathology and include soft palate, tongue and stomatognathic function exercises and facial as well as muscle exercises [12]. Upper airway exercise treatment could be considered as a new therapy for OSAS and snoring because of its direct action on oral motility. The myofunctional therapy includes the correction of functions by means of functional exercises (respiratory, suction, swallowing and chewing), use of the stomatognatic structures and muscular exercises with the aim of increasing the tonus and mobility of the oral and cervical structures [12, 13]. Currently, only a few studies have recognized the effectiveness of oropharyngeal exercises in pediatric patients with OSAS - a reduction in mouth breathing, nasal obstruction and snoring [12]. However, there is still an open question of the possibility of using these exercises as a simple method for treatment of mild to moderate obstructive sleep apnea syndrome and for the residual OSAS in pediatric population. In adult patients with moderate OSAS, oropharyngeal exercises improved subjective measurements of snoring, daytime sleepiness, sleep quality and objective measurements of OSAS. These studies confirmed that upper airway exercises can achieve subjective and objective improvement of symptoms and PSG abnormalities in patients with mild to moderate OSAS and so can be considered as complementary therapy to AT to effectively treat pediatric OSAS [12, 13].

5.2.4. Orthodontic Therapy

Orthodontists now play an important role in the management of obstructive sleep apnea syndrome. The theme of craniofacial and orthodontic abnormalities associated with sleep disordered breathing in children have still not been thoroughly discussed. A narrow upper airway with maxillary constriction and some degree of mandibular retrusion is a common phenotype of OSAS in the pediatric population and children in such cases are typically described as having a narrow, long face [16]. Orthodontic treatment is a relatively new therapeutic modality in selected groups of children with OSAS and malocclusion [39]. This therapy using oral devices is considered to represent a potential or supplementary treatment. Oral appliances may improve upper airway patency during sleep by enlarging the upper airway and by decreasing collapsibility of upper airway, thereby improving upper airway muscle tone. Rapid maxillary expansion (RME), mandibular retropositioning and modified monoblock (MM) are the available treatment options in the pediatric population [16]. Rapid maxillary expansion (RME) is a dentafacial orthodontic procedure used in young patients (starting after the age of 4-when deciduous dentition is complete) with constricted maxillary arches. There are three RME methods: orthodontic, orthosurgical and surgical expansion. Indication depends on the degree of deformity. Orthodontic expansion, also know as a RME, is performed using a fixed oral appliance with expansion screws anchored on selected teeth. The expansion screw is periodically activated to open the midpalatal suture, which results in the maxillary bones diverging from each other. The RME is usually removed after 12 months and patient undergo monthly follow-up assessments until the therapy ends [16, 21, 39]. There are only a few studies using this type of therapy in selected groups of pediatric population. There was a significant improvement in symptoms and signs of OSAS as well as PSG parameters. In summary, rapid maxillary expansion is an orthodontic technique that holds promise as an alternative treatment of OSAS in children with malocclusion [31, 39, 40, 41].

5.2.5. Lifestyle Changes

There are some lifestyle changes, which may be very effective in mitigating the symptoms of obstructive sleep apnea syndrome. Nowadays, the prevalence of childhood obesity is increasing [26]. An intensive weight reduction program is an important first-line step for obese or overweight pediatric patients. Weight loss has been recommended on the basis that it should decompress the upper airway and promote its patency, particularly if weight gain has coincided with worsening of the symptoms [34]. OSAS may aggravate gastroesophageal reflux or vice versa. Children with significant sleep apnea should avoid eating large amounts just before bedtime, especially in the case of children who are being treated with CPAP, which can lead to air swallowing and gastric distension. However, there is a lack of data regarding the effects of weight loss on OSAS in children and adolescents. Finally, along with many other health-related benefits, achieving weight loss and increasing exercise and dietary management seems to be beneficial for OSAS and should be recommended along with other interventions for OSAS in the obese pediatric population [21, 38]. Other life style modifications are designed to improve sleep hygiene, which is very important for any individual. These include measures to improve the sleep environment (child's bedroom should be cool, quiet and comfortable), improving the sleep-wake patterns, increasing physical activity during the day, preparation for sleep by mentally winding down in the evenings and avoiding daytime naps and avoiding caffeinated drinks in the evening and other stimulants dinks. Avoidance of alcohol and drugs that suppress respiratory reflexes is also important in adolescents because of the supporting relaxation of pharyngeal muscles allowing the pharyngeal walls to collapse more easily. Also smoking results in irritation and swelling of the pharyngeal space, increasing the likelihood of snoring and OSAS. There have been only a few clinical studies in the adult population on sleep hygiene, but sleep deprivation has been shown to increase the collapsibility of the upper airway. However, it remains uncertain how effective they are in reducing symptoms and if they are effective especially in the pediatric population with OSAS [34, 35].

5.2.6. Position Therapy

Although several retrospective studies evaluated the effect of body position during sleep on OSAS in the pediatric population, these studies had conflicting results. One study found that young children had an increased AHI in the supine position; another study did not find a positional change in AHI [6, 44]. No study evaluated the effect of changing body positions or the feasibility of maintaining a child in a certain position overnight. Therefore, at the present, there are no recommendations that can be made with regard to positional therapy for OSAS in children [21].

Conclusion

Early identification of obstructive sleep apnea syndrome is desirable, because it is a high prevalence disorder and accurate diagnosis and treatment can result in alleviation of current symptoms, improved quality of life, prevention of sequelaes, education of parents and decreased health care utilization. Interventions for pediatric OSAS are multidisciplinary. AT remains the first-line of treatment for children with hypertrophy of the lymphoid tissues and OSAS. CPAP is recommended as treatment if an AT is not performed or if OSAS persists postoperatively. Weight loss is recommended in addition to other therapy in children, who are obese or overweight. Pharmacological therapy is usually used for mild forms of OSAS and in children with associated allergic diseases. Special orthodontic treatment and oropharyngeal exercises are a relatively new therapeutic modality used in selected groups of children with OSAS.

Acknowledgments

This work was supported by project Grant UK 198/2014, project "Centre of Experimental and Clinical Respirology" and co-financed by EU sources.

References

[1]   Alexopoulos, E.I.; Kaditis, A.G.; Kalampouka, E.; et al. (2004). Nasal corticosteroids for children. *Pediatr Pulmonol*, 38 (2): 161-67.

[2] Al-Ghamdi, S.A.; et al. (1997). Do systemic corticosteroids effectively treat obstructive sleep apnea secondary to adenotonsillar hypertrophy? *Laryngoscope*, 107 (10): 1382-87.

[3] Aurora, RN.; Zak, R.S.; Karippot, A.; Lamm, C.I.; et al. (2011). Practice Parameters for the Respiratory Indications for Polysomnography in Children. *SLEEP*, 34 (3): 379-85.

[4] Bhattacharjee, R.; Kheirandish-Gozal, L.; Spruyt, K.; et al.(2010). Adenotonsillectomy outcomes in treatment of obstructive sleep apnea in children: a multicenter retrospective study. *Am J Respir Crit Care Med*, 182 (5): 676-83.

[5] Celenk, F.; Bayazit, Y.A.; Yilmaz, M.; et al. (2008). Tonsillar regrowth following partial tonsillectomy with radiofrequency. *Int J Pediatr Otorhinolaryngol*, 72 (1): 19–22.

[6] Dayyat, E.; Maarafeya, M.M.; Capdevila, O.S.; et al. (2007). Nocturnal body position in sleeping children with and without obstructive sleep apnea. *Pediatr Pulmonol*, 42 (4): 374–79.

[7] Downey, R.; Perkin, R.M.; Mac Quarrie, J. (2000). Nasal continuous positive airway pressure use in children with obstructive sleep apnea younger than 2 years of age. *Chest*, 117 (6): 1608-12.

[8] Eviatar, E.; Kessler, A.; Shlamkovitch, N.; et al. (2009). Tonsillectomy vs. partial tonsillectomy for OSAS in children—10 years post-surgery follow-up. *Int J Pediatr Otorhinolaryngol*, 73 (5): 637-40.

[9] Goldbart, A.D.; Goldman J.L; Veling M. C.; et al. (2005). Leukotriene modifier therapy for mild sleep-disordered breathing in children. *Am J Respir Crit Care Med*, 172 (3): 364-70.

[10] Goldbart, A.D.; Veling M.C.; Goldman J.L; et al. (2005). Glucocorticoid receptor subunit expression in adenotonsillar tissue of children with obstructive sleep apnea. *Pediatr Res*, 57: 232-36.

[11] Guilleminault, C.; Huang, Y.S.; Monteyrol, P.J.; et al. (2013). Critical role of myofascial reeducation in pediatric sleep-disordered breathing. Sleep Med, 14 (6): 518-525.

[12] Guimaraes, K.C.; Drager, L. F.; Genta, P.R.; et al. (2009). Effects of Oropharyngeal Exercises on Patients with Moderate Obstructive Sleep Apnea Syndrome. *Am J Respir Crit Care Med*, 179 (10): 962-66.

[13] Hill, C.A.; Litvak, A.; Canapari, C.; et al. (2011). A pilot study to identify pre- and peri-operative risk factors for airway complications following adenotonsillectomy for treatment of severe pediatric OSA. *Int J Pediatr Otorhinolaryngol*, 75 (11): 1385-90.

[14] Chan, J.; Edman, J.C.; Koltai, P.J.; et al. (2004). Obstructive Sleep Apnea in Children. *Am Fam Physician.*, 69 (5): 1147-54.

[15] Kheirandish-Gozal, L.; Gozal, D. (2008). Intranasal budesonide treatment for children with mild obstructive sleep apnea syndrome. *Pediatrics,* 122 (1): 149 -55.

[16] Kheirandish-Gozal, L.; Gozal, D. (2012). Sleep Disordered Breathing in Children. A Comprehensive Clinical Guide to Evaluation and Treatment. Humana Press. ISBN 978-1-60761-724-2.

[17] Koontz, K.L.; Slifer, K.J.; Cataldo, M.D.; et al. (2003). Improving pediatric compliance with positive airway pressure therapy: the impact of behavioral intervention. *Sleep*, 26 (8): 1010-15.

[18] Kryger, M.H.; Roth, T.; Dement, W.C. (2011). *Principles and Practice of SLEEP MEDICINE*. 5th ed. Missouri: Elsevier. ISBN 978-1-4377-0731-1.

[19] Lipton, A.J., Gozal, D. (2003). Treatment of obstructive sleep apnea in children: do we really know how? *Sleep Medicine Reviews*. 7 (1): 61-80.

[20] Marcus, C.L.; Rosen, G.; Ward, S.L.D.; et al. (2006). Adherence to and effectiveness of positive airway pressure therapy in children with obstructive sleep apnea. *Pediatrics*, 117: 442-51.

[21] Marcus, S.L. 2012. Diagnosis and Management of Childhood Obstructive Sleep Apnea Syndrome. Clinical Practise Guideline. *Pediatrics*, 130 (4): 576-84.

[22] McGinley, B.; Halbower, A.; Schwartz, A.R.; et al. (2009). Effect of a high-flow open nasal cannula system on obstructive sleep apnea in children. *Pediatrics*, 124: 179-88.

[23] Mindell, J.A.; Owens, J.A. (2010). A Clinical Guide to Pediatric SLEEP: Diagnosis and Management of Sleep Problems. Philadelphia. ISBN 978-1-60-54-7389-5.

[24] Muzumdar, H., Arens, R. (2008). Diagnostic Issues in Pediatric Obstructive Sleep Apnea. *Proc Am Thorac Soc*, 5 (2): 263-73.

[25] Nanaware, S.K.V.; Gothi, D.; Joshi, J.M. (2006). Sleep Apnea. *Indian Journal of Pediatrics*, 73: 597-01.

[26] Ogden, C.L.; Carroll, M.D.; Curtin, L.R.; et al. (2004). Prevalence of overweight and obesity in the United States. *JAMA*, 295 (13): 1549-55.

[27] O´Donnell, A.R.; Bjornson C.L.; Bohn, S.G.; et al. (2006). Compliance rates in children using noninvasive continuous positive airway pressure. *SLEEP*, 29 (5): 651-58.

[28] Peeke, K.; Hershberger, M.; Marriner, J. (2006). Obstructive Sleep Apnea Syndrome in Children. *Pediatric Nursing,* 32 (5): 489-94.

[29] Pereira, K.D.; Roebuck, J.C.; Howell, L. (2005). The effect of body position on sleep apnea in children younger than 3 years. *Arch Otolaryngol Head Neck Surg*, 131 (11): 1014-16.

[30] Powell, S.; Kubba, H.; Brien, C.H.; et al. (2010). CLINICAL REVIEW: Paediatric obstructive sleep apnoea. *BMJ*, 340 (14): 1018-23.

[31] Pirelli, P.; Saponara, M.; Guilleminault, C. 2004. Rapid maxillary expansion in children with obstructive sleep apnea syndrome. *SLEEP*, 27 (4): 761-66.

[32] Ravesloot, M.J.L.; Maanem, J.P.; Vries, N. (2012). The undervalued potential of positional therapy in position-dependent snoring and obstructive sleep apnea-a review of the literature. *Sleep Breath,* 17 (1): 39-49.

[33] Sanders, J.C.; King, M.A.; Mitchell, R.B.; et al. (2006). Perioperative complications of adenotonsillectomy in children with obstructive sleep apnea syndrome. *Anesth Anal,* 103 (5): 1115-21.

[34] Shneerson, J.; Wright, J. (2009). Lifestyle modification for obstructive sleep apnoea. Cochrane Database Syst Rev.1:CD002875.

[35] Sujanska, A.; Durdik, P.; Banovcin, P. (2012). The Recent View on the Obstructive Sleep Apnoea Syndrome in Children. *Acta Medica Martiniana,* 12 (3):

[36] Tauman, R.; Gozal, D. (2011). Obstructive Sleep Apnea Syndrome in Children. *Expert Review of Respiratory Medicine*, 3 (5): 425-40.

[37] Uong, E.C.; Epperson, M.; Bathon, S.A.; et al. (2007). Adherence to nasal positive airway pressure therapy among school-aged children and adolescents with obstructive sleep apnea syndrome. *Pediatrics*, 120 (5): 1203 -11.

[38] Verhulst, S.L.; Franckx, H.; Van Gaal, L.; et al. (2009). The effect of weight loss on sleep-disordered breathing in obese teenagers. *Obesity*, 17 (6):1178-83.

[39] Villa, M.P.; Malagola, C.; Pagani, J.; et al. (2007). Rapid maxillary expansion in children with obstructive sleep apnea syndrome: 12-month follow-up. *Sleep Med*, 8 (2): 128-34.

[40] Villa, M.P.; Rizzoli, A.; Miano, S.; et al. (2011). Efficacy of rapid maxillary expansion in children with obstructive sleep apnea syndrome: 36 months of follow-up. *Sleep Breath*, 15 (2): 179-184.

[41] Villa, M.P.; Paolino, M.C.; Castaldo, R.; et al. (2013). Sleep clinical record: an aid to rapid and accurate diagnosis of pediatric sleep disordered breathing. *Eur Respir J*, 41 (6): 1355-61.

[42] Ye, J.; Liu, H.; Zhang, G.; et al. (2009). Postoperative respiratory complications of adenotonsillectomy for obstructive sleep apnea syndrome in older children: prevalence, risk factors, and impact on clinical outcome. *J Otolaryngol Head Neck Surg*, 38 (1): 49-58.

[43] Zagólski, O. (2010). Why do palatine tonsils grow back after partial tonsillectomy in children? *Eur Arch Otorhinolaryngol*, 267 (10): 1613-17.

[44] Zhang, X.W.; Li, Y.; Zhou, F.; et al. (2007). Association of body position with sleep architecture and respiratory disturbances in children with obstructive sleep apnea. *Acta Otolaryngol*, 127 (12): 132.

Reviewed by:

Assoc. Prof. Milan Kuchta, M.D., Ph.D. – Department of Pediatrics, Centre for Sleep Medicine, Faculty of Medicine, P.J. Safarik University, Children University Hospital, Kosice, Slovakia

In: Advances in Respiratory Therapy Research
Editor: Miloš Jeseňák

ISBN: 978-1-63463-004-7
© 2015 Nova Science Publishers, Inc.

Chapter 7

Animal Models to Assess the Efficacy and Safety of Chest Physiotherapy Techniques for Critically Ill Patients

Talitha Comaru[1,4]*, Joan Daniel Martí[1,2]
and Gianluigi Li Bassi[1,2,3]

[1]Division of Animal Experimentation, Department of Pulmonary and Critical Care
Medicine, Thorax Institute, Hospital Clínic, Barcelona, Spain
[2]Centro de Investigación Biomédica En Red-Enfermedades Respiratorias,
Mallorca, Spain
[3]Institut d'Investigacions Biomèdiques August Pi i Sunyer, Barcelona, Spain
[4]CNPq Fellow, Brasil

Abstract

Mucociliary clearance impairment is common in critically ill patients on invasive mechanical ventilation, resulting in retention of airway secretions, lung collapse and pulmonary infections. Endotracheal intubation, patient positioning, impaired cough and prolonged immobilization are the main risk factors for mucus retention. Chest physiotherapy techniques are often applied in these patients to improve clearance of mucus, preserve airway patency, and optimize gas exchanges. As for the most commonly applied interventions, clapping and shaking are used to prevent or treat retention of airway secretions through bronchial oscillations; postural drainage is used to drain mucus through gravity; manual chest compressions and pulmonary hyperinflation propel mucus outward through the interaction of airflows with the mucus layer, namely the two-phase gas-liquid flow mechanism. The effects of these techniques have not been comprehensively evaluated, mainly because of methodological limitations in assessing

---

* Corresponding Author address: Division of Animal Experimentation, Department of Pulmonary and Critical Care Medicine, Thorax Institute, Hospital Clínic, Barcelona, Spain, e-mail: talithacomaru@hotmal.com.

mucus clearance in clinical settings. This has led to uncertainties on indications, efficacy and safety of the interventions.

Therefore, animal models are pivotal to advance knowledge in this field and to allow translational research. In particular dogs, pigs, sheep and rabbits have been largely used in respiratory research, because they present close similarities to humans in airway structure and physiology. Excellent methods to track mucus clearance rate have been developed in these models. Thus, several chest physiotherapy techniques such as postural drainage, percussion, clapping, chest compressions, vibrations, and manual hyperinflation have been assessed in these animals.

The aim of this chapter is to perform a critical analysis of experimental studies to assess efficacy and safety of chest physiotherapy techniques, identify challenges in the assessment of mucus clearance *in-vivo,* and call attention to the areas within the field that require further investigations.

Keywords: Animal Model, Chest Physiotherapy, Critically Ill Patient, Mucociliary clearance

1. Introduction

Mucus retention is highly prevalent in tracheally intubated patients on prolonged mechanical ventilation (MV), which can result in potential respiratory complications [1]. In particular, endotracheal intubation [2], insufficient humidification of respiratory gases [3], sedation and analgesia [4], positioning of the patient [5], and muscular weakness caused by prolonged immobility [6] are risk factors for mucus clearance impairment.

Chest physiotherapy (CPT) is often used in the intensive care unit (ICU) to improve clearance of mucus, preserve airway patency, and optimize gas exchanges in critically ill patients [7]. A great variety of CPT techniques have been developed to prevent and treat retention of airway secretions [8-9]. These CPT interventions greatly differ based on the applied methods, indications and affected pulmonary regions. Indeed, clapping and postural drainage are commonly implemented to improve mucus clearance in the proximal and distal airways through bronchial oscillations and gravitational force, respectively. Whereas, the forced expiratory technique, manual chest compressions and pulmonary hyperinflation improve outward clearance of mucus from the main airways through the two-phase gas-liquid flow mechanism [10-13].

The efficacy and safety of CPT techniques in the critically ill patients still lacks of clear evidence [14]. This is partially due to the absence of methods to reliably assess movement of mucus in clinical settings. Thus, in studies evaluating CPT techniques, often surrogate endpoints are used, i.e. volume of aspirated mucus, pulmonary mechanics parameters, gas exchange [14]. Thus, in this field of investigation animal models play a key role in advancing knowledge. Several animal models have been developed, i.e. dogs, pigs, sheep and rabbits [15-18], to assess mucus clearance and test efficacy of CPT methods [19].

In the next sections we describe the most important experimental studies to assess efficacy and safety of CPT techniques. We also highlight challenges in the assessment of mucus clearance *in-vivo,* and call attention to the areas within this field of investigation that require further investigations.

2. Animal Models to Evaluate CPT Techniques

In the last 4 decades a few laboratory studies in animals were published to assess the efficacy and safety of CPT techniques. These studies differ based on the animal models, study design, applied CPT techniques and outcomes. The majority of these studies evaluated techniques frequently used in clinical settings. As reported in table 1, dogs [20-23], sheep [24, 25], rabbits [26, 27, 28], Wistar rats [29] and pigs [30] are the species most commonly used in these studies. Unfortunately, several of these studies present limitations, i.e. surrogate outcomes; safety of the techniques is rarely reported; finally a few studies used very small populations. Of note, only a few studies [20-22, 30] evaluated mucus clearance rate; this highlights methodological limitations of this field of investigation. Nevertheless, despite aforementioned limitations, several interesting findings are reported, which could have important applications in laboratory and clinical settings, and lead to future advancement in the field.

Table 1. Animal models to assess efficacy and safety of chest physiotherapy techniques

Study, Year of Publication	Animal Model (Body Weight, Kg)	Chest Physiotherapy Technique	Main Outcomes	Conclusions
Chopra et al., 1977	10 Mongrel Dogs (15-28)	Postural Drainage, Chest percussion	Tracheal Mucus Clearance Rate.	Postural drainage and chest percussion (combined or alone) improve mucus clearance rate. Dehydration causes impairment of mucus clearance rate, which reverted to normal with rehydration.
King et al., 1983	9 Dogs (25-35)	High Frequency Chest Wall Compression	Tracheal Mucus Clearance Rate	High frequency chest wall compressions (5-17 Hz) enhance tracheal mucus clearance rate
Gross et al., 1985	17 Dogs (21-35)	High Frequency Chest Wall Compression	Tracheal Mucus Clearance Rate, Distal Airways Mucus Clearance Rate	High frequency chest wall compressions are effective in improving both distal airways and tracheal mucus clearance rate
Zidulka et al., 1989	20 Mongrel Dogs (22-29)	Clapping, Chest Percussion	Lung ventilation, Lung Structure, Oxygenation	Gas exchange improve toward the end of the percussion or clapping period. Clapping causes pulmonary atelectasis.
Unoki et al., 2003	41 Japanese White Rabbits (3.4±0.5)	Manual Rib-Cage Compressions, Body Positioning	Oxygenation, Ventilation, Dynamic pulmonary compliance	Chest compressions are unable to opening collapsed lung; prone position improves oxygenation in rabbits with induced atelectasis
Anning et al., 2003	9 Sheep (39.5±1.6)	Manual Hyperinflation	Hemodynamics	Manual hyperventilation produces significant hemodynamic changes

Table 1. (Continued)

Study, Year of Publication	Animal Model (Body Weight, Kg)	Chest Physiotherapy Technique	Main Outcomes	Conclusions
Wong et al., 2003	2 Merino Sheep (37.9 and 38.4)	Clapping, Vibration,Shaking	Frequency of Application and Forces generated by Physiotherapist, Pulmonary Parameters, Hemodynamics	Clapping, vibration and shaking can be consistently applied by physiotherapists; these techniques are significantly associated with physiotherapist's characteristics, particularly clinical experience; they do not cause significant hemodynamic effects
Unoki et al., 2004	28 Japanese White Rabbits (2.8±0.2)	Manual Rib-Cage Compressions	Oxygenation, Ventilation	Following induced lung atelectasis, neither chest compressions alone, nor combined with endotracheal suctioning improve oxygenation, ventilation, dynamic compliance or mucus clearance. The alveolar and airway collapse is probably exacerbated by chest compressions
Zhang et al., 2005	23 Japanese White Rabbits (from 2.5 to 3)	Manual Hyperinflation, Chest Squeezing	Hemodynamics Oxygenation, Ventilation	The combination of exogenous surfactant lavage and chest physiotherapy (squeezing) improves respiratory disturbance in meconium aspiration syndrome.
Lima et al., 2008	24 Wistar Rats (0.200-0.250)	Unilateral Chest Compressions (Flow Direction)	Histology features	Following pulmonary atelectasis, unilateral chest compressions (flow direction) are not efficient in reopening atelectatic areas
Marti et al., 2013	9 Large White– Landrace Pigs (27-37)	Manual Rib-Cage Compressions	Expiratory flow, Mucus clearance	Hard manual rib cage compression improves mucus clearance rate in animals positioned in a model of the semi-recumbent position. The technique appeared to be safe. Conversely, soft manual rib cage compression was not effective and potentially unsafe.

3. Effects of CPT on Tracheal and Peripheral Mucus Movement

The effects of CPT on mucus movement were evaluated in 4 studies [20-22, 30]. Chopra and colleagues [20], evaluated in dogs the effects of postural drainage, percussion or a concomitant use of both techniques. The authors instilled into the distal trachea albumin microspheres with a diameter of 5-7 μm, labeled with technetium-99m and/or indium 113m. Then, they tracked these microspheres through a gamma camera to compute mucus clearance. They found that mucus clearance velocity increased by 7.7±1.78 mm/min applying postural drainage, in comparison with baseline values, and by 8.2±1.2 mm/min with chest percussion. Finally, with concurrent application of the two techniques, they found an increase of 9.5±0.32 mm/min vs. baseline values.

In a later report by King and colleagues [21], the effects of high frequency chest wall compression (HFCWC) on mucus clearance were studied. They used in dogs oscillatory tidal volumes between 25 and 100 mL and frequencies of 3-17 Hz. As for the methods to assess mucus clearance rate, they insufflated charcoal particles into the distal trachea through a bronchoscope. Then, they continuously tracked these particles through the bronchoscope. Mucus clearance rate was computed as the distance travelled by the particle toward the proximal trachea, divided by the elapsed time. They found that applying frequencies higher than 3 Hz, mucus clearance rate progressively increased. Yet, most significant improvements were associated with frequencies between 11 and 15 Hz. In particular, with a frequency of 13 Hz, mucus clearance rate increased from 8.2±5.6 mm/min to 27.6 ± 13.8 mm/min. Gross and collaborators [22] also evaluated benefits of HFCWC in dogs. Differently than previous report, the authors were able to analyze peripheral mucus clearance through nebulization of technetium-99m sulfur colloid into the lungs during mechanical ventilation. Clearance of the isotope was monitored through a gamma camera. They found that HFCWC at 13 Hz, with pressures of 50-60 cmH$_2$O significantly enhanced tracheal mucus clearance and peripheral mucus clearance index, without any associated adverse effect.

In a recent report by our group [30], the effects of two types of manual rib cage compressions on mucus clearance velocity were tested in pigs on mechanical ventilation up to three days and kept in a model of the semi-recumbent position. Tantalum disks, 0.1-mm thick and with a diameter of 1.0 mm, were instilled into the trachea through a bronchoscope, and tracked through sequential lateral fluoroscopic images. Stronger manual compressions, applied early during the expiratory phase, significantly enhanced mucus clearance rate to 1.01 ± 2.37, in comparison with -0.28±0.61 mm/min without any treatment, and -0.15±0.95 mm/min with softer manual compressions, applied during the late expiratory phase. Of note, aforementioned negative values indicate abnormal mucus clearance rate toward the lungs. Indeed, 87.5% and 44.4% of the disk moved toward the lungs during no intervention and soft compression, respectively. This was mainly caused by the semirecumbent position, which led to tracheal orientation above horizontal [5]. Conversely, when hard compressions were applied mucus moved toward the lungs only in 30% of the cases.

Importantly, several of the studies mentioned above [21, 22, 30] demonstrated a strong association between expiratory flow rate and mucus clearance. This is in line with earlier physiology studies that clearly corroborated that expiratory flow plays a major role in propelling retained mucus toward the glottis [11, 12, 31-33]. Some of the above-mentioned techniques, i.e. HFCWC or chest compressions, specifically enhance the expiratory flow rate and this lead to the improvement in mucus clearance. Other CPT do not alter expiratory flow rate. In particular, postural drainage clears mucus through gravitational force. Whereas, in HFCWC, the alteration of mucus crosslink [34], enhanced airflow-interaction [35] and ciliary beating could be the major mechanisms for the improvement in mucus clearance. Finally, theoretically all CPT techniques could also trigger autonomic reflexes, or activate lung mediators that activate and heighten cilia function [36].

4. Hemodynamic Effects of CPT

The hemodynamic effects of chest physiotherapy techniques were evaluated in four studies [24, 25, 28, 30]. In one study, the effects of clapping, vibration and shaking were evaluated in sheep [25]; while, the effects of bag-squeezing were evaluated in rabbits [28], in a model of meconium aspiration syndrome. No significant hemodynamic effects were found in both studies. Conversely, in a study on the effects of manual hyperinflation in healthy sheep [24], investigators found reduced cardiac output, increased systemic vascular resistance, and a drop in mean arterial pressure during and after application of the technique. Moreover, in a more recent study in pigs positioned in a model of the semi-recumbent position [30], the hemodynamic effects of manual rib cage compression were studied. Firm compressions, applied at the beginning of expiration for a very brief period did not impact hemodynamic parameters. Conversely, gentle squeezing of the thoracic cage, from the mid-expiratory phase up to the end of the exhalation, slightly worsened cardiac output.

5. Effects of CPT on Oxygenation and Ventilation

The effects of CPT techniques in oxygenation and ventilation were evaluated in five studies [23, 26-28, 30]. In the model of meconium aspiration syndrome in rabbits [28], significant improvement in blood gas analysis parameters was found up to three hours after manual hyperventilation associated with bag-squeezing. A model of atelectasis in rabbits was developed by Unoki et al. [26], to test the effects of manual rib cage compression and, interestingly, no major enhancement in gas exchange was found, according with a later study in pigs [30]. Yet, it is important to emphasize that in both studies, secretions were not aspirated after the technique, and this could have limited potential associated benefits. Of note, in one of these studies [26], the investigators used positive end-expiratory pressure of 5 cmH_2O; these setting were associated with a significant enhancement of gas exchange during application of the technique. Unfortunately, this improvement was short-lasting, since gas exchange rapidly returned to worse baseline values, after the CPT session was completed. Also, a transient increase in arterial partial pressure of O_2 and decrease in arterial partial pressure of CO_2 were found in healthy dogs, during and immediately after the application of clapping and percussion [23]. In another study in rabbits, blood gas did deteriorate when rib cage compressions were applied without positive end expiratory pressure [27]. In conclusion, it is important to highlight that the effects of CPT techniques on oxygenation and ventilation are understudied; thus, there is a strong need for additional pathophysiology studies to understand how CPT techniques impact oxygen consumption, carbon dioxide production, pulmonary shunt, alveolar dead space and ultimately lead to an improvement or deterioration of blood gases.

6. Pulmonary Mechanics During CPT

Modulation of airflows during CPT was evaluated in several studies. In a study in pigs by our group [30], both soft chest compressions applied at late expiration, and hard compressions applied during the very early expiratory phase affected the expiratory flow rates. Specifically, the soft compressions prolonged the expiratory phase, whereas hard compressions significantly increased the peak expiratory flow. Thus, both techniques produced an expiratory-inspiratory flow bias. Changes in peak expiratory flow rates were also assessed in two studies evaluating high frequency chest wall compressions in dogs [21, 22]. High frequency chest wall compressions always increased the mean peak expiratory-inspiratory flow ratio, irrespective of the applied frequencies. Theoretically, these maneuvers could have significant benefits in the management of patients with retained secretion, because previous in vitro [12, 31] and animal studies [33] reported a strong association between peak expiratory flow and mucus clearance.

Among the studies evaluating pulmonary mechanics during CPT techniques, in a study in rabbits with pulmonary atelectasis, no improvement in dynamic compliance associated with the use of chest compressions were found [26]. Additionally, in a different study [27], when chest compressions were applied without concomitant use of positive end-expiratory pressure dynamic compliance worsened. Whereas, in a study in pigs [30], when soft ribcage compressions were applied at the end of expiration, static lung elastance slightly worsened; conversely no change in static lung elastance were associated with the use of hard compressions, applied at early expiration.

The effects of CPT on expiratory volumes were evaluated in aforementioned study in pigs, in which prolongation of expiration through soft ribcage compressions caused a significant increase in expiratory volume, which led to a decrease in positive end expiratory pressure [30]. Interestingly, the reduction in positive end expiratory pressure was associated with the expiratory time. Finally, chest vibration significantly increased the expired tidal volume in anesthetized sheep [25], without changes in the expiratory peak flow.

In research settings, esophageal pressure is commonly used as an estimate of the pleural pressure [37]. The effects of CPT on esophageal pressure were evaluated in four studies [23, 25, 26, 30]. In two studies [23-25] esophageal pressure was used to estimate the intensity of the force applied by physiotherapists. In particular, clapping increased esophageal pressure by 12.0 ± 6.8 cm H_2O [25]. In another study, clapping at a frequency of 4-7 Hz was applied in animals and this caused an increase in esophageal pressure of 6-17 cmH$_2$O [23]. Similarly, chest percussions, at a frequency of 10-16 Hz, increased esophageal pressure by 10-17 cmH$_2$O [23]. Conversely, the lowest increase in esophageal pressure was generated by chest vibration and shaking, 1.0 ± 0.4 cm H_2O, and 1.9 ± 1.0cmH$_2$O, respectively [25]. In a study in pigs an association between esophageal pressure and mean expiratory flow was found during manual ribcage compressions [30]. Finally, the esophageal pressure was evaluated during application of ribcage compressions [26]; accordingly with aforementioned studies, an increase during the expiratory phase was found. Thus, the esophageal pressure seems a reliable parameter, which could be used in research and clinical settings, to estimate intra-thoracic pressures generated during CPT, and estimate the associated increase in expiratory flow.

Conclusion

In conclusion several animal models are available in medium and large animals to appraise efficacy and safety of CPT techniques. Unfortunately, throughout the years, critical features and effects of CPT techniques have been understudied; thus, these models should be used in comprehensive pathophysiology studies to evaluate efficacy, indication and safety of CPT techniques. In particular, one of the main advantages of these models is the possibility to assess mucus clearance rate *in-vivo*; rather than use surrogate endpoints, with limited specificity, such as gas exchange or pulmonary mechanics. To date, the most common methods to quantify mucus clearance rate are through the use of markers instilled into the trachea or radioisotopes nebulized into the airways. Most of these methods were developed decades ago; thus, there is an important need for new methods to evaluate mucus clearance in patients and laboratory settings, which could lead to major advancement in this field.

References

[1]   Konrad F, Schreiber T, Brecht-Kraus D, Georgieff M. Mucociliary transport in ICU patients. *Chest* 1994; 105(1):237-41.
[2]   Sackner M, Hirsch J, Epstein S. Effect of cuffed endotracheal tubes on tracheal mucous velocity. *Chest* 1975; 68(6): 774-7.
[3]   Kilgour E, Rankin N, Ryan S, Pack R. Mucociliary function deteriorates in the clinical range of inspired air temperature and humidity. *Intensive Care Med* 2004; 30(7): 1491-4.
[4]   Wang L, Tiniakov RL, Yeates DB. Peripheral opioidergic regulation of the tracheobronchial mucociliary transport system. *J Appl Physiol* 2003; 94(6): 2375-83.
[5]   Bassi GL, Zanella A, Cressoni M, Stylianou M, Kolobow T. Following tracheal intubation, mucus flow is reversed in the semirecumbent position: Possible role in the pathogenesis of ventilator–associated pneumonia. *Crit Care Med* 2008; 36(2): 518-25.
[6]   De Jonghe B, Sharshar T, Lefaucheur J-P, Authier F-J, Durand-Zaleski I, Boussarsar M, et al. Paresis acquired in the intensive care unit: a prospective multicenter study. *JAMA* 2002; 288(22): 2859-67.
[7]   Norrenberg M, Vincent JL. A profile of European intensive care unit physiotherapists. *Intensive Care Med* 2000 Jul; 26(7): 988-994.
[8]   Branson RD. Secretion management in the mechanically ventilated patient. *Respir Care* 2007; 52:1328-1342.
[9]   Lewis RM. Airway clearance techniques for the patient with an artificial airway. *Respir Care* 2002; 47:808-817.

[10] Benjamin RG, Chapman GA, Kim CS, et al. Removal of bronchial secretions by two-phase gas-liquid transport. *Chest* 1989; 95:658-663.7.

[11] Kim CS, Rodriguez CR, Eldridge MA, et al. Criteria for mucus transport in the airways by two-phase gas-liquid flow mechanism. *J Appl Physiol* 1986; 60:901-907.

[12] Kim CS, Iglesias AJ, Sackner MA. Mucus clearance by two-phase gas-liquid flow mechanism: asymmetric periodic flow model. *J Appl Physiol* 1987; 62:959-971.

[13] Li Bassi G, Saucedo L, Marti JD, et al. Effects of duty cycle and positive end-expiratory pressure on mucus clearance during mechanical ventilation. *Crit Care Med* 2012; 40: 895–902.

[14] Stiller K. Physiotherapy in intensive care: An updated systematic review. *Chest* 2013; 144(3): 825–847.

[15] Tomkiewcz R, Albers G, De Sanctis G, et al. Species differences in the physical and transport properties of airway secretions. *Can J Physiol Pharmacol* 1994; 73:165-71.

[16] Felicetti SA, Wolff RK, Muggenburg BA. Comparison of tracheal mucous transport in rats, guinea pigs, rabbits, and dogs. *J Appl Physiol* 1981; 51:1612-7.

[17] Boucher RC, Bromberg PA, Gatzy JT. Airway transepithelial electric potential in vivo: species and regional differences. *J Appl Physiol* 1980; 48:169-76.

[18] Plopper CG, Mariassy AT, Lollini LO. Structure as revealed by airway dissection. A comparison of mammalian lungs. *Am Rev Respir Dis* 1983; 128(2 Pt 2):S4-7.

[19] Li Bassi G. Airway secretions and suctioning. In: Tobin MJ (editor). Principles and Practice of Mechanical Ventilation. 3rd edition. New York. McGraw-Hill. 2013.1213-36.

[20] Chopra SK, Taplin GV, Simmons DH, Robinson GD, Elam D, Coulson A. Effects of hydration and physical therapy on tracheal transport velocity. *Am Rev Respir Dis* 1977; 115:1009-14.

[21] King M, Philips DM, Gross D, Vartian V, Chang HK, Zidulka A. Enhanced tracheal mucus clearance with high frequency chest wall compression. *Am Rev Respir Dis*1983; 128:511-15.

[22] Gross D, Zidulka A, O'Brien C, Wight D, Fraser R, Rosenthal L, King M. Peripheral mucociliary clearance with high-frequency chest wall compression. *J ApplPhysiol* 1985;58(4):1157-63.

[23] Zidulka A, Chrome J, Wight D, Burnett S, Bonnier L, Fraser R. Clapping or percussion causes atelectasis in dogs and influences gas exchange.*J Appl Physiol*1989;66(6):2833-38

[24] Anning L, Paratz J, Wong WP, Wilson K. Effect of manual hyperinflation on haemodynamics in an animal model. *Physiother Res Int*. 2003;8(3):155-63

[25] Wong W, Paratz J, Wilson K, Burns Y. Hemodynamic and ventilatory effects of manual respiratory physiotherapy techniques of chest clapping, vibration, and shaking in an animal model. *J Appl Physiol*. 2003;95(3):991-8

[26] Unoki T, Mizutani T, Toyooka H. Effects of expiratory rib cage compression and/or prone position on oxygenation and ventilation in mechanically ventilated rabbits with induced atelectasis. *Respir Care*. 2003;48(8):754-62.

[27] Unoki T, Mizutani T, Toyooka H. Effects of expiratory rib cage compression combined with endotracheal suctioning on gas exchange in mechanically ventilated rabbits with induced atelectasis. *Respir Care*. 2004;49(8):896-901.

[28] Zhang E, Hiroma T, Sahashi T, Taki A, Yoda T, Nakamura T. Airway lavage with exogenous surfactant in an animal model of meconium aspiration syndrome. *Pediatr Int.* 2005;47(3):237-41.

[29] Lima J, Reis L, Moura F, Souza C, Walchan E, Bergmann A. Compressão Manual Torácica em um modelo experimental de atelectasia em ratos Wistar. *Fisioterapia em Movimento.* 2008;21(3):77-82.

[30] Martí JD, Li Bassi G, Rigol M, Saucedo L, Ranzani OT, Esperatti M, Luque N, Ferrer M, Vilaró J, Kolobov T, Torres A.Effects of Manual Rib Cage Compressions on Expiratory Flow and Mucus ClearanceDuring Mechanical Ventilation.*Crit Care Med* 2013; 41:850–856.

[31] Volpe MS, Adams AB, Amato MB, et al: Ventilation patterns influence airway secretion movement. *Respir Care* 2008; 53:1287–1294.

[32] King M, Zidulka A, Phillips DM, Wight D, Gross D, and Chang HK. Tracheal mucus clearance in high-frequency oscillation: effect of peak flow rate bias. *Eur Respir J* 3: 6–13, 1990.

[33] Benjamin RG, Chapman GA, Kim CS, et al: Removal of bronchial secretions by two-phase gas-liquid transport. *Chest* 1989; 95:658–663.

[34] King M, Gilboa A, Meyer FA, Silberberg A. On the transport of mucus and its rheologic simulants in clliated systems. Am Rev Resp Dis 1974; 110:740-45.

[35] Scherer PW, Burtz L. Fluid mechanical experiments relevant to coughing. J Biomech 1978; 11: 183-87.

[36] Wanner A. Does Chest Physiotherapy Move Airway Secretions? *Am Rev Respir Dis* 1984; 130:701-02.

[37] Akoumianaki, Evangelia, *American journal of respiratory and critical care medicine 2014;* 189: no. 5: doi:10.1164/rccm.201312-2193CI.

Reviewed by: Jaroslav Fabry, M.D., Ph.D. – Department of Pediatric Pneumology and Phthiseology, Srobar's Institute for Children Tuberculosis and Respiratory Diseases, Dolny Smokove, High Tatras, Slovakia

Index

B

C

F

G

Q

R

S

T